# ALZHEIMER'S DISEASE

*Problems, Prospects,
and Perspectives*

# ALZHEIMER'S DISEASE

*Problems, Prospects, and Perspectives*

Edited by

# Harvey J. Altman

*Director, Department of Behavioral Animal Research*
*Lafayette Clinic and*
*Assistant Professor, Department of Psychiatry*
*Wayne State University School of Medicine*
*Detroit, Michigan*

PLENUM PRESS • NEW YORK AND LONDON

Library of Congress Cataloging in Publication Data

National Conference on Alzheimer's Disease and Dementia: Problems, Prospects, and Perspectives (1986: Detroit, Mich.)
Alzheimer's disease.

"Proceedings of a National Conference on Alzheimer's Disease and Demen-
tia: Problems, Prospects, and Perspectives, held April 10–12, 1986, in Detroit,
Michigan"—T.p. verso.
Includes bibliographies and index.
1. Alzheimer's disease—Congresses. I. Altman, Harvey, J. II. Title. [DNLM:
1. Alzheimer's Disease—congresses. WM 220 N2755a 1986]
RC523.N38   1986                          618.97'683                          87-15374
ISBN 0-306-42662-5

Proceedings of a National Conference on Alzheimer's Disease and Dementia:
Problems, Prospects, and Perspectives, held April 10–12, 1986,
in Detroit, Michigan

© 1987 Plenum Press, New York
A Division of Plenum Publishing Corporation
233 Spring Street, New York, N.Y. 10013

Dedicated to my wife Barbara and my three
children, Jill, Paul, and Stefanie

PREFACE

Alzheimer's disease is a primary neurodegenerative disease whose incidence and prevalence is rapidly approaching epidemic proportions. A major reason for this is that man is living longer than he has ever lived before and the likelihood of contracting the disease is significantly greater within the elderly portion of the population. The problem becomes even more acute in the light of recent estimates which predict that the number of people living beyond the age of 65 is expected to continue to increase. The impact of these statistics on the family and the health care industry in terms of time, effort and cost are staggering. A recent report issued by the Michigan Task Force on Alzheimer's Disease and Related Conditions (1987) effectively underscores this last point. "Each person with a dementing disease requires an average of seven years of care, either at home or in a residential care facility. Care provided at home is estimated to cost about $12,000 annually, for a total of $84,000 per person. This is a conservative figure, however, because many persons with dementia spend their last few years in a nursing home at an average cost of $22,000 per year, and some spend from 10 to 15 years in a nursing home, for a total cost of $220,000 to $330,000. The human cost cannot be calculated so easily, because it includes exhausted caregivers and shattered families as well as depleted financial assets."

Although there has been and continues to be a significant amount of research conducted with respect to this disease, no clear consensus as to the etiology, pathophysiology or means of treatment or prevention has yet to emerge. That is not to say that advances in our understanding of what this disease is and how it can be treated have not been forthcoming. To the contrary, a significant number of advances have been and continue to be made. However, much more needs to be accomplished and with great urgency.

The hallmark of the disease is a progressive and insidious deterioration in recent memory and cognition. However, loss of memory and cognition are not the only functions to be affected by this disease. The disease also results in a significant deterioration in many aspects of normal daily functioning. Frequently, significant shifts in affect and/or personality are also reported; developing either as a result of the neurodegenerative process of the disease itself or independently as a consequence of other neurological or psychological problems. Eventually, the disease robs the individual of all conscious contact with the outside world; leaving the afflicted individual bed ridden and entirely dependent on those around him for all of his or her daily care and needs.

Invariably, at some point during the course of the disease, the family or whoever it is that is left with the responsibility of caring for such an individual will be faced with the often times painful decision of whether or not it would be in the best interests of all involved (caregiver(s) and patient alike) to have such an individual institutionalized. This decision is further complicated by a whole gamut of financial, legal and ethical issues revolving around third party payments, patient's rights, competency, and the appropriateness of legal representation (both with respect to the patient and his personal property). At some point changes will have to be made at the State and Federal level. Some of these have already begun to emerge. Additional progress is clearly needed.

The purpose of the conference and this book is to provide a comprehensive overview of the broad spectrum of issues and problems which will have to be addressed if this disease and the impact it is having on society is ever to be brought under control. Unlike most of the previous conferences and books on this subject, an attempt was made to foster the exchange and integration of ideas and view points across widely divergent areas and disciplines (e.g., research, professional health care and management, the family, legal and ethical issues and public policy). In so doing, it is hoped that the problems being faced by professionals and family members alike would better be appreciated and this would, in turn, foster the development of more effective methods of dealing with this disease.

Harvey J. Altman, Ph.D.

Director,
Department of Behavioral Animal Research
Lafayette Clinic
        and
Assistant Professor,
Department of Psychiatry
Wayne State University School of Medicine
Detroit, Michigan

ACKNOWLEDGEMENTS

The editor of this book would like to take this opportunity to thank each member of the Conference Coordinating Committee for their help and input in organizing this year's conference. It was only through the concerted effort of all of the members of the Committee that this conference became such a success.

The editor would also like to graciously acknowledge the generous contributions of the following institutions for their support of the conference on which this book is based:

The Department of Psychiatry
Wayne State University School of Medicine

Alzheimer's Disease and Related Disorders Association
Detroit Area Chapter

The LeVine Institute on Aging
of the Jewish Home For Age

Astra Läkemedel AB

Ciba-Geigy Company

Hoescht-Roussel Pharmaceutical, Inc.

Janssen Pharmaceutica Company

Lederle Laboratories

The UpJohn Company

Warner-Lambert Company

Department of Family Medicine
Wayne State University School of Medicine

Neurosciences Program
Wayne State University School of Medicine

Stroh Brewing Company

Perry Drugs, Inc.

CONTENTS

PRIMARY CARE/PHYSICIANS

NURSING

## THE FAMILY

## PUBLIC POLICY/LEGAL AND ETHICAL ISSUES

BEHAVE-AD: A CLINICAL RATING SCALE FOR THE ASSESSMENT OF
PHARMACOLOGICALLY REMEDIABLE BEHAVIORAL SYMPTOMATOLOGY IN
ALZHEIMER'S DISEASE

Barry Reisberg,
Jeffrey Borenstein,
Emile Franssen,
Stacy Salob,
Gertrude Steinberg,
Emma Shulman,
Steven H. Ferris and
Anastase Georgotas

Department of Psychiatry
New York University Medical Center
New York, New York

INTRODUCTION

The clinical characteristics of Alzheimer's disease have only begun to
be described in detail over the course of the past few years.   In our
laboratory, we initially described three broad clinical phases of the
progression of the disease (Reisberg, 1981; Schneck et al., 1982).   Subsequently, we published detailed descriptions of seven, clinically identifiable global stages in the progression from normal aging to most severe
Alzheimer's disease (Reisberg et al., 1982).   Corresponding levels of
cognitive abilities in terms of assessments of concentration, recent memory,
past memory, orientation, and functioning and self-care have also been
described (Reisberg et al., 1983a; Reisberg et al., 1984; Reisberg et al.,
1985a) as has the stage-specific longitudinal outcome of subjects with normal aging and has progressive Alzheimer's disease (Reisberg et al., 1986).

Mood changes are less constant features of the progression of
Alzheimer's disease than the changes in areas reflecting cognitive abilities
and functioning. Nevertheless, such changes tend to occur in a somewhat
characteristic pattern with the progression of Alzheimer's disease (Reisberg
et al., 1983b). More specifically, the earliest clearly definable stage of
Alzheimer's disease, the fourth Global Deterioration Scale stage (GDS = 4)
is most frequently marked by a flattening of affect and withdrawal from
previously challenging situations. In the fifth GDS stage tearful episodes
are a frequent occurrence, as is the flattening of affect observed earlier
in the illness. In the sixth GDS stage overt symptoms of agitation and
psychosis are frequently noted, whereas in the final stage of Alzheimer's
disease--the seventh stage--a pathologic passivity frequently replaces the
agitation and psychosis which may have been observed earlier in the illness.

The behavioral symptoms of Alzheimer's disease, in particular the
agitation and psychosis referred to above, are an enormous source of anguish
for caregivers of victims of the disease. Our research indicates that

concerns about these symptoms, and with regard to medications which are prescribed to treat these symptoms, are the most frequently voiced by caregivers in support groups settings (Shulman and Steinberg, 1984). Issues with respect to these agitation symptoms are also the one's most frequently cited by caregivers for placing their beloved spouses or relatives in institutional settings (Ferris et al., 1985).

Despite the importance of these symptoms, and the frequent use of psychotropic medications by physicians to treat these symptoms, very few studies have examined the utility of psychotropic medications in treating these symptoms in Alzheimer's patients. Apparently only two reports have been published with regard to the treatment of affective symptoms (depression) in Alzheimer's patients. One was a study of minaprine, a compound which is not marketed in the United States, in the treatment of Alzheimer's patients (Passeri et al., 1985). The other was of some cases of Alzheimer's disease with depression who successfully responded to monoamine oxidase inhibition treatment (Jenike, 1985). Only one study, described further below, has specifically examined the treatment of agitation and psychotic symptomatology in Alzheimer's patients (Borenstein et al., 1986). A few other studies have examined these treatment issues in diverse dementia patient groups which have included patients with specifically diagnosed Alzheimer's disease (Petrie et al., 1982; Barnes et al., 1982; Helms, 1985).

Before adequate investigations can proceed, the nature of potentially remediable behavioral symptomatology in Alzheimer's patients must be described and appropriate rating instruments for measuring such symptoms must be available.

NATURE OF PHARMACOLOGICALLY REMEDIABLE SYMPTOMATOLOGY

The recent work, alluded to above, which has described in detail the nature of the primary cognitive symptomatology in Alzheimer's disease, has permitted the separation of remediable symptoms which are not part of this core syndrome. The nature of these symptoms in the Alzheimer's patient appear to be the result of two primary interacting processes: (1) the characteristic neurotransmitter changes which occur in the brains of the Alzheimer's patient, and (2) the cognitive changes occurring in the Alzheimer's patient.

With respect to neurotransmitter changes in Alzheimer's disease, deficits in choline acetyltransferase have been repeatedly observed in the brains of Alzheimer's patients and have been shown to correlate with the severity of the illness process (Davies and Maloney, 1976; Perry et al., 1977; Perry et al., 1978a; Bowen et al., 1979). Other deficits in the cholinergic system (Perry et al., 1978b; Marsh et al., 1985) and other central neurotransmitter systems (Francis et al., 1985; Rossor et al., 1984) have been noted to occur in Alzheimer's patients. Notable amongst these are noradrenergic deficits (Bondareff et al., 1982), and perhaps decrements in serotonergic (Bowen et al., 1983) and glutamate (Greenamyre et al., 1985) cerebral neuronal functioning. Increments in MAO-B activity have also been noted to occur centrally and peripherally in Alzheimer's patients (Adolfsson, et al., 1980). Collectively, these changes are likely to produce characteristic neurochemical milieus of pharmacologic relevance in the brains of Alzheimer's patients. Indeed, the oft-cited cholinergic deficits are frequently posited to mitigate against the utility of psychotropic substances with prominent anticholinergic effects.

In addition to neurochemical changes, the essential cognitive disturbances accompanying Alzheimer's disease are likely to be of relevance with respect to behavioral syndromes. For example, it has been noted that

2

Alzheimer's patients frequently have the delusions, that "people are stealing things from them," that "the spouse is an imposter" and that their "house is not their home" (Reisberg and Ferris, 1985). It is possible that the delusional tendencies in these patients are manifested by symptomatology, the specific nature of which is colored by the cognitive deficit. For example, with increasing cognitive deficit, Alzheimer's patients no longer remember where they have placed things as well as formerly. Consequently, when they become delusional, they may have a tendency to develop the delusion that people are stealing things from them. Similarly, with the evolution of cognitive deficit, Alzheimer's patients no longer recognize their spouse or their home environment with the same facility. Accordingly, when they develop delusional tendencies, these may frequently be manifested in content as the false belief that their spouse is not truly their spouse or that they are not, in actuality, in their domicile.

Another behavioral syndrome frequently noted in the Alzheimer's patient is purposeless activity or cognitive abulia (literally, a loss of will power resulting from decreased cognitive abilities). Decreased cognition results in decreased ability to channel one's energy in specific, goal-oriented, behavior. Since motoric functioning is relatively well-preserved until the very last substages of the illness, Alzheimer's patients begin to exhibit purposeless behavior such as pacing. In severe Alzheimer's disease abrading is common. The patient may scratch themselves, tear at a sofa, etc.

In order to develop more information about the precise nature and incidence of potentially remediable behavioral symptoms in outpatients with specifically diagnosed Alzheimer's disease, we conducted a retrospective chart review (Borenstein et al., 1986).

Fifty-seven patients with a diagnosis of Alzheimer's disease and Global Deterioration Scale (GDS) scores of 4 or greater were studied. The mean age of the patients was $75 \pm 9.1$ years (range = 55-93 years) and they consisted of 24 men and 33 women.

The records of these patients were reviewed in detail with particular reference to the incidence of psychotic and depressed symptoms. Specifically, for each patient visit or telephone contact, the nature of any behavioral symptoms as documented in the patient records was noted. Patients were characterized as having behavioral symptoms associated with primarily psychotic or depressive symptomatology. The severity of illness, as reflected by GDS scores was also noted for all subjects. Additionally, pharmacologic interventions to remediate these behavioral symptoms were examined in detail with respect to medication, dosage, side effects and response. A positive response was noted if specific mention of this was made in the patient's record or if the treatment protocol was indicative of improved behavior (e.g., a steady state dose was maintained or medication dose was decreased for reasons other than side effects).

Thirty-three of the 57 (58%) patients with Alzheimer's disease were noted to have had psychotic and/or depressive symptoms at some point in their assessment. These subjects did not differ significantly from those without behavioral symptomatology in either age or sex. Twenty-six of the subjects showed symptoms of a psychotic nature only, six manifested depressive symptomatology which was subsequently followed by psychotic symptoms, and one patient showed depressive symptoms only. The single patient who manifested symptoms of depression without psychosis was not followed subsequently.

Forty-seven percent of patients in the 4th GDS stage (mild Alzheimer's disease, e.g., decreased ability to handle finances) had psychotic symptoms, 43% of patients in the 5th stage (moderate Alzheimer's disease, e.g., decreased ability to choose proper clothing) had psychotic symptoms, and 68% of patients in the 6th stage (moderately severe Alzheimer's disease, e.g., decreased ability to dress, bathe and toilet) had psychotic symptoms.

Of the six patients with depressive symptomatology who were seen subsequently, half presented in the 4th GDS stage and half in the 5th GDS stage; all developed symptoms of primarily a psychotic nature one GDS stage later.

The specific nature of the symptoms can be seen in Table 1. The most frequent symptoms noted were the delusion that "people are stealing things" from the patient and agitation of a non-specific nature. Forty-eight percent of all subjects who displayed behavioral symptoms were noted to have each of the above symptoms. The next most frequently observed were day/night disturbances (42%), purposeless activity or cognitive abulia (36%), violence (30%), and verbal outbursts (24%). The most frequent affective symptom noted was tearful episodes (24%).

Table 1. Nature and Incidence of Behavioral Symptoms
Noted in Thirty-Three Alzheimer's Patients

| Symptoms | Na | %b |
|----------|-----|-----|
| **PSYCHOTIC** | | |
| "People are stealing things" | 16 | 48 |
| Agitation | 16 | 48 |
| Day-night Disturbance | 14 | 42 |
| Purposeless Activity (cognitive abulia) | 12 | 36 |
| Violence | 10 | 30 |
| Verbal Outbursts | 8 | 24 |
| "One's house is not one's house | 7 | 21 |
| Delusion of Abandonment | 7 | 21 |
| Suspiciousness | 7 | 21 |
| Paranoia | 7 | 21 |
| Visual Hallucinations | 4 | 12 |
| Hallucinations (unspecified type) | 4 | 12 |
| Delusions (unspecified type) | 4 | 12 |
| "Spouse is an imposter" | 3 | 9 |
| Threats | 3 | 9 |
| Fearfulness | 3 | 9 |
| Compulsive Behavior | 2 | 6 |
| Wandering | 1 | 3 |
| **DEPRESSIVE** | | |
| Tearful Episodes | 8 | 24 |
| Anxiety | 4 | 12 |
| Decreased Appetite | 3 | 9 |
| Mood Fluctuations | 1 | 3 |
| Flattened Affect/Withdrawn | 1 | 3 |

aTotal number of patients exhibiting particular symptom.

bPercentage of patients with behavioral (psychotic and/ or depressive) symptomatology who were noted to exhibit the symptom.

Of the 33 subjects with behavioral symptomatology, 23 were treated for these symptoms with thioridazine for intervals of two weeks to 22 months (mean treatment interval = $7.8 \pm 6.8$ months), with dosages ranging from 10 to 250 mg (mean maximum dose = $54.6 \pm 46.2$ mg.). Fifteen (56%) subjects showed a positive response to the thioridazine regimen and five subjects (19%) showed no response. Seven of the subjects (26%) were not followed long enough to determine response.

NEED FOR A NEW CLINICAL RATING SCALE

Standardized and widely utilized clinical rating instruments are currently available for assessment of the magnitude of depressive symptomatology (Hamilton, 1960; Zung, 1965; Yesavage et al., 1983) psychotic symptomatology (Overall and Gorham, 1962), so-called "psychogeriatric symptomatology" (Shader et al., 1974), dementia symptomatology (Blessed et al., 1968; Folstein et al., 1975; Jacobs et al., 1977; Kahn et al., 1960; Pfeiffer, 1975; Reisberg et al., 1983a, 1983b), and Alzheimer's symptomatology (Reisberg et al., 1982; Reisberg et al., 1984; Reisberg et al., 1985a). All of these assessments have serious deficiencies in terms of their ability to assess the magnitude of pharmacologically remediable behavioral symptomatology in the Alzheimer's patient.

Self-rating depression scales such as those of Zung and Yesavage et al. are clearly inappropriate for the patient with Alzheimer's disease whose recall is seriously impaired and in whom denial is a major defense mechanism (Reisberg et al., 1985b). Even when tearful episodes, sleep disturbance, agitation or other depressive or depression-like symptoms do occur in the Alzheimer's patient, the patient is not a reliable informant as to the nature or magnitude of such symptoms both because of their cognitive deficit and because of the significant denial of symptomatology. Indeed, whereas depressed patients have often been noted to exaggerate the magnitude of their symptoms, this is not true of the Alzheimer's patient, even when family members or other close contacts note the presence of depressive symptoms such as those enumerated above.

Depression scales such as the Hamilton scale, are also inappropriate for the Alzheimer's patient for several reasons. Most fundamentally the depressive syndrome of Alzheimer's disease is different in its symptomatology and course from the unipolar and bipolar major affective disorders (APA, 1980) which the Hamilton scale is designed to measure. Major affective disorder may, or may not, be accompanied by psychosis. The depressive syndrome of Alzheimer's disease generally evolves into, and is ultimately replaced by, a psychotic or psychosis-like syndrome marked by agitation, repetitive wakenings over the course of the evening, suspiciousness, delusional ideation, and, less frequently, hallucinations.

Certain Hamilton scale items are clearly inappropriate for the Alzheimer's patient with impaired cognitive and functional abilities. Notable among these are Hamilton items 7, 8, 17, and 19, assessing "work and activities," "retardation," "insight," and "depersonalization and derealization," respectively. The presence of dementia itself is of course invariably associated with a decrement in occupational and other abilities. Additionally, early dementia is associated with a flattening of affect and a decrease in activities. Insight, too, by definition is altered by dementia, although denial also plays a role in altering responses to queries designed to measure insight (Reisberg et al., 1985b). Psychomotor slowing is also frequently noted in the patient with Alzheimer's disease, apparently resulting from the more general cognitive decrement (Reisberg et al., 1983b). This slowing in dementia patients may be entirely independent of affective changes. Finally "depersonalization" and "derealization" are inappropriate queries for the patient with Alzheimer's disease or, indeed, other forms of dementia.

The remaining Hamilton items are not particularly evocative of the depressive syndrome of Alzheimer's disease. This tends to be marked by

5

transient episodes of tearfulness, but not pervasive dysphoria. It also tends to be marked by a sleep disturbance associated with a decrease in diurnal cues, and hence a tendency to nap during the day with frequent wakenings in the evening. The origins and character of this sleep disturbance is somewhat different from that of a major depressive episode. Weight loss, suicidal ideation, and diurnal variations in mood are very uncommon in the depressive syndrome of Alzheimer's disease (see Table 1).

For all of the above reasons, present rating instruments for the magnitude of affective disorder are inappropriate for the depressive syndrome of Alzheimer's disease. Because this syndrome appears to exist in a continuum with the psychotic syndrome of Alzheimer's disease, a rating instrument designed to assess this syndrome should probably incorporate both phases of the continuum, while being independent of the magnitude of cognitive symptomatology.

Currently available clinical rating instruments for assessing the magnitude of psychotic symptomatology are also inappropriate for the Alzheimer's patient. The Brief Psychiatric Rating Scale (BPRS; Overall and Gorham, 1962) is the most widely utilized scale for the assessment of psychotic symptomatology and its pharmacologic remediation, irrespective of etiology. The scale consists of 18 items, each assessed on a seven-point magnitude of severity rating. Of these 18 items, those reflecting emotional withdrawal (lack of spontaneous interaction, isolation, deficiency in relating to others); blunted affect (reduced emotional tone, reduction in normal intensity of feeling, flatness); and disorientation (confusion or lack of proper association for person, place, or time--items 3, 16, and 18, respectively), are clearly inappropriate in the assessment of possibly remediable affective and psychosis-like symptomatology in the Alzheimer's patient. Other items such as Item 4, conceptual disorganization (thought processes confused, disconnected, disorganized, disrupted) and Item 13, motor retardation (slowed weakened movements or speech, reduced body tone), are confounded for assessment purposes either directly, as in the case of Item 4, or indirectly, in the case of Item 13, by the cognitive symptomatology of Alzheimer's disease. Many of the remaining items are not particularly evocative of the potentially remediable behavioral affective and psychotic symptomatology in Alzheimer's disease. For example, Items 7, 8, and 15 assessing mannerisms and posturing (peculiar, biazrre, unnatural motor behavior), grandiosity (exaggerated self-opinion, arrogance, conviction of unusual power or abilities), and unusual thought content (unusual, odd, strange, bizarre thought content), all occur rarely, if ever, in Alzheimer's patients. Of the remaining ten items, those reflecting somatic concerns and guilt feelings (Items 1 and 5) are very uncommonly seen even in the affective syndrome of Alzheimer's disease. This leaves eight items on the BPRS which are to a variable extent potential measures of the remediable behavioral syndrome of Alzheimer's disease. However, even these measures are not ideal assessments of this characteristic syndrome.

The psychogeriatric scales, of which the Sandoz Clinical Assessment Geriatric (SCAG; Shadar et al., 1974) is probably the most widely utilized, also suffer from many of the same deficiencies as the BPRS, namely (1) the prominent inclusion of items reflecting cognitive symptomatology which is presently, unfortunately, not remediable in the Alzheimer's patient, and which exists invariably in the Alzheimer's patient and is independent of the behavioral syndrome, and (2) items reflecting behavioral changes which either do not occur in Alzheimer's disease, or are not ideally evocative of the potentially pharmacologically remediable behavioral syndrome in Alzheimer's disease. Of the 19 SCAG items, five reflect cognitive dysfunction and three reflect withdrawal (Salzman, 1983). These eight items are not useful in regard to assessing the behavioral syndrome of Alzheimer's disease. Five items reflect "mood depression." One of these "dizzyness", commonly relates to inner ear disturbance, orthostatic hypotension and other cardiovascular disturbances, but is unrelated to Alzheimer's disease or, more particularly, to the affective changes in Alzheimer's disease. Another item in this mood depression "orthogonal factor," "fatigue," also has little or no relationship to Alzheimer's disease. Appetite decrement is very uncommon in Alzheimer's disease. This leaves only the SCAG items "mood depression" and "anxiety" to assess the affective elements in the Alzheimer's behavioral syndrome. Tearfulness, the most common affective symptom in Alzheimer's patients is not assessed in the SCAG and not mentioned as a descriptor of any SCAG item. Neither is the other commonly observed affective symptom, frequent nighttime wakenings, alluded to in the SCAG, although, early wakening is mentioned as a component of the mood depression item.

The SCAG's "agitation irritability" orthogonal factor does contain items which occur in the behavioral syndrome of Alzheimer's disease. The major problem is that these items: "emotional lability," "irritability," "hostility," "bothersomeness," and "uncooperativeness," lack specific severity criteria useful in Alzheimer's patients and hence tend to all be assessed on the same, somewhat arbitrary continuum. Suspiciousness and delusions--the most common and prominent features of the behavioral syndrome of Alzheimer's disease--are not assessed on the SCAG.

Mental status assessments such as the commonly utilized assessments alluded to above (Folstein et al., 1975; Jacobs et al., 1977; Kahn et al., 1960; Pfeiffer, 1975), do not incorporate emotional or behavioral assessments. Other scales assessing the magnitude of dementia symptomatology such as the Blessed Dementia Scale (Blessed et al., 1968) and the Brief Cognitive Rating Scale (BCRS; Reisberg et al., 1983a, 1983b) incorporate some emotional change measures. The Blessed Dementia Scale has a section assessing "changes in personality, interests, drive." However, as has been true of many of the measures which have been discussed above, many of these items are the secondary resultants of cognitive changes in the patient with Alzheimer's disease (increased rigidity; coarsening of affect; diminished emotional responsiveness; hobbies relinquished; and diminished initiative or growing apathy). The remaining six items frequently have no relationship to the clinical syndrome of Alzheimer's disease (increased egocentricity, impairment of regard for feelings of others, hilarity in inappropriate situations, and sexual misdemeanor). This leaves only two all-or-none assessments in the Blessed scale of relevance, namely "impairment of emotional control" and "purposeless hyperactivity." Clearly these two items do not in and of themselves evoke the behavioral syndrome described in Table 1. Similarly, the single BCRS axis assessing progressive mood changes accompanying the evolution of progressively more severe Alzheimer's disease is an insufficient description of the behavioral syndrome in the disease as are global and functional changes reflecting the progression of the disease (GDS, Reisberg et al., 1982; FAST, Reisberg et al., 1984).

DESCRIPTION OF THE BEHAVIORAL PATHOLOGY IN ALZHEIMER'S DISEASE RATING SCALE (BEHAVE-AD)

The Behavioral Pathology in Alzheimer's Disease Rating Scale (BEHAVE-AD) can be found in Table 2. It differs from the rating measures discussed in the previous section in several important ways. Specifically: (1) all assessment measures are designed to specifically reflect and measure the characteristic behavioral symptoms which commonly occur in the Alzheimer's patient; (2) all assessment measures are largely independent of the primary, presently unremediable, cognitive symptomatology of Alzheimer's disease; (3) all assessment measures reflect behaviors which are frequently disturbing to caregivers of the Alzheimer's patient, and (4) all assessment measures re-

flect behaviors which present clinical and research experience indicates
are potentially remediable in the Alzheimer's patient, through pharmacologic
and perhaps other interventions. Collectively, these advantages should
enable clinical investigators to utilize this quantified assessment tool in
prospectively designed studies of pharmacologically remediable symptoms in
the Alzheimer's patient. Since virtually no such prospective studies have
yet been conducted, this would appear to be an opportune time for the introduction of such a measure. It should be noted that this scale incorporates
information and experience from a previous measure designed by us which we
found to be underinclusive (Reisberg and Ferris, 1985).

The separation of unremediable cognitive symptomatology from the
BEHAVE-AD permits investigators to examine the stage-specific nature of
behavioral symptomatology in Alzheimer's disease. As briefly discussed
earlier in this paper, on the basis of current data there does appear to be
a tendency for behavioral symptoms to occur in a relatively stage-specific
time-course in Alzheimer's patients. The further identification of these
stage-specific aspects is of relevance for clinicians in the treatment of
Alzheimer's patients and the counseling of their families. Such issues can
now be examined independently. Alzheimer's patients can be assessed as to
their degree of cognitive impairment on the GDS, on Part I of the BCRS, on
mental status assessments, and on neuropsychological tests, independently of
their behavioral assessment, except to the extent to which agitation
delusions, or other behavioral aspects directly interfere with cognitive
measures. In the majority of cases the latter caveat does not appear to be
a major problem.

The separation of cognitive and behavioral features of Alzheimer's
disease, also permits investigators to independently examine the effects of
pharmacologic agents which improve BEHAVE-AD symptomatology on cognitive
functioning. Some of the agents which present clinical experience indicates
may be most effective in remediating BEHAVE-AD symptoms, such as
thioridazine and amitriptylene, are frequently said to exert anticholinergic
effects which interfere with cognitive abilities. Whether, in the dosages
which are therapeutically useful in Alzheimer's patients, these anticholinergic effects are indeed of clinical relevance and indeed interfere
with cognition, is not presently clear. This question, and similar ones,
are now amenable to investigation.

The relative specificity of the BEHAVE-AD with regard to remediable
symptomatology in Alzheimer's disease should make it particularly useful in
studies in this patient population. Behaviors which are relatively common
in these patients, which might otherwise be overlooked are specifically
graded, in part serving the clinician and caregiver by alerting them to
potentially remediable symptomatology. Also, the tendency evident in some
previous scales toward clustering of ill-defined symptoms should be avoided
utilizing the BEHAVE-AD except in cases where such symptoms indeed occur
together.

Table 2. Behavioral Pathology in Alzheimer's Disease Rating Scale
(BEHAVE-AD)*

---

Part I: Symptomatology

Assessment Interval: Specify: _____ wks.
Total Score: _____

(continued)

A. Paranoid and Delusional Ideation

1. "People are Stealing Things" Delusion
   (∅)  Not present
   (1)  Delusion that people are hiding objects
   (2)  Delusion that people are coming into the home and hiding or stealing objects
   (3)  Talking and listening to people coming into the home

2. "One's House is Not One's Home" Delusion
   (∅)  Not present
   (1)  Conviction that the place in which one is residing is not one's home (e.g., packing to go home; complaints, while at home, of "take me home")
   (2)  Attempt to leave domiciliary to go home
   (3)  Violence in response to attempts to forcibly restrict exit

3. "Spouse (or Other Caregiver) is an Imposter" Delusion
   (∅)  Not present
   (1)  Conviction that spouse (or other caregiver) is an imposter
   (2)  Anger toward spouse (or other caregiver for being an imposter)
   (3)  Violence towards spouse (or other caregiver) for being an imposter

4. "Delusion of Abandonment" (e.g. to an institution)
   (∅)  Not present
   (1)  Suspicion of caregiver plotting abandonment or institutionalization (e.g. on telephone)
   (2)  Accusation of a conspiracy to abandon or institutionalize
   (3)  Accusation of impending or immediate desertion or institutionalization.

5. "Delusion of Infidelity"
   (∅)  Not present
   (1)  Conviction that spouse and/or children, and/or other caregivers, are unfaithful
   (2)  Anger toward spouse, relative or other caregiver for their infidelity
   (3)  Violence toward spouse, relative or other caregiver for their supposed infidelity

6. "Suspiciousness/Paranoia" (other than above)
   (∅)  Not present
   (1)  Suspicious (e.g. hiding objects which they later may be unable to locate)
   (2)  Paranoid (i.e. fixed conviction with respect to suspicions and/or anger as a result of suspicions)
   (3)  Violence as a result of suspicions
   Unspecified?_____
   Describe_____
   _____
   _____

7. Delusions (other than above)
   (∅)  Not present
   (1)  Delusional
   (2)  Verbal emotional manifestations as a result of delusions
   (3)  Physical actions or violence as a result of delusions
   Unspecified?_____
   Describe_____
   _____
   _____

B. Hallucinations

    8. Visual Hallucinations
      (Ø) Not present
      (1) Vague: not clearly defined
      (2) Clearly defined hallucinations of objects or persons (e.g. sees other people at the table)
      (3) Verbal or physical actions or emotional responses to the hallucinations

    9. Auditory Hallucinations
      (Ø) Not present
      (1) Vague: not clearly defined
      (2) Clearly defined hallucinations of words or phrases
      (3) Verbal or physical actions or emotional responses to the hallucinations

    10. Olfactory Hallucinations
      (Ø) Not present
      (1) Vague: not clearly defined
      (2) Clearly defined
      (3) Verbal or physical actions or emotional responses to the hallucinations

    11. Haptic Hallucinations
      (Ø) Not present
      (1) Vague: not clearly defined
      (2) Clearly defined
      (3) Verbal or physical actions or emotional responses to the hallucinations

    12. Other Hallucinations
      (Ø) Not present
      (1) Vague: not clearly defined
      (2) Clearly defined
      (3) Verbal or physical actions or emotional responses to the hallucinations
      Unspecified?_____
      Describe_____
      _____
      _____


C. Activity Disturbances

    13. Wandering: away from home or caregiver
      (Ø) Not present
      (1) Somewhat, but not sufficient as to necessitate restraint
      (2) Sufficient as to require restraint
      (3) Verbal or physical emotional responses to attempts to prevent wandering

    14. Purposeless activity (cognitive abulia)
      (Ø) Not present
      (1) Repetitive purposeless activity (e.g. opening and closing pocketbook; packing and unpacking clothing; repeatedly putting on and removing clothing; opening and closing drawers; insistent repeating of demands or questions)
      (2) Pacing or other purposeless activity sufficient to require restraint
      (3) Abrading or physical harm resulting from purposeless activity

15. Inappropriate Activity
    (∅) Not present
    (1) Inappropriate activities (e.g. storing and hiding objects in inappropriate places such as throwing clothing in wastebasket or putting empty plates in the oven; inappropriate sexual behavior such as inappropriate exposure)
    (2) Present and sufficient to require restraint
    (3) Present, sufficient to require restraint and accompanied by anger or violence when restrained

D. Aggressivity

16. Verbal outbursts
    (∅) Not present
    (1) Present (including unaccustomed use of foul or abusive language)
    (2) Present and accompanied by anger
    (3) Present, accompanied by anger, and clearly directed at other persons

17. Physical threats and/or violence
    (∅) Not present
    (1) Threatening behavior
    (2) Physical violence
    (3) Physical violence accompanied by vehemence

18. Agitation (other than above)
    (∅) Not present
    (1) Present
    (2) Present with emotional component
    (3) Present with emotional and physical component
    Unspecified?_____
    Describe_____
    _____
    _____

E. Diurnal Rhythm Disturbances

19. Day/Night Disturbance
    (∅) Not present
    (1) Repetitive wakenings during night
    (2) 5∅ to 75% of former cycle at night
    (3) Complete disturbance of diurnal rhythm (i.e. less than 5∅% of former sleep cycle at night)

F. Affective Disturbances

2∅. Tearfulness
    (∅) Not present
    (1) Present
    (2) Present and accompanied by clear affective component
    (3) Present and accompanied by affective and physical component (e.g., "wrings hands" or other gestures)

21. Depressed Mood: Other
    (∅) Present
    (1) Present (e.g. occassional statement "I wish I were dead," without clear affective concomitants)
    (2) Present with clear concomitants (e.g. thoughts of death)

(3)   Present with emotional and physical concomitants (e.g. suicide gestures)

Unspecified? _____

Describe _____

_____

_____

G.   Anxieties and Phobias

22.   Anxiety regarding upcoming events (Godot syndrome)
(Ø)   Not present
(1)   Present:  Repeated queries and/or other activities regarding upcoming appointments and/or events
(2)   Present and disturbing to caregivers
(3)   Present and intolerable to caregivers

23.   Other anxieties
(Ø)   Not present
(1)   Present
(2)   Present and disturbing to caregivers
(3)   Present and intolerable to caregivers

Unspecified? _____

Describe _____

_____

_____

24.   Fear of being left alone
(Ø)   Not present
(1)   Present:  fear of being alone is voiced
(2)   Vocalized and sufficient to require specific action on part of caregiver
(3)   Vocalized and sufficient to require patient to be accompanied at all times

25.   Other phobias
(Ø)   Not present
(1)   Present
(2)   Present and of sufficient magnitude to require specific action on part of caregiver
(3)   Present and sufficient to prevent patient activities

Unspecified? _____

Describe _____

_____

_____

Behavioral Pathology in Alzheimer's Disease Rating Scale

(BEHAVE - AD)

Part 2:   Global Rating

With respect to the above symptoms, they are of sufficient magnitude as to be:

(Ø)   Not at all troubling to the caregivers or dangerous to the patient

(1) Mildly troubling to the caregiver or dangerous to the patient
(2) Moderately troubling to the caregiver or dangerous to the patient
(3) Severely troubling or intolerable to the caregiver or dangerous to the patient

CONCLUSION

The rationale and development of a new clinical rating scale designed to assess the presence and magnitude of potentially remediable behavioral symptomatology in Alzheimer's patients have been presented herein.  The scale, the BEHAVE-AD, enables clinicians to sensitively and accurately assess behavioral symptoms in Alzheimer's patients, independent of untreatable cognitive features of the illness.  We believe the scale will be useful in pharmacologic investigations into the treatment of affective and psychotic aspects of Alzheimer's disease.

Acknowledgements

This work was supported in part by a grant from the Hurd Foundation and the Beckman Research Institute of the City of Hope and U.S. Public Health Service grants AG03051, MH38275, and MH29590.

REFERENCES

Adolfsson, R., Gottfries, C.G., Oreland, L. et al.,  Increased activity of brain and platelet monoamine oxidase in dementia of the Alzheimer type, Life Sciences, 27:1029-1034.

American Psychiatric Association Diagnostic and Statistical Manual of Mental Disorders, 3rd Edition, 1980, Washington:  American Psychiatric Association, 1980.

Barnes, R., Veith, R., Okimoto, J., Raskind, M. & Gumbrecht, G., 1982, Efficacy of antipsychotic medication in behaviorally disturbed dementia patients,  American Journal of Psychiatry, 139: 1170-1174.

Blessed, G., Tomlinson, B.E., & Roth, M., 1968, The association between quantitative measures of dementia and senile change in the cerebral gray matter of elderly subjects,  British Journal of Psychiatry, 114:797-811.

Bondareff, W., Mountjoy, C.Q. & Roth, M., 1982,  Loss of neurons of origin of the adrenergic projection to cerebral cortex (nucleus locus ceruleus) in senile dementia, Neurology, 32:164-168.

Borenstein, J., Reisberg, B., Salob, S. & Ferris, S.H., 1986, Behavioral symptomatology in patients with Alzheimer's disease:  Phenomenology and treatment.  Society of Biological Psychiatry, Forty-First Annual Convention and Scientific program, (Abstract), p. 325.

Bowen, D.M., Allen, S.J., Benton, J.S. et al., Biochemical assessment of serotonergic and cholinergic dysfunction and cerebral atrophy in Alzheimer's disease, Journal of Neurochemistry, 41:266-272.

Bowen, D.M., Spillane, J.A., Curzon, G., Meier-Ruge, W., White, P., Goodhardt, M.J., Iwangoff, P & Davison, A.N., 1979, Accelerated aging or selective neuronal loss as an important cause of dementia, Lancet, 1:11-14.

Davies, P. & Maloney, A.J.F., 1976, Selective loss of central cholinergic neurons in Alzheimer's disease, Lancet, 1976, 2:1403.

Ferris, S.H., Steinberg, G., Shulman, E., Kahn, R. & Reisberg, B., 1985, Institutionalization of Alzheimer's patients: Reducing precipitating factors through family counseling. Archives of the Foundation of Thanatology, 12:7.

Folstein, M.F., Folstein, S.E., & McHugh, P.R., 1975, Mini-mental state: A practical method of grading the cognitive state of patients for the clinician, Journal of Psychiatric Research, 12:189-198.

Francis, P.T., Palmer, A.M., Sims, N.R., Bowen, D.M., Davison, A.N., Esiri, M.M., Neary, D., Snowden, J.S., Wilcock, G.K., 1985, Neurochemical studies of early-onset Alzheimer's disease: Possible influence on treatment. New England Journal of Medicine, 313:7-11.

Greenamyre, J.T., Penney, J.B., Young, A.B., D'Amato, C.J., Hicks, S.P. & Shoulson, I., 1985, Alterations in L-glutamate binding in Alzheimer's and Huntington's diseases. Science, 227:1496-1499.

Hamilton, M., 1960, A rating scale for depression, Journal of Neurology, Neurosurgery and Psychiatry, 1960, 23:56-62.

Helms, P.M., 1985, Efficacy of antipsychotics in the treatment of the behavioral complications of dementia: A review of the literature. Journal of the American Geriatrics Society, 33:206-209.

Jacobs, J.W., Bernhard, M.R., Delgado, A. & Strain, J.F., 1977, Screening for organic mental syndromes in the mentally ill, Annals of Internal Medicine, 80:40-46.

Jenike, M.A., 1985, Monoamine oxidase inhibitors as treatment for depressed patients with primary degenerative dementia (Alzheimer's disease), American Journal of Psychiatry, 142:763-764.

Kahn, R.L., Goldfarb, A.I., Pollack, M., & Peck, A., 1960, Brief objective measures for the determination of mental status in the aged, American Journal of Psychiatry, 117:326-328.

Marsh, D.C., Flynn, D.D. & Potter, L.T.,1985, Loss of M2 muscarinic receptors in the cerebral cortex in Alzheimer's disease and experimental cholinergic denervation, Science, 227:1115-1117.

Overall, J.E. & Gorham, D.R., 1982, The brief psychiatric rating scale, Psychological Reports, 10:799-812.

Passeri, M., Cucinotta, D., DeMello, M., Storchi, G., Roncucci, R. & Biziere, K., 1985, Minaprine for senile dementia. Lancet, 1:824.

Perry, E.K., Perry, R.H., Blessed, G. & Tomlinson, B.E., 1977, Necropsy evidence of central cholinergic deficits in senile dementia, Lancet, 1:189.

Perry, E.K., Perry, R.H., Blessed, G., et al., 1978b, Changes in brain cholinesterases in senile dementia of the Alzheimer type. Neuropath. Appl. Neurobiology, 4:273-277.

Perry, E.K., Tomlinson, B.E., Blessed, G., Bergmann, K., Gibson, P.H. & Perry, R.H., 1978a, Correlation of cholinergic abnormalities with senile plaques and mental test scores in senile dementia, British Medical Journal, 2:1457-1459.

Petrie, W.M., Ban, T.A., Berney, S., et al., 1982, Loxapine in psychogeriatrics: A placebo- and standard-controlled clinical investigation, Journal of Clinical Psychopharmacology, 2:122.

Pfeiffer, E.A., 1975, Short portable mental status questionnaire for the assessment of organic brain deficit in the elderly, Journal of the American Geriatric Society, 23:433-441.

Reisberg, B., 1981, Brain failure: An Introduction to Current Concepts of Senility, New York: Macmillan, (Published in paperback as, A Guide to Alzheimer's Disease, New York: The Free Press/Macmillan 1983).

Reisberg, B. & Ferris, S.H., 1985, A clinical rating scale for symptoms of psychosis in Alzheimer's disease, Psychopharmacology Bulletin, 21: 101-104.

Reisberg, B., Ferris, S.H., Anand, R., de Leon, M.J., Schneck, M.K., Buttinger, C. & Borenstein, J., 1984, Functional staging of dementia of the Alzheimer's type, Annals of the New York Academy of Sciences, 1984, 435:481-483.

Reisberg, B., Ferris, S.H., de Leon, M.J. & Crook, T., 1982, The global deterioration scale for assessment of primary degenerative dementia. American Journal of Psychiatry, 139:1136-1139.

Reisberg, B., Ferris, S.H., & Franssen, E., 1985a, An ordinal functional assessment tool for Alzheimer's type dementia. Hospital & Community Psychiatry, 36:593-595.

Reisberg, B., Ferris, S.H., Shulman, E., Steinberg, G., Buttinger, C., Sinaiko, E., Borenstein, J., de Leon, M.J. & Cohen, J., 1986, Longitudinal course of normal aging and progressive dementia of the Alzheimer's type: A prospective study of 106 subjects over a 3.6 year mean interval, Prog. Neuro Psychopharmacol. & Biol. Psychiat., 10:571-578.

Reisberg, B., Gordon, B., McCarthy, M., Ferris, S.H. & de Leon, M.J., 1985b, Insight and denial accompanying progressive cognitive decline in normal aging and Alzheimer's disease, in: B. Stanely Ed., Geriatric Psychiatry: Ethical and Legal Issues, Washington: American Psychiatric Press, pp 37-79.

Reisberg, B., London, E., Ferris, S.H., Borenstein, J., Scheier, L. & de Leon, M.J., 1983b, The Brief Cognitive Rating Scale: Language, motoric, and mood concomitants in primary degenerative dementia, Psychopharmacology Bulletin, 19:702-708.

Reisberg, B., Schneck, M.K., Ferris, S.H., Schwartz, G.E. & de Leon, M.J., 1983a, The brief cognitive rating scale (BCRS): Findings in primary degenerative dementia (PDD). Psychopharmacology Bulletin, 19:47-50.

Rossor, M.N., Iversen, L.L., Reynolds, G.P., et al., 1984, Neurochemical characteristics of early and late onset types of Alzheimer's disease, British Medical Journal, 288:961-964.

Salzman, L., 1983, The Sandoz clinical assessment geriatric scale. in:

"Assessment in Geriatric Psychopharmacology, T. Crook, S.Ferris, and R. Bartus, eds., Mark Powley Associates, New Canaan, CT, pp. 53-58.

Schneck, M.K., Reisberg, B. & Ferris, S.H., 1982, An overview of current concepts of Alzheimer's disease. *American Journal of Psychiatry*, 139:165-173.

Shader, R.I., Harmatz, J.S., Salzman, C., 1974, A new scale for clinical assessment in geriatric populations: Sandoz Clinical Assessment-Geriatric (SCAG). *Journal of the American Geriatrics Society*, 22: 107-113.

Shulman, E., and Steinberg, G., 1984, Emotional reactions of Alzheimer's caregivers in support group settings. *Gerontologist*, (Special Issue).

Yesavage, J.A., Brink, T.L., Rose, T.L. & Adey, M., 1983, The geriatric depression rating scale: Comparison with other self-report and psychiatric rating scales. in: "Assessment in Geriatric Psycho-pharmacology," T. Crook, S.H. Ferris, and R. Bartus, eds., Mark Powley Associates, Inc., New Canaan, CT, pp. 153-165.

Zung, W.W.K., 1965, A self-rating depression scale. *Archives of General Psychiatry*, 12:63-70.

# DIAGNOSIS OF ALZHEIMER'S DISEASE

## BY DERMATOGLYPHIC DISCRIMINANTS

Herman J. Weinreb

Department of Neurology
New York University Medical Center
New York, N.Y.

Laboratory of Bacteriology and Immunology
The Rockefeller University
New York, N.Y.

## INTRODUCTION

The operation of a genetic factor in the etiology of Alzheimer's disease (AD) is most strongly supported by multiple levels of association between AD an Down's syndrome (DS). An excess frequency of DS among the first-degree relatives probands with autopsy-proven AD was first uncovered by the extensive pedigree studies of Heston and his colleagues (1976; 1981; 1982), and had recently been independently confirmed by Heyman (1983). Virtually all individuals with DS surviving to the fourth decade manifest the neuropathologic changes of sporadic AD, both qualitatively and quantitatively (Olson and Show, 1969; Ellis et al., 1974; Ball and Nuttall, 1980; Mann et al., 1984; Wisniewski et al., 1985). Amino acid sequence analyses indicate extensive homologies between the cerebrovascular and plaque amyloid fibril proteins of adult DS and sporadic AD brains (Glenner and Wong, 1984; Masters et al., 1985).

Recently, another level of genetic association between AD and DS has been identified in the correspondence of their dermatoglyphic patterns (Weinreb, 1985). Dermatoglyphics is the systematic classification and study of the epidermal ridge patterns on the fingers, palms, and soles (Cummings and Midlo, 1943; Alter, 1966; Schaumann and Alter, 1976; Loesch, 1983). The morphology of dermatoglyphic patterns is genetically determined, but the mode of inheritance is unknown and the genetic mechanisms involved are obscure (Cummins and Midlo, 1943; Schaumann and Alter, 1976). Once fully developed by the sixth prenatal month, these patterns remain unaltered throughout the lifespan (Cummins and Midol, 1943; Walker, 1957; Schaumann and Alter, 1976).

A group of AD patients, when compared to a sample of non-demented patients with other neurological diseases, was observed to have a significantly higher frequency of a particular dermatoglyphic pattern--the ulnar loop--on their fingertips (Weinreb, 1985). This finding was significant because an elevated frequency of ulnar loops is the most salient dermatoglyphic trait in DS patients, and is one of the traits most useful in discriminating DS patients from controls (Cummins and Midlo, 1943; Alter, 1966; Rosner et al., 1967; Schaumann and Alter, 1976).

Prior to the establishment of karyotyping as the definitive procedure for confirming DS, discriminant schemes were devised for this diagnosis, based upon the relative frequencies of specific dermatoglyphic traits in DS and matched normals. These schemes efficiently separated these two populations by dermatoglyphic discriminants and supplemented clinical judgement (Walker, 1957; Reed et al., 1970; Bolling et al., 1971; Borgaonkar et al., 1971; Penrose and Leoesch, 1971; Deckers et al., 1973a; Deckers et al., 1973b; Deckers et al., 1973c). For example, the Hopkins score, proposed by Borgaonkar and colleagues (1971), is based upon predictive discriminant weights assigned to thirty pattern areas on both hands and feet; the summated score discriminates between trisomic DS and karyotypically normal controls with 97% accuracy, and is also able to detect cases of translocation DS and mosaic DS.

The present study surveyed a sample of patients with presumed AD and matched controls, examining for the frequency of those dermatoglyphic traits which are prominent in DS and robust in discriminating DS patients from normals. These traits are the fingertip patterns, interdigital area III patterns, the palmar flexion creses, the palmar hypothenar patterns, and hallucal region patterns (Walker, 1957; Reed et al., 1970; Bolling et al., 1971; Borgaonkar et al., 1971; Penrose and Loesch, 1971; Ceckers et al., 1973c; Schaumann and Alter, 1976). A simple discriminant scheme is devised, based upon an analysis of the relative frequencies of common patterns in these areas.

## METHODS

Patient Selection. Fifty patients comprised the AD group; they fulfilled recent recommendations for the research diagnosis of probable AD (McKhann et al., 1984). Their mean age was 72.1 years. Controls consisted of one hundred randomly sampled patients who were age 50 years or older with other medical or neurological illnesses. Their mean age was 71.7 years. They had no diagnosis of dementia and had no history of an acute or chronic encephalopathy in the year prior to evaluation. Each AD patient was matched to two control patients by age (to the nearest half-decade), sex, and racial background. The matching of sex and race minimizes the small but potentially significant confounding influence of these variables on the frequency of dermatoglyphic patterns (Cummins and Midlo, 1943; Schaumann and Alter, 1976), while age matching minimizes cohort effects.

Excluded from this analysis were patients with diagnosis of Parkinson's disease, with or without dementia; patients in whom limb trauma prevented accurate assessment; and patients with genetic defects or a history of mental retardation.

Dermatoglyphic analysis. Dermatoglyphic patterns were recorded from the fingers, palms, and feet by non-invasive inkless methods (Schaumann and Alter, 1976). Five pattern areas were analyzed: fingertip patterns, interdigital area III patterns, palmar flexion crease, hypothenar region patterns, and hallucal region patterns. These patterns were classified into standard categories following commonly accepted criteria (Cummins and Midlo, 1943; Alter, 1966; Penrose, 1968; Schaumann and Alter, 1976). Due to the relatively small size of the AD sample, the frequencies of dermatoglyphic traits were combined for the sexes, races, and for the right and left limbs.

## RESULTS

Fingerprint patterns. Fingerprint pattern types are classified into four categories: ulnar loops (opening toward the ulnar side of the hand), whorls, and arches. Table 1 tabulates the percentage frequencies of these patterns in the AD patients and in the controls. In contrast to the control group, the frequency of ulnar loops is globally increased in AD patients. This increase in ulnar loops is globally increased in AD patients. This increase in ulnar loop is complemented by a reciprocal decrease in the frequency of whorls; the frequency of arches is also diminished, but to a much lesser extent. In order of relative magnitude, the increase in ulnar loops is greatest for digits II, I, IV, III, and V. Chi-square analyses support associations between AD and the overall frequency of ulnar ($X2 =$ 27.7, df = 1, p < 0.0001), the frequency of ulnar loops on digit I ($X2 =$ 16.6, df = 1, p < 0.001), and the frequency of ulnar loops on digit II ($X2 =$ 11.6, df = 1, p < 0.001). The frequency of radial loops varies in a minor way between the two groups. Radial loops on digits IV and V are slightly more prevalent among AD patients, but their frequency is not significantly different from controls (p < 0.10).

This increase in the ulnar loop frequency in AD is commensurate with the median percentage frequency of ulnar loops in DS patients (78.3) versus controls (56.8) reported in other studies (Schaumann and Alter, 1976). In contrast to AD patients, DS patients exhibit a much greater decrement in their frequency of radial loops; these are far more likely to appear on digits IV and V. Ulnar loops on all ten fingers were present in 22% of the AD sample and 2% of the controls. Significant associations exist between AD and a total ulnar loop count of seven or greater ($X2 = 14.1$, df =1, p < 0.001) and eight or greater ($X2 = 16.1$, df = 1, p < 0.001).

Interdigital III patterns. AD patients did not differ remarkably from the controls in their frequency of whorl/loop patterns (26.0% versus 23.5%, respectively) in this region (p < 0.10). In DS patients, the frequency of these patterns in this region is consistently elevated above controls (Walker, 1957; Schaumann and Alter, 1976; Loesch, 1983).

Palmar creases. The two common variants of the major palmar flexion creases are the Simian crease and the Sydney line. Simian creases and Sydney lines are more prevalent in AD, and were observed in 11% and 10% of AD hands, respectively. In the controls, the frequency of these creases was 4% and 7%, respectively. This association is significant for Simian creases ($X2 = 4.38$, df =1, p < 0.05), but not for Sidney lines (p > 0.10). Both Simian creases and Sydney lines are consistently more common in DS palms than in control palms (Plato et al., 1973).

Palmar hypothenar patterns. Only whorls and loops are considered to be 'true' patterns in this region. Loops are further designated as radical, ulnar, or carpal in relation to the aspect of the palm towards which they open (Cummins and Midlo, 1943). Simple arches and open fields are not classified as true patterns. Table 2 indicates that true hypothenar patterns, and radial loops in particular, are more frequent in AD patients and are observed in 50% of their palms, as opposed to 26% of control patients palms. Further, true hypothnar patterns occur on both hands in 44% of the AD patients, while only 18% of control patients manifest this trait. There are significant associations between AD and the frequency of true hypothenar patterns ($X2 = 16.0$, df = 1, p < 0.001) the frequency of radial loops ($X2 = 16.9$, df = 1, p < 0.001) and the frequency of patients with bilateral true hypothenar patterns ($X2 = 10.8$, df = 1, p < 0.01). True patterns were noted on 58.4% of palms in a survey of DS subjects by Plato et al., (1973), and these were often bilateral and symmetrical. In sharp contrast to the AD patients, however, the hypothenar patterns in DS were mostly ulnar loops: radial loops were extremely rare.

Table 1. Percentage frequencies of finger patterns in AD
patients and controls, right and left hands combined*

### Pattern Type

| Digit | | Ulnar Loop | Radial Loop | Whorl | Arch |
|---|---|---|---|---|---|
| I | Thumb | | | | |
| | AD | 73.0 | 0.0 | 26.0 | 1.0 |
| | Controls | 47.5 | 0.5 | 46.5 | 5.5 |
| II | Index | | | | |
| | AD | 52.0 | 20.0 | 24.0 | 4.0 |
| | Controls | 31.0 | 21.5 | 38.5 | 9.0 |
| III | Middle | | | | |
| | AD | 83.0 | 1.0 | 13.0 | 3.0 |
| | Controls | 73.5 | 2.0 | 20.0 | 4.5 |
| IV | Ring | | | | |
| | AD | 65.0 | 2.0 | 32.0 | 1.0 |
| | Controls | 57.0 | 0.0 | 41.5 | 1.5 |
| V | Little | | | | |
| | AD | 87.0 | 1.0 | 11.0 | 1.0 |
| | Controls | 80.5 | 0.5 | 18.5 | 0.5 |
| All digits | | | | | |
| | AD | 72.0 | 4.8 | 21.2 | 2.0 |
| | Controls | 57.9 | 5.0 | 33.0 | 4.0 |

*AD indicates Alzheimer's disease

Table 2.  Percentage frequencies of hypothenar patterns in AD
          patients and controls, right and left combined*

Pattern Type

|       | Open/Arch | Radial | True Patterns Loops | Other** | Bilateral | Unilateral |
|-------|-----------|--------|---------------------|---------|-----------|------------|
| Group |           |        |                     |         |           |            |
| AD       | 50 | 42 | 8 | 44 | 10 |
| Controls | 74 | 21 | 5 | 18 | 16 |

*AD indicates Alzheimer's disease
**ulnar loops, carpal loops, and whorls

Table 3.  Percentage frequencies of hallucal region patterns,
          right and left feet combined

Pattern Type

|          | Large Distal  Loop | Small Distal Loop | Whorl | Other |
|----------|--------------------|-------------------|-------|-------|
| AD*      | 55.0 | 3.0 | 27.0 | 15.0 |
| Controls | 38.0 | 0.5 | 44.0 | 17.5 |

*AD indicates Alzheimer's disease
**proximal arches, tibial loops, and fibular loops

21

Hallucal region patterns. Table 3 tabulates the distribution of these
patterns in the present sample. Distal loops are subdivided into large and
small variants, depending upon the number of ridges present: Large distal
loops have ridge counts of 20 or greater (Reed et al., 1970). AD patients
have an increased frequency of both large and small distal loops, while
control patients, in contrast, tend to have more whorl patterns, followed by
large distal loops. Chi-square confirms the association between large
distal loops and AD ($X2 = 7.2$, df = 1, p < 0.01). Large distal loops on
both feet were more frequent in AD patients (50%) than in controls (34%),
but this trend was not significant (p > 0.01). In DS, and arch tibial
pattern dominates the hallucal region, accounting for over 50% of the
patterns in several studies. Small distal loops comprise the second
commonest pattern in this region in DS subjects, followed by large distal
loops and fibular loops (Schaumann and Alter, 1976).

Discriminant analysis. In constructing a discriminant scheme that
would best distinguish between the AD and the Control patients by dermatoglyphic traits, it is important to emphasize that: (1) only in terms of the
relative frequencies of particular traits in comparable sampled populations
(Smith and Berg, 1976); (2) traits combined into a single score ideally
should be obtained from uncorrelated pattern regions (Bolling et al., 1971;
Smith and Berg, 1976); (3) the combination of traits with differing degrees
of specificity can be optimized by weighing them according to their
discriminant efficiency (Smith and Berg, 1976); and (4) the direct
application of discriminant schemes with high accuracy in distinguishing
trisomic DS from normals to AD patients might yield misleading results since
this would not take into account the important differences between the
categories and frequencies of specific patterns in AD and in DS (e.g., the
elevated prevalence of radially oriented hypothenar patterns in AD vis a vis
the ulnar oriented hypothenar patterns in DS).

Penrose and Smith (1966) proposed an index of discrimitive efficiency
which is simple in computation, yet powerful in identifying those
dermatoglyphic traits which best differentiate affected patients from
controls. This index is essentially the product of the difference between
the frequency of a trait in two populations and the natural logarithm of the
relative likelihood of the trait to be associated with a particular
diagnosis. When this methods is applied to the roster of dermatoglyphic
traits sampled above, a table of probability scores favoring the diagnosis
of AD can be constructed, based upon the discriminative power of specific
dermatoglyphic traits (Table 4). These probability scores can be summed,
according to the presence or absence of these particular dermatoglyphic
traits, to yield an overall score for an individual patient. Note that
traits significantly associated with AD, such as the presence of Simian
creases, are too infrequent in both AD patients and in controls to be of
sufficient discriminative power to justify inclusion on this list.

This discriminant scheme has been applied to the present data sample,
and the frequency distribution of scores are displayed in Figure 1. The
mean score obtained by the AD patients (1.23) is significantly higher than
that of controls (-.47) (t = 7.05, df = 148, p < 0.0001 two tailed). A
score above zero, indicating a preponderance of dermatogylphic traits in the
direction of AD, separates 78% of the AD patients for 62% of the controls.
Thus, this scoring scheme can detect AD with a sensitivity and specificity
of 78% and 62%, respectively; the predictive value of a positive score for
the diagnosis of AD is 67%; while a score below zero has a predictive value
of 73% in excluding AD. Figure 2 schematically illustrates pertinent
dermatoglyphic findings in an autopsy-confirmed case of Alzheimer's disease:
by the method outlined above, this patient obtained a discriminant score of
2.57. Two other patients in the AD group with subsequent neuropathological
confirmation of AD obtained scores of .72 and .89 by this method.

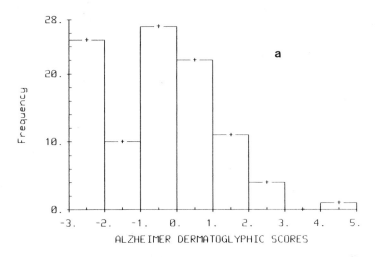

+    HALF-INTERVAL = .5

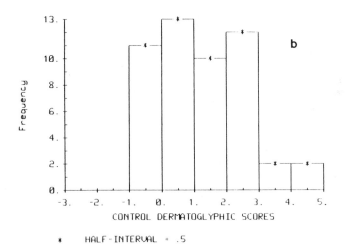

*    HALF-INTERVAL = .5

Figure 1. Frequency distributions discriminant dermatoglyphic scores, displayed as histograms: (a) AD patients: (b) control patients. Vertical dotted lines indicate mean score for each group.

Table 4. Discriminant Weights of Selected Dermatoglyphic Traits

| | Probability score | Efficiency index* |
|---|---|---|
| **Fingertips:** | | |
| 10 ulnar loops | (+)2.40 | .52 |
| 9 ulnar loops | (+)1.49 | .59 |
| 8 ulnar loops | (+) .88 | .53 |
| 7 ulnar loops | (+) .57 | .44 |
| 6 or less | (−) .80 | .44 |
| **Hypothenar:** | | |
| bilateral patterns present | (+) .89 | .38 |
| bilateral patterns absent | (−) .64 | .15 |
| **Hallucal:** | | |
| bilateral loops present | (+) .80 | .15 |
| bilateral loops absent | (−) .74 | .15 |

*computational method of Smith and Berg (1976)

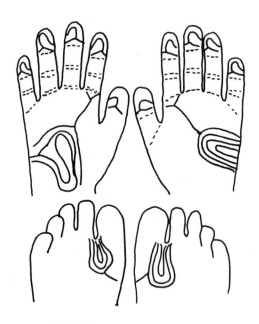

RIGHT        LEFT

Figure 2. Sample dermatoglyphic analysis. Patient
PG (male): literature professor with progressive
dementia beginning age 52, culminating in myoclonus and
vegetative state. Severe Alzheimer's disease confirmed
by autopsy at age 60. History of senile-onset dementia
in mother and maternal grandfather. Right hand: ulnar
loops on digits I-III; radial loops on digits IV and V;
large S-pattern whorl present in hypothenar region.
Left hand: ulnar loops on all digits; large ulnar loop
present in hypothenar reegion. Large distal loops
present in hallucal region of both sides.

DISCUSSION

This present study extends a prior investigation by identifying further congruence between the dermatoglyphic features peculiar to DS and those in a sample of AD patients (Weinreb, 1985). Discriminant scores assigned to dermatoglyphic traits on the fingertips, hypothenar, and hallucal region are modestly sensitive in distinguishing AD patients from a sample of matched control patients. While it could be argued that, in general, an increase in the prevalence of loop patterns succinctly characterizes the dermatoglyphic correspondence between DS and AD, important distinctions remain. Radial loops on digits IV and V are common in DS, but infrequent in AD. Interdigital III region loops are not increased in AD. Hypothenar loop patterns, while present frequently in both AD and DS, are usually of radial orientation in AD, while in DS these loops are virtually always of the ulnar variety. Arch tibial patterns and small distal loops are frequent hallucal region findings in DS, but the former pattern is rare in all non-DS populations and the latter pattern is present only as a trend in AD. It is reasonable to conclude that, when measured on a hypothetical scale of dermatoglyphic 'distance,' AD patients as a group are closer at the DS phenotype than a matched set of control patients.

The dermatoglyphic attributes common to AD and DS are denominators unique to these two entities; they have not been reported in other genetic disorders involving autosomal, sex chromosome, or single gene aberrations, nor in other neurological diseases (Barbeau et al., 1965; Alter, 1966; Rosner et al., 1967; Schaumann and Alter, 1976; Schaumann and Mayersdorf, 1979; Garruto et al., 1983). Dermatoglyphic features resembling those found in DS have thus far been detected in one other intriguing group of persons: the first-degree relatives of DS patients, especially their mothers (Penrose, 1954; Priest, 1969; Priest et al., 1973; Ayme et al., 1979; Loesch, 1981; Rodewald et al., 1982; Schmidt et al., 1981). The aggregate conclusions of dermatoglyphic studies in the parents of DS children support the conclusion that, on the hypothetical scale of dermatoglyphic 'distance' alluded to earlier, the parents (particularly the mothers) of DS children are closer to DS phenotype than AD patients, who in turn are closer to the DS phenotype than controls. The genesis of DS, in the majority of cases, is felt to depend upon the mother's age at the time of conception, and is ascribed to non-disjunction during oogenesis due to an age-related malfunction of the meiotic cell division apparatus (Smith and Berg, 1976; Hansson and Mikkelson, 1978). Of corollary relevance is the observation that, in families in which DS and AD cluster, the patients with DS are usually related to the AD probands through their mothers, and in these families the probands develop AD at an earlier age and have a more severe form of the disease (Heston, 1976; Heyman et al., 1983). There is no evidence to suggest that parents of DS children are at any increased risk of developing AD.

While it might be conjectured that the genetic factors governing the development of epidermal ridge patterns are linked to other genes controlling the propensity of meiotic non-disjunction or the predilection to develop AD, an equally plausible and more compelling hypothesis is that a common genetic factor modulates: (1) the growth patterns of epidermal anlage during prenatal development, resulting in dermatoglyphic features resembling the DS phenotype; (2) cytokinetic events during gametogenesis, resulting in an increased probability of meiotic non-disjunction with aging; (3) neuronal metabolism during senescence, resulting in a negative trophic effect upon neuronal viability and the accelerated degeneration of susceptible neurotransmitter- and neuromodulator-specific systems.

Further dermatoglyphic studies encompassing larger, stratified samples of AD patients and controls, with necropsy follow-up, will codify other

latent dermatoglyphic trends in this disorder, thereby enhancing the
presently primitive specificity of dermatoglyphics as a useful research
technique in AD. Dermatoglyphic data, in conjunction with clinico-
pathological correlations, are a useful adjunct to pedigree studies of the
transmission of AD, and offer the potential to classify younger asymptomatic
individuals along an ordinal scale of risk for AD. Epidermal ridges are a
unique non-neural tissue, reflecting the outcome of a multifaceted genetic
process completed well before birth. It may be said with confidence that
the dermatoglyphic phenotype precedes the development of AD in every case.
The eventual value of dermatoglyphic studies in AD will lie in the screening
and identification of individuals at increased risk of developing AD, and
ultimately, in the prevention of Alzheimer's disease and related disorders.

ACKNOWLEDGEMENTS

Dr. Clark T. Randt provided enthusiasm and counsel. Jason Brown, M.D.,
Michael Serby, M.D., and Elisa Violi, R.N., referred suitable patients.

REFERENCES

Alter, M., 1966, Dermatoglyphic analysis as a diagnostic tool, Medicine,
    46:35-66.
Ayme, S., Mattei, M.G., Mattei, J.F., Auran, Y., Giraud, F., 1979,
    Dermatoglyphics in parents of children with trisomy 21, Clin. Genet.,
    15:78-84.
Ball, M.D., Nuttall, K., 1980, Neurofibrillary tangles, granulovacuolar
    degeneration, and neuron loss in Down syndrome: Quantitative
    comparison with Alzheimer dementia, Ann. Neurol., 7:462-65.
Barbeau, A., Trudeay, J., Coiteux, C., 1965, Fingerprint patterns in
    Huntington's chorea and Parkinson's disease, Canad. Med. Ass. J.,
    92:514-16.
Bolling, D.R., Borgaonkar, D.S., Herr, H.M., Davis, M., 1971, Evaluation of
    dermal patterns in Down's syndrome by predictive discrimination, Clin.
    Genet., 2:163-69.
Borgaonkar, D.S., Davis, M., Bolling, D.R., Herr, H.M., 1971, Evaluation of
    dermal patterns by predictive discrimination. Preliminary analysis
    based on frequencies of patterns, John Hopk. Med. J., 28:141-52.
Cummins, H., Midlo, C., 1943, "Finger prints, palms and soles," The
    Blakiston Co., Philadelphia.
Deckers, J.F.M., Oorthuys, A.M.A., Doesburg, W.H, 1973, Dermatoglyphics in
    Down's syndrome. I. Evaluation of discriminating ability of pattern
    areas, Clin. Genet., 4:311-17.
Deckers, J.F.M., Oorthuys, A.M.A., Doesburg, W.H., 1973, Dermatoglyphics in
    Down's syndrome. II. Evaluation of scoring methods, Clin. Genet.,
    4:318-27.
Deckers, J.F.M., Oorthuys, A.M.A., Doesburg, W.H., 1973, Dermatoglyphics in
    Down's syndrome. III. Proposal of a simplified scoring method, Clin.
    Genet., 4:381-87.
Ellis, W.G., McCulloch, J.R., Corley, C.L., 1974, Presenile dementia in
    Down's syndrome: Ultrastructural identity with Alzheimer's disease,
    Neurology, 24:101-06.
Garruto, R.M., Plato, C.C., Myrianthopolous, N.C., Schanfield, M.S.,
    Gajdusek, D.C., 1983, Blood groups, immunoglobulin allotypes and derma-
    toglyphic features of patients with amyotrophic lateral sclerosis and
    Parkinsonism-dementia of Guam, Am. Jour. Med. Genet., 14:289-98.
Glenner, G.G., Wong, C.W., 1984, Alzheimer's disease and Down's syndrome:
    sharing of a unique cerebrovascular amyloid fibril protein, Biochem.
    Biophys. Res. Commun., 122: 1131-35.

Hansson, A., Mikkelson, M., 1978, The origin of the extra 21 chromosome in Down's syndrome, Cytogen. Cell. Genet., 20:194-203.

Heston, L.L., 1976, Alzheimer's disease, trisomy 21, and myeloproliferative disorders: Associations suggesting a genetic diathesis, Science, 196:322-23.

Heston, L.L., 1982, Alzheimer's dementia and Down's syndroms: Genetic evidence suggesting as association, in: "Alzheimer's disease, Down's syndrome, and aging," F.M. Sinex and R.H. Myers, eds., New York Academy of Sciences, New York.

Heyman, A., Wilkinson, W.E., Hurwitz, B.J., et al., 1983, Alzheimer's disease: Genetic aspects and associated clinical disorders, Ann. Neurol., 14:507-15.

Loesch, D.Z., 1981, Dermatoglyphic studies in the parents of trisomy 21 children, Hum. Hered., 31:201-07.

Mann, D.M.A., Yates, P.O., Maryniuk, B., 1984, Alzheimer's presenile dementia, senile dementia of Alzheimer type and Down's syndrome in middle age from an age-related continuum of pathological changes, Neuropath. Appl. Neurobiol., 10:185-207.

Masters, C.L., Simms, G., Weinman, N.A., Multhaup. G., McDonald, B.L., Beyreuther, K., 1985, Amyloid plaque core protein in Alzheimer disease and Down syndrome, Proc. Natl. Acad. Sci. USA, 82:4245-49.

McKhann, G., Drachman, D., Folstein, M., Katzman, R., Price, D., Stadlan, E.M., 1984, Clinical diagnosis of Alzheimer's disease: Report of the NINCDS-ADRDA Work Group under the auspices of the Department of Health and Human Services Task Force on Alzheimer's disease, Neurology, 34:939-44.

Olson, M.I., Shaw, C.M., 1969, Presenile dementia and Alzheimer's disease in mongolism, Brain, 92:147-56.

Penrose, L.S., 1954, The distal triradius t on the hands of parents and sibs of mongol imbeciles, Ann Hum Genet., 19:10-27.

Penrose, L.S., Smith, G.F., 1966, Down's anomaly, J & A Churchill Ltd., London.

Penrose, L.S., Loesch, D., 1971, Dermatoglyphic patterns and clinical diagnosis by discriminant function, Ann. Hum. Genet., 35:51-60.

Plato, C.C., Cureghino, J.J., Steinberg, F.S., 1973, Palmar dermatoglyphics of Down's syndrome: Revisited, Pediatr. Res., 7:111-18.

Priest, J.H., 1969, Parental dermatoglyphics in age-independent mongolism, J. Med. Genet., 6:304-09.

Reed, T.E., Borgaonkar, D.S., Conneally, P.M., Yu, P., Nance, W.E., Christian, J.C., 1970, Dermatoglyphic nomogram for the diagnosis of Down's syndrome, J. Pediatr., 77:1024-32.

Rodewald, A., Bar, M., Zankl, M., Zankl, H., Reicke, S., Zang, K.D., 1982, Dermatoglyphic studies in parents of children with trisomy 21: Detection of hidden mosaicism and its role in genetic counselling, in: "Progress in dermatoglyphic research," C.S. Bartsocas, ed., Alan R. Liss, Inc., New York.

Rosener, F., Steinberg, F.S., Spriggs, H.A., 1967, Dermatoglyphic patterns in patients with selected neurological disorders, Am. J. Med. Sci., 254:137-50.

Schaumann, B., Alter, M., 1976, "Dermatoglyphics in medical disorders," Springer-Verlag, New York.

Schaumann, B., Mayersdorf, A., 1979, Dermatoglyphics in epilepsy, in: "Dermatoglyphics - fifty years later. Birth defects: Original Article Series," W. Wertelecki and C. Plato, eds., Alan R. Liss Inc., New York.

Schmidt, R., Dat, H., Nitowsky, W., 1981, Dermatoglyphic and cytogenetic studies in parents of children with trisomy 21, Clin. Genet., 20:203-10.

Smith, G.F., Berg, J.M., 1976, "Down's anomaly," Churchill Livingstone, New York.

Walker, N.F., 1957, The use of dermal configurations in the diagnosis of mongolism, J. Pediatr., 50:19-26.

Weinreb, H.J., 1985, Fingerprint patterns in Alzheimer's disease, <u>Arch Neurol.</u>, 42:50-54.

Wisniewski, K.E., Wisniewski, H.M., Wen, G.Y., 1985, Occurrence of neuropathological changes and dementia of Alzheimer's disease in Down's syndrome, <u>Ann. Neurol.</u>, 17:278-82.

DEMENTIA, DEPRESSION, AND PSEUDODEMENTIA

Barry Siegel[1] and Samuel Gershon[2]

[1]Department of Geriatrics
Lafayette Clinic
Detroit, Michigan

[2]Professor and Chairman
Department of Psychiatry
School of Medicine
Wayne State University
Director, Lafayette Clinic

INTRODUCTION

There has been an increasing interest in the varieties of dementia and particularly their differentiation from pseudodementia (Terry and Katzman, 1983;  Bulbena and Berrios, 1985).  This should not be surprising since dementia and depression are the most prevalent mental disorders of the elderly whose proportion of the population in every developing country is growing rapidly (Butler and Lewis, 1982;  OTA, 1985).

At age 65, one is a survivor, with an average life span ahead of almost 15 years for men and 19 for women (Eisdorfer et al., 1981;  Butler and Lewis, 1982).  Although the majority of older persons can expect to have good mental health, epidemiological studies show that the incidence of psychopathology is an increasing risk with advancing age (Rowe, 1984) affecting up to 30 percent of the elderly population (Wasylenki, 1980).

Despite increased awareness amongst physicians, it has been estimated that from 11-57% of those initially diagnosed as suffering from dementia are shown to be affected by some other disorder, usually depression (Garcia et al., 1981).  Cognitive changes observed during normal aging and cognitive impairment caused by potentially treatable disorders are often misdiagnosed as a progressive, deteriorating, and irreversible de-mentia (NIA, 1980).  The diagnosis of dementia of the Alzheimer type thus can be made excessively, while other possibly reversible or at least potentially treatable conditions can be missed (Cummings, 1986).

DEMOGRAPHICS

The percentage of those over 65 in the United States has almost tripled since the beginning of this century.  The average life expectancy was 47 years in 1980 and only 4% of the population was 65 and older (OTA, 1985).  By 1983 the average life expectancy at birth had increased by more than 50% and had reached 74 years with almost 12% of the population, an estimated 27 million people, over the age of 65 years.

Within the next fifty years about 50 million or 1 in 5 Americans could be over 65 (Wells, 1981; OTA, 1985). The proportion of the elderly population over 85 years of age which has doubled in the last 75 years could double again in the next 50 to 75 years (Brody, 1982; OTA, 1985). So far, such projections of the number of older persons have turned out to be underestimations (Butler and Lewis, 1982; OTA, 1985).

## DEMENTIA

The significant extension of the average human life has resulted in a rising prevalence of chronic diseases. Dementing illnesses, such as dementia of the Alzheimer type have become major health problems. Although originally the term "dementia" referred to a syndrome associated with a progressive inevitable decline, this concept has undergone considerable change. Today it is seen as a syndrome consisting of a constellation of symptoms characterized by an acquired loss of intellectual abilities of sufficient severity to interfere with social and occupational functioning (APA, 1980). Global impairment of intellect without a disturbance in consciousness is the central and essential feature, manifest as difficulty with memory, attention, thinking and comprehension. It is almost always of long duration, usually progressive, and often irreversible when the result of a neurodegenerative disorder such as dementia of the Alzheimer type, but these latter features are not included as part of the definition. Considerations of prognosis and etiology are excluded from the current definition since a variety of disorders are subsumed (Lishman, 1978).

Potentially reversible somatic and psychiatric conditions can cause cognitive dysfunction in a significant number of patients presenting with dementia. A wide variety of disorders are potentially treatable including metabolic disturbances, intoxications, tumors, deficiency disorders, normotensive hydrocephalus, sensory deprivation, vascular disorders and the consequence of trauma. There may be as many as 50 different causes of dementia, and perhaps 10%-33% of all dementias are secondary to treatable causes (Hasse, 1977; Katzman, 1981; Cummings and Benson, 1983; McAllister, 1983). It has been estimated that as many as two thirds of patients in whom a reversible cause of dementia is found could show partial or full cognitive recovery (Rabins, 1983). Once the syndrome has been identified, it should challenge clinicians to search for ultimate causes (NIA, 1980).

## SENILE DEMENTIA OF THE ALZHEIMER TYPE

The most prevalent type of dementia is dementia of the Alzheimer type (DAT) (Schneck et al., 1982).

DAT is the major cause of irreversible dementia, affecting between 1.2 million and 4 million Americans (OTA, 1985). As the disorder progresses, all the patient's functioning declines. Eventually contact is lost with the outside world, and often he enters a nursing home or other long term care. Thirty to fifty percent of nursing home residents suffer from DAT and it is the most frequent cause of admission to facilities for long term care. Although patients do not die directly of this disorder, its appearance reduces life expectancy by 50%. DAT has been estimated to be the fourth most common cause of death of the elderly (Kerzner, 1974).

The risk for DAT increases with age and the progressive cognitive dysfunction develops usually over a period of years. The nature of the cognitive and behavioral symptoms depends upon the stage of the disease. Reisberg has described 7 clinically identifiable and ratable stages in the evolution of dementia (Reisberg et al., 1982). According to his findings, if the initial diagnosis is correct, then progression through each of these stages in a typical order is inevitable.

## GENETICS OF DEMENTIA

There is evidence for a significant genetic component in the etiology of Alzheimer's disease. Evidence has come from individual pedigrees, family studies, and twin studies (Matsuyama, 1983). Morbidity risks in first degree relatives of probands ranges from 3 to 15 percent and for parents from 2 to 20 percent for siblings (Matsuyama, 1983; Terry and Katzman, 1983; Kerzner, 1984).

## EPIDEMIOLOGY OF DEMENTIA IN THE ELDERLY

Of the 27 million Americans more than 65 years of age, about 5% are afflicted by severe dementia to the extent that they are unable to care for themselves (Mortimer, 1983). Up to 20% of those over 65 could be suffering from mild to moderate degrees of dementia (Gurland et al., 1980). Dementia may reach epidemic proportions in the near future; its prevalence tripling within the lifetime of our grandchildren (Katzman, 1981).

## COGNITIVE IMPAIRMENT IN THE ELDERLY

The cognitive changes associated with normal aging also resemble some aspects of the memory impairments seen in progressive idiopathic dementia (Weingartner et al. 1981). Forgetfulness is by far the most common and an almost universal complaint of humans as they grow older (Benson, 1984). Aging results in reduced memory function, but impairments are neither uniform nor extensive (Botwinick, 1977; Craik, 1977; Cummings and Benson, 1983). Normal elderly have little difficulty with "immediate" or "remote" recall, but often do worse than younger adults on tests of "recent" memory (LaRue, 1982). Normal elderly perform as well as young adults on tests of vocabulary and tests of general information and digit span gives stable results with increasing age (or else are only slightly diminished by aging) (Eisdorfer et al., 1981; LaRue, 1982).

Kral introduced the terms benign and malignant senescent forgetfulness to denote two types of memory impairment that he observed among groups of elderly subjects in mental hospitals and retirement homes (Kral, 1978). The malignant form of forgetfulness probably corresponds to what is currently called primary degenerative dementia and the benign form to normal aging changes. Kral's data fail to demonstrate that benign forgetfulness is not simply a milder form of malignant amnestic syndrome (LaRue, 1982). No measures currently exist to distinguish persons with benign senescent forgetfulness who subsequently develop dementia from those who do not. Mild and apparently benign disturbances in a sample of elderly community residents were found to be associated with the development of symptoms of dementia after a period of 4 years (Botwinick, 1977). LaRue and Jarvik (1980) found that deficits in performance on intelligence tests were predictive of the development of dementia some 20 years later.

## DEPRESSION IN THE ELDERLY

Depressive episodes and grief reactions increase in frequency and depth in the advanced years of life (Busse, 1983). Two out of three elderly patients coming to psychiatric attention in different clinical settings suffer from a depressive illness (Straker, 1984). It is therefore

Table 1.  Medical Conditions Associated with Symptoms of
          Depression (Blumenthal, 1980;  Finlayson, 1982;
          Ban, 1984;  Lazarus, 1985).

| | |
|---|---|
| Collagen Diseases | CNS Disorders |
| Endocrinopathies | Metabolic disorders |
| Major Organ Failure | Malignancies |
| Nutritional Disorders | Viral Infections |
| Intoxications | |

not surprising that depressive disorders are the most frequent psychiatric disturbances in the elderly (Finlayson, 1982; Busse, 1983;  Georgotas, 1983).  However, affective disorders are not only the most commonly encountered psychiatric illness, but those most often untreated (Eisdorfer et al., 1981).

The depressions of old age are extremely variable in their presentation, and can often be missed or misdiagnosed (Busse, 1983).  Symptoms of depression may be associated with physical illness and medications (Table 1 and 2).

Often the symptoms of depression are difficult to differentiate from normal aging (Wasylenki, 1980;  Kramer, 1982).  Much of what is called depression in the elderly may actually represent decreased life satisfaction and periodic episodes of grief secondary to physical, social and economic difficulties encountered by aging individuals in the community (Good, 1981).  Loss of support systems, mobility, income, sensory inputs, and self-worth along with the general decrease in adaptiveness may predispose and contribute to the development of depression in the elderly (Butler and Lewis, 1982).

Some researchers have stated that the elderly depressed patient often voices complaints typical of depressives of all ages (Hirshfield, 1979).  Signs and symptoms of depression in the geriatric age group would then be similar to those of younger individuals and diagnosis could

Table 2.  Medications Associated with Symptoms of Depression
          (Blumenthal, 1980;  Finlayson, 1982;  Gerner, 1985).

| | |
|---|---|
| Analgesics | Antianxiety Agents |
| Antiarthritic agents | Antibiotics |
| Anticancer agents | Anticonvulsants |
| Antihypertensives | Antiparkinsonian drugs |
| Antipsychotics | Appetite suppressants |
| Cardiovascular drugs | CNS depressants |

Miscellaneous:
    alcohol, choline, oral contraceptives, ethambuto,
    corticosteroids, disulfiram, physostigmine, methyl
    mercury, organic pesticides, Cimetidine

reliably be made using the DSM III criteria (Spar and LaRue, 1983). However, others feel that diagnosis is more difficult in the elderly as some symptoms are seen more often and others less frequently than in younger age groups (Blumenthal, 1980; Janowsky, 1982; Finlayson and Martin, 1982; Georgotas, 1983; Charatan, 1985). More specific diagnostic criteria are needed in a population in which depressive illness can be present with features different from typical symptomatology (Georgotas, 1983). The elderly are more likely to mask their depression than individuals at earlier stages in the life cycle (Blazer and Williams, 1980). Mood disturbances are often denied and the elderly patient appears anxious and irritable, rather than sad. Crying is not as common as in younger age groups. The depressed elderly often have the appearance of self-neglect. Disturbances of appetite resulting in significant weight loss and insomnia are particularly common. Somatic complaints predominate, usually focusing on the chest and abdomen. Psychotic features, including somatic delusions and paranoid ideation, are more common than in younger patients.

Cases of depression in which there is a predominance of somatic or cognitive complaints may be overlooked, especially if depression is mild. On the other hand, scales that place a great deal of weight on physical symptoms, as in the Zung or Hamilton scales may improperly identify persons suffering from physical illness as suffering from depression (Blazer and Williams, 1980).

In recent years it has been emphasized repeatedly that depression may present in the elderly as a predominately intellectual impairment which can be easily misdiagnosed as dementia (Wells, 1979). In elderly patients, cognitive impairment is frequently associated with pure depressive illness and the cognitive deficit may be extremely severe (McAllister and Price, 1982). The cognitive impairment is of a diffuse, global nature, although deficits in memory and verbal learning may predominate. However, there is no pattern of deficits specific to depressive illnesses as compared with dementia (McAllister, 1983). The cognitive deficits tend to be reversible with the resolution of the depressive illness (McAllister, 1981).

EPIDEMIOLOGY OF DEPRESSION

Because of variation in diagnostic criteria, differences in diagnostic terminology, and other variables, studies of depression in this age group are often difficult to interpret and evaluate (Wasylenki, 1980; Busse, 1983). The use of standardized criteria (such as DSM-III) in studies in the elderly improves reliability and comparability of results; but results in decreased sensitivity. Cases of masked depression might be overlooked, especially if a subject does not describe a dysphoric affect but exhibits mainly by physiologic symptoms (Blazer and Williams, 1980).

Depressive disorders most easily diagnosed by psychiatrists present between the ages of 25 and 65 (Kramer, 1980). However, 50% of depressed geriatric patients experience their first depressive episode after age 60 (Ban, 1978). Studies have shown that clinical symptoms of depression may increase past the age of 65 (Eisdorfer et al., 1981). The risk of depression increases with age, with women at higher risk than men, until after the age of 65, when the risks become equal or even reverse (Wasylenki, 1980). Life-time risks of depression have been estimated to be 8.5% for men and 17.7% for women up to age 80. The prevalence of depression declines sharply in persons (without physical illness) over 80 (Ban, 1984). Estimates of the incidence and prevalence of depression among the aged of the US vary greatly. Reported prevalence rates in the elderly range from 10% ot 65%, depending on the population surveyed and criteria used (Blazer and Williams, 1980; Gerner, 1985). However, when stricter criteria are used (DSM III), prevalence rates decrease significantly for major affective disorders to about 1-3% (Finlayson and Martin, 1982). Prevalence rates from other countries with different social-cultural structures, such as Japan, are as low as 0.9% (Hasegawa, 1985).

Table 3. Differentiating Dementia from Pseudodementia[a]

| Dementia | Pseudodementia |
| --- | --- |
| Clinical Course and History | |
| Family often unaware of dysfunction and its severity | Family usually aware of dysfunction and its severity |
| Insidious onset | Acute onset |
| Onset can be dated only within broad limits | Onset can be dated with some precision |
| Slow progression of symptoms throughout course | Rapid progression of symptoms after onset |
| History of previous psychiatric dysfunction uncommon | History of previous psychiatric dysfunction common |
| Behavior | |
| Patient minimizes cognitive loss | Patient exaggerates cognitive loss |
| Patients' complaints of cognitive dysfunction usually vague | Patients' complaints of cognitive dysfunction usually detailed |
| Patients conceal disability | Patients emphasize disability |
| Patients delight in accomplishments, however trivial | Patients highlight failures |
| Patients struggle to perform tasks | Patients make little effort to perform even simple tasks |
| Patients rely on notes, calendars, etc. to keep up | Patients don't try to keep up |
| Patient often appear unconcerned | Patients usually communicate strong sense of distress |
| Affect usually labile and shallow | Affect change often pervasive |
| Social skills often retained | Loss of social skills often early and prominent |
| Behavioral disability equals cognitive loss | Behavior better than cognitive loss would predict |
| Noctural accentuation of dysfunction common | Noctural accentuation of dysfunction uncommon |

Table 3.  Differentiating Dementia from Pseudodementia[a] (cont'd)

| Dementia | Pseudodementia |
|---|---|

### Clinical Features Related to Memory, Cognition and Intellect

| Dementia | Pseudodementia |
|---|---|
| "Near miss" answers frequent | "Don't know" answers typical |
| Memory loss for recent events usually more severe than for remote events | Memory loss for recent and remote events usually equally severe |
| Consistently poor performance on tasks of similar difficulty | Marked variability in performance on tasks of similar difficulty |

[a] Modified from Wells, C. E., 1979,  Pseudodementia, Am. J. Psychiatry, 136:895.

Among the institutionalized aged or those with significant medical illnesses, depressive episodes are considerably more frequent (Eisdorfer et al., 1981).  Manifestations of depression are present in more than 50% of patients age 60 to 70 hospitalized for mental disorder (Ban, 1984). There is a close connection between physical illness and depression in the geriatric population:  30-50% of the  elderly who have physical diseases also have affective disorders (Wasylenki, 1980; Gershon and Herman, 1982).

SUICIDE AND THE ELDERLY

The high rate of suicide of the aged reflects the existence of significant depression in this group (Ban, 1984).  Although people over 65 constitute only about 10-11% of the population, they account for 25% of all suicides (Blumenthal, 1980).  The suicide rate for white males increases progressively from age 15 and peaks in the ninth decade;  while for women, the peak suicide rate occurs between 40 to 60 years of age, followed by a gradual decline.  In the USA elderly, divorced, white males in the seventh decade are 4 times as likely to commit suicide as the rest of the population (Finlayson and Martin, 1982).

PSEUDODEMENTIA

The syndrome of pseudodementia has been the subject of increasing attention and interest due to the diagnostic challenges it presents (McAllister, 1983).  The term "pseudodementia" has an inprecise nosological meaning (Arie, 1983), some authors claiming that it does not exist and that the concept should be abandoned (Shraberg, 1978;  Reifler, 1982; Mahandra, 1984).  The initial experience of 'pseudodementia' came from the recognition that certain patients diagnosed as demented were observed to be suffering from depression.  Many features of their clinical course differed from those of the majority of demented patients suffering from progressive and terminal illnesses (Mahandra, 1985).

Although the relationship between depression and dementia has been noted since antiquity it still eludes precise understanding (Mahandra, 1985).  By 1883 there was already awareness of the fact that severe affective disorder could lead to cognitive impairment (Berrios, 1985). Reports of reversible dementia had been explained by postulating the

Table 4.  Disorders Associated with Dementia (Lishman, 1978;
Wells, 1979; Kiloh, 1961; Marsden and Harrison, 1972;
Nott and Fleminger, 1975; Smith and Kiloh, 1981;
Mahandra, 1985)

| | |
|---|---|
| Ganser syndrome | Malingering |
| Compensation neurosis | Post-traumatic disorder |
| Sensory deprivation | Depression |
| Mania | Obsessive disorders |
| Anxiety states | Paraphrenia |
| Shoplifting | Bizarre hypochondriasis |
| Chronic pain | Thyrotoxicosis |
| Drug toxicity | |
| Conversion and dissociative reactions | |
| Schizophrenia and schizophreniform conditions | |

existence of "vesanic" dementia, that is dementia caused by functional
psychosis.  Mairet used the term "melancholic dementia" to point out the
association between severe depression, cognitive impairment and the
potential for recovery.

Madden et al. (1952) were the first to use the term 'pseudodementia.'
Their study of 300 patients reported that symptoms "ordinarily considered
to indicate dementia (disorientation, defects of recent memory, retention,
calculation and judgement)" could be reversed with appropriate psychiatric
interventions.  Such pseudodementia was not uncommon with psychoses
associated with cerebrovascular disease, presenile depressions and
involutional psychoses.

Ten years later, Kiloh (1961) published a comprehensive review of
pseudodementia.  He reported 10 cases in which initially "the picture of
dementia may be very closely mimicked" but the subsequent courses of the
illness is such as to be incompatible with the diagnosis of dementia.
His use of the term was purely descriptive.

Post (1962) felt that even experienced clinicians could not always
discern whether they were dealing with an emotional disorder or cerebral
dysfunction when the onset was acute.  He emphasized that functional
psychoses rarely have an abrupt onset and usually have prodromal affective
symptoms.  Of diagnostic importance in his formulation was the order of
the appearance of symptoms, as well as the presence of a past history of
psychiatric illness in differentiating depression from dementia.

Wells (1979) described 10 cases in which cognitive impairment was
judged to be due to functional psychiatric illness.  She defined the syndrome as one in which "dementia is mimicked or rather caricatured by
functional psychiatric illness."  The syndrome could be associated with a
variety of primary psychiatric illnesses, including personality disorders
and posttraumatic neuroses, and in his study population its association
with primary affective disorders was not as high as in other reports.
Whereas previous papers did not focus on clinical features which could be
used to differentiate pseudodementia from "true" dementia, he outlined
clinical features that taken together could help distinguish pseudodementia
from dementia (Table 3).

Caine (1981) attempted to define pseudodementia as a neuropsychiatric
syndrome and established preliminary diagnostic criteria (Table 4).  He
suggested that the pattern of intellectual impairment seen is a "subcortical"
one (Cummings and Benson, 1983), sparing higher cortical functions.  In

Table 5. Criteria to define and diagnose pseudodementia
(Caine, 1981)

Intellectual impairment in a patient with a primary
psychiatric disorder

The features of the syndrome resemble those induced by
degenerative CNS disorders

The intellectual compromise is reversible

The patient has no primary identifiable neurologic disease
that can account for the cognitive changes


his study 6 of 11 patients had major depressive disorders, 2 others had
other disorders with major depressive features.

All authors point out that the term 'pseudodementia' refers to a
variety of conditions where the presenting clinical picture resembles
organic dementia but which is due to functional psychiatric illness. It
does not relate specifically to one psychiatric disorder (Table 5)
although it does occur more commonly in older depressed patients
(McAllister, 1983). Pseudodementia is not a homogeneous syndrome, the
underlying psychiatric disorder influences the clinical presentation and
therapy (McAllister, 1983). The patients' clinical picture of profound,
progressive cognitive impairment may be indistinguishable from that seen
in progressive, irreversible degenerative disorders (McAllister and
Price, 1982).

The literature on pseudodementia is confusing, in part, since some
studies refer only to persons suffering from affective disorders, while
others include all functional psychiatric disorders which give rise to a
clinical picture of dementia. Moreover there has been no consensus as to
its definition, so that estimates of the incidence and prevalence of
pseudodementia will vary. Since the majority of authors refer to
pseudodementia associated with affective disorders, further discussion
will focus on this disorder.

An important issue in the concept of "pseudodementia" is that some
authors treat this disorder as a misdiagnosis of dementia, while others
see it as a potentially treatable dementia. This further confuses the
interpretation of epidemiologic studies.

EPIDEMIOLOGY OF PSEUDODEMENTIA

Pseudodementia can occur at any age (Cavenar, 1979; McAllister,
1983). While anecdotal and single case reports suggest that it is the
elderly who present most with 'pseudodementia,' the evidence from several
reported series suggests a wider range (Mahandra, 1985). Depressive
'pseudodementia' also occurs in middle age with an average age of 50 in
one of series patients (McAllister, 1983). Its occurrence is not necessarily,
or preferentially limited to the senium (Mahandra, 1985). Still it is
believed to be present in 10 to 57 percent of the geriatric population
initially diagnosed as demented (Table 6). 8-15% of those initially
diagnosed as demented are later judged to be suffering from depressive
illness (Marsden and Harrison, 1972; Nott and Fleminger, 1975; Ron et
al., 1979; Gershon and Herman, 1982).

Wells (1979) reported an age range between 33 and 69, and 7 of his

Table 6. Frequency of Misdiagnosis of Dementia
(i.e., prevalence of pseudodementia)

| Study | Number of Cases | % Misdiagnosed |
|-------|-----------------|----------------|
| Madden et al. (1952) | 300 | 10% |
| Marsden and Harrison (1972) | 106 | 15% |
| Kendal (1974) | 98 | 8.2% |
| Nott and Fleminger (1975) | 35 | 57% |
| Freemon (1976) | 60 | 30% |
| Bergman (1977) | 66 | 20% |
| Ron et al. (1979) | 51 | 31% |
| Smith and Kiloh (1981) | 200 | 10% |

10 patients were in their fifties or sixties. Smith and Kiloh (1981) showed in their series of 200 demented patients that 'pseudodementia' accounted for 10% of all dementias under 45 and for 13.6% of dementias between the ages of 45 and 64 years, but only for 1.8% of dementias over 65 years. McAllister's (1983) pooled data yielded a mean of 60.5 years, with a range between 22 and 85 years.

PROBLEMS IN DIFFERENTIATING BETWEEN DEMENTIA AND DEPRESSION

The diagnosis of a depressive pseudodementia is especially difficult in the older patient because of the complexity of psychological, somatic and social factors (Straker, 1984). When depression is not a complaint and physical signs and symptoms dominate the clinical picture, the likelihood of making diagnostic blunders is enhanced (Good, 1981). Confusion regarding the clinical diagnosis is due not only to the enormous overlap in the performance deficits noted between elderly depressive and demented populations but also the many variations in the clinical picture of depression which occur in old age (Straker, 1984). In elderly patients, the cognitive impairment associated with a purely depressive illness may be extremely severe, and can be the presenting complaint of an unrecognized depressive illness (McAllister and Price, 1982). Moreover older patients show a marked tendency for the depressed affect to be replaced by "somatic equivalents" and physical complaints (NIA, 1980). It may be impossible to differentiate the two even in conjunction with sophisticated neurodiagnostic testing (McAllister, 1982).

Both Wells (1979) and Rabins et al. (1984) attempted to delineate those findings which would differentiate patients suffering from dementia related to depression from "true" dementia. Rabins et al. (1984) concluded that a past history of depression, self reports of depressed mood, self blaming, nihilistic and somatic delusions, appetite disturbance, and subacute onset served to differentiate the "depressed-demented" patients from the ones with progressive dementia.

There has not been general agreement as to the utility of ancillary tests in distinguishing pseudodementia from "true" dementia (i.e., depression from neuropathological degenerative disorders). While both

Kiloh (1961) and Wells (1979) felt that ancillary diagnostic tools were not helpful others found them to be of assistance. Procedures reported as potentially useful included psychometric testing (Ron et al., 1979; Rabins, 1983), diagnostic inventories (Cummings and Benson, 1986), electroencephalogram (Ron et al., 1979), dexamethasone suppression testing (Grunhaus et al., 1983), sleep studies (Reynolds et al., 1985), brain blood flow and oxidative metabolism measurements (Hoyer et al., 1984), and the use of sodium amylobarbitone (Ward et al., 1978).

In many clinical situations, the problem is not to decide between an organic dementia or a depressive disorder, but to sort out the complex admixtures of both of these variables (Straker, 1984). Feinberg and Goodman (1984) described four typical patterns of patients with combinations of depression and dementia. The most characteristic case has depression presenting as dementia. On the other hand, in "the depression syndrome of dementia" as described by Folstein et al. (1975), the dementia is secondary to a recognized depressive disorder.

Some patients present with both affective disorder and dementing process which converge in equal measure toward the final clinical pathway (Straker, 1984). A major affective disorder or an organic affective disorder can develop in a patient whose brain function is also compromised by pre-existing neuropathologically-determined dementias, by certain medications, or by metabolic derangement. When a 'functional' psychiatric illness is superimposed on an 'organic' disorder, neurological deficits can be enhanced (Mahandra, 1985) and only treatment of depression may reveal the underlying organic dementia (Shraberg, 1978; Devanand and Nelson, 1985). A considerable number of Alzheimer cases develop one or more longer-lasting episodes with typical symptomatology of an endogenous depression (Kral, 1983) or may present with depression (Mahandra, 1985). Depression was noted in 15% of patients in one series in which Alzheimer's disease was clinically diagnosed (Kral, 1983). Moreover, depression and dementia are not uncommon features of Parkinson's disease and Huntington's chorea (Mahandra, 1985).

Finally dementia may present as depression. Gustafson (1975) reported that 30% and Liston (1977) that 25% of patients ultimately having dementia had depression as the reason for referral. Kral (1983) reported on 22 patients (16 women, 8 men; age range 62-78 with a mean of 76.5 years) diagnosed as suffering from pseudodementia. The patients were followed up from 4-18 years (average of 8). At the end of the period, 20 had developed senile dementia of the Alzheimer type (pathologically proven in 3).

The severe cognitive impairment seen in pseudodementia associated with depression occurs in a disorder that has been shown to have numerous indications or markers of associated diffuse CNS dysfunction.
There may be an unmasking by the depression of certain structural brain pathologies (Rabins et al., 1984). This suggests that depressive illness can induce a "true" organic mental disorder (McAllister, 1983).

PROGNOSIS

Cognitive deficits may resolve completely after an associated psychopathology is diagnosed and treated. However, the dementia does not always recede when the depressive component in a depressive 'pseudodementia' is removed by treatment (McAllister and Price, 1982; Rabins et al., 1984).

In general coexisting cognitive impairment and depression are not predictive of a more severe illness, high relapse rate or unmasking of a dementing illness (McAllister, 1983; Rabins et al., 1984).

## TREATMENT OF PSEUDODEMENTIA ASSOCIATED WITH DEPRESSION

The presence of substantial cognitive impairment does not appear to hold any specific implications for somatic treatment approaches (McAllister, 1983). Treatment is one of the underlying disorder, which is usually depression.

Antidepressant medication is most effective for moderate to severe depressions (Lazarus et al., 1985). If grief or mourning are suspected, a trial of psychotherapy is indicated. Even if the diagnosis is major depression, the combination of psychotherapy and antidepressant medication is superior than either alone (Weisman, 1970).

The decision as to which medication is used will depend on previous experience by the patient or a family member with a particular medication, the clinical picture (whether there is agitation or psychomotor retardation, the sensitivity to particular side effects, and the concomitant use of other drugs) (Stern et al., 1980). As in the younger age groups, tricycles, MAO inhibitors, lithium and ECT have all been found to be effective in particular cases (Ban, 1984; Charatan, 1985; Gerner, 1985).

## CLINICAL VIGNETTE

The following clinical case adapted from McAllister and Price (1983) shows both the difficulty with the diagnosis and the potential for response to treatment.

Ms. A., a 61 year old housewife, was referred for evaluation of agitation, social withdrawal, and pronounced memory deficits of several months' duration. Her past history was notable for a hospital admission 20 years prior to the present assessment. At the time she was diagnosed as suffering from schizophrenia, but after discharge had functioned normally for 20 years.

On admission she appeared disheveled. General and neurologic examination were within normal limits except for buccal-lingual dyskinesia and some pelvic thrusting. During the mental status examination she was unable to give history of her current illness, was oriented only to person, knew none of the presidents, was unable to perform simple calculations, and had a marked imprinting deficit. She had a full range of affect, and she did not appear nor did she complain of being depressed. There was no evidence of a thought disorder.

Results of extensive ancillary testing were all normal. EEG showed bilateral slowing with no focal or lateralizing features. Formal neuropsychological testing could not be carried out because of the patient's profound cognitive impairment.

Because of her past history of psychiatric illness and the acuteness of onset and short duration of her symptoms, she was given electroconvulsive therapy (ECT) for possible depressive pseudodementia. After nine treatments she was discharged to her home.

She was given formal neuropsychological testing, following her second ECT treatment. On repeated testing two and a half months later she showed a striking improvement on both the WAIS and the Halstead-Reitan battery.

CONCLUSION

Diagnostic clarity decreases in the elderly. Old age is associated with expected physiological changes and an increase in the appearance of multiple chronic health conditions, all of which may impair cognitive functioning. Depression, a potentially treatable disorder, is disproportionately prevalent in the elderly as exemplified by the high rate of suicide in this age group. Its clinical presentation often resembles that of another disorder causing cognitive impairment and particularly prevalent in the elderly, dementia. These two disorders are not mutually exclusive and may appear together, the symptoms of either predominating.

The need to distinguish between the usually progressive and irreversible dementia and the potentially treatable depression has given rise to the term pseudodementia. Pseudodementia is not a diagnostic category on its own, but rather an operational concept in the differential diagnosis of dementia. It underscores that accurate diagnosis may result in more effective treatment. While a diagnosis of dementia usually commits the patient and family to a life with dismal prospects and the need for costly long term care, the successful treatment of depression may enable to elderly to live more dignified and independent lives.

REFERENCES

A P A, 1980, "Diagnostic and Statistical Manual of Mental Disorders (Third Edition)," A P A, Washington, DC.

Arie, T., 1983, Pseudodementia, Br. Med. J., 286:1301.

Ban, T. A., 1984, Chronic disease and depression in the geriatric population, J. Clin. Psychiatry, 45:18.

Ban, T. A., 1978, The treatment of depressed patients, Am. J. Psychother., 32:93.

Benson, D. F., 1984, Neuropathology of memory disorders, Psychosomatics, 25:12.

Berrios, G. E., 1985, "Depressive pseudodementia" or "Melancholic dementia": a 19th centry view, J. Neurol. Neurosurg. Psychiatry, 48:393.

Blazer, D., and Williams, C., 1980, Epidemiology of dysphoria and depression in an elderly population, Am. J. Psychiatry, 137:439.

Blum, F., 1979, Dementia: An approaching epidemic, Nature, 279:373.

Blumenthal, M. D., 1980, Depressive illness: getting behind the mask, Geriatrics, 35:34.

Botwinick, J., 1977, Intellectual abilities, in, "Handbook of the Psychology of Aging," Birrin, J. E., and Schaie, K. W., ed., Van Nostrand Reinhold, New York.

Brody, J. A., 1982, An epidemiologist views senile dementia: facts and fragments, Am. J. Epidemiol., 115:155.

Bulbena, A., and Berrios, G. E., 1985, Pseudodementia: facts and figures, Br. J. Psychiatry, 148:87.

Busse, E., and Simpson, D., 1983, Depression and antidepressants in the elderly, J. Clin. Psychiatry, 44:35.

Butler, R. N., and Lewis, M. I., 1982, "Aging and Mental Health: Positive Psychosocial and Biomedical Approaches," C.V. Mosby Company, Toronto.

Caine, E. D., 1981, Pseudodementia, Arch. Gen. Psychiatry, 38:1359.

Carroll, B. J., 1985, Dexamethasone suppression test: a review of contemporary confusion, J. Clin. Psychiatry, 46:13.

Cavenar, J. O. J., Maltbie, A. A., and Austin, L., 1979, Depression simulating organic brain disease, Am. J. Psychiatry, 136:521.

Charatan, F. B., 1985, Depression and the elderly: Diagnosis and treatment, Psychiatr. Annals, 15:313.

Craik, F. I., 1977, Age differences in human memory, in: "Handbook of the Psychology of Aging," Birren, J. E., and Schaie, K. W., ed., Van Nostrand Reinhold, New York.

Cummings, J. L., 1986, Dementia of the Alzheimer Type: An inventory of diagnostic clinical., J. Am. Geriatr. Soc., 34:12.

Cummings, J. L., and Benson, F. D., 1983, Dementia: Clinical appraoch, Butterworths, Boston.

Devanand, D. P., and Nelson, J. C., 1985, Concurrent depression and dementia: Implications for diagnosis and treatment. J. Clin. Psychiatry, 46:389-396.

Eisdorfer, C., Cohen, D., and Veith, R., 1981, "The Psychopathology of Aging," Upjohn Company.

Feinberg, T., and Goodman, B., 1984, "Affective illness, dementia, and pseudodementia,"

Finlayson, R. E., and Martin, L. M.. 1982, Recognition and management of depression in the elderly, Mayo Clin. Proc., 57:115.

Folstein, M. F., Folstein, S. E., and McHugh, P. R., 1975, "Minimental state": A practical method for grading the cognitive state, J. Psychiatr. Res., 12:189.

Freemon, F., 1976, Evaluation of patients with progressive intellectual deterioration, Arch. Neurol., 33:658.

Garcia, C. A., Reding, M. J., and Blass, J. P., 1981, Overdiagnosis of dementia, J. Am. Geriatr. Soc., 29:407.

Georgotas, A., 1983, Affective disorders in the elderly: diagnostic and research considerations, Age Ageing, 12:1.

Gerner, R. H., 1985, Present status of drug therapy of depression in late life, J. Affective Dis., Suppl 1:S23.

Gershon, S., and Herman, S. P., 1982, The differential diagnosis of dementia, J. Am Geriatr. Soc., 30 (suppl):S58.

Good, M. I., 1981, Pseudodementia and physical findings masking significant psychopathology, Am. J. Psychiatry, 138:

Grunhaus, L., Dilsaver, S., Greden, J. F., and Carroll, B. J., 1983, Biol. Psychiatry, 18:215.

Gurland, B., Dean, L., Cross, P., and Golden, R., 1980, The epidemiology of depression and dementia in the elderly: the use of multiple indicators of these conditions, in: "Psychopathology of the Aged," Cole, J. O., and Barrett, J. E., eds., Raven Press, New York.

Gustafson, L., 1975, Psychiatric symptoms in dementia with onset in the presenile period, Acta Psychiatr. Scand., 247 (suppl):7.

Hasse, G. R., 1977, Diseases presenting as dementia, in: "The Dementias," Wells, C.E., ed.

Hasegawa, K., 1985, The epidemiological study of depression in late life, J. Affect. Dis., Suppl 1:S3.

Hirshfield, N., and Klerman, G. L., 1979, Treatment of depression in the elderly, Geriatrics, 34:

Hoyer, S., Oesterreich, K., and Wagner, O., 1984, Depression in old age and its relation to primary dementia: variations in brain blood flow and oxidative metabolism, Monogr. Neural Sci., 11:187.

Janowsky, D. S., 1982, Pseudodementia in the elderly: differential diagnosis and treatment, J. Clin. Psychiatry, 43:19.

Katzman, R., 1981, Early detection of senile dementia, Hosp. Pract., 16:61.

Kendell, R., 1974, The stability of psychiatric diagnosis, Br. J. Psychiatry, 124:352.

Kerzner, L. J., 1984, Diagnosis and treatment of Alzhiemer's disease, Advancs in Intern. Med. 447.

Kiloh, L. G., 1961, Pseudo-dementia, Acta Psychiatr. Scand., 37:336.

Kral, V. A., 1978, Benign senescent forgetfulness, in, "Alzheimer's Disease: Senile Dementia and Related Disorders" Katzman, R., Terry, R. D., and Bick, K., ed., Raven Press, New York.

Kral, V. A., 1983, The relationship between senile dementia (Alzheimer type) and depression, Can. J. Psychiatry, 28:304.

Kramer, B. A., 1982, Depressive pseudodementia, Compr. Psychiatry, 23:538.

Kramer, M., 1980, The diagnosis of depression in the elderly, J. Am. Geriatr. Soc., 28:52.

LaRue, A., 1982, Memory loss and aging. Distinguishing dementia from benign senescent forgetfulness and depressive pseudodementia, Psychiatr. Clin. North Am., 5;89.

LaRue, A., and Jarvik, L., 1980, Reflections on biological changes in the psychological performance of the aged, Age, 3:29.

Lazarus, L. W., Davis, J. M., and Dysken, M. W., 1985, Geriatraic depression: A guide to successful therapy, Geriatrics, 40:43.

Lishman, W. A., 1978, "Organic Psychiatry," Blackwell Scientific, Oxford.

Liston, E. J. J., 1977, Occult senile dementia, J. Nerv. Ment. Dis., 164:263.

Madden, J. J., Luhan, J. A., and Kaplan, L. A., 1952, Nondementing psychoses in older persons, JAMA, 150:1567.

Mahendra, B., 1984, Pseudodementia: abandon the term? [letter], Am. J. Psychiatry, 141:471.

Mahendra, B., 1985, Depression and dementia: the multi-faceted relationship, Psychol. Med. 15:227.

Marsden, C. D., and Harrison, M. J. G., 1972, Outcome of investigation of patients with presenile dementia, Br. Med. J., 2:249.

Masters, C., Gajdusek, C., and Biggs, C. J. J., 1981, The familial occurrence of Creutzfeldt-Jakob disease and Alzheimer disease, Brain, 104:535.

Matsuyama, S. S., 1983, Genetic factors in dementia of the Alzheimer type, in: "Alzheimer Disease: The Standard Reference," Reisberg, B., ed., The Free Press, New York.

McAllister, T. W., 1983, Overview: Pseudodementia, Am. J. Psychiatry, 140:528.

McAllister, T. W., 1981, Cognitive functioning in the affective disorders, Compr. Psychiatry, 22:572.

McAllister, T. W., and Price, T. R., 1982, Severe depressive pseudodementia with and without dementia. Am. J. Psychiatry, 139:626.

Mendels, J., 1981, Antidepressants, in: "Physicians Handbook on Psychotherapeutic Drug Use in the Aged," Crook, T., and Cohen, G. D., ed., Mark Powley Associates Inc., New Canaan.

Mortimer, J. A., 1983, Alzheimer's disease and senile dementia: prevalence and incidence, in: "Alzheimer Disease: The Standard Reference," Reisberg, B., ed., The Free Press, New York.

Mortimer, J. A., Schuman, L. M., and Frenech, L. R., Epidemiology of dementing illness, in: "The Epidemiology of Dementia," Mortimer, J. A., and Schuman, L. M., ed., Oxford University Press, New York.

N I A Task Force, 1980, Senility reconsidered: Treatment possibilities for mental impairment in, JAMA, 244:259.

Nott, P. N., and Fleminger, J. J., 1975, Presenile dementia: the difficulties of early diagnosis, Acta Psychiatr. Scand., 51:210.

OTA, 1985 "Technology and Aging in America," U. S. Government Printing Office, Washington, D. C.

Post, F., 1962, "The Significance of Affective Symptoms in old Age," Oxford University Press.

Rabins, P. V., 1981, The prevalence of reversible dementia in a psychiatric hospital, Hosp. Community Psychiatry, 32:490.

Rabins, P. V., 1983, Reversible dementia and the misdiagnosis of dementia: A review, Hosp. Community Psychiatry, 34:830.

Rabins, P. V., Merchant, A., and Nestadt, G., 1984, Criteria for diagnosing reversible dementia caused by depression, Br. J. Psychiatry, 144:488.

Reifler, B. V., 1982, Arguments for abandoning the term pseudodementia, J. Am. Geriatr. Soc., 30:665.

Reisberg, B., 1985, Alzheimer's Disease Update, Psychiatr. Annals, 15:319.

Reisberg, B., 1983, An overview of current concepts of Alzheimer disease, senile dementia, and age-associated cognitive decline, in: "Alzheimer

Disease: The Standard Reference," Reisberg, B., ed., The Free Press, New York.

Reisberg, B., Ferris, S., De Leon, M. J., and Crook, T., 1982, The global deterioration scale for the assessment of primary degenerative dementia, Am. J. Psychiatry, 139:1136.

Reynolds, C. F., Kupfer, D. J., Taska, L. S., Hoch, C. C., Spiker, D. G., Sewitch, D. E., Zimmer, B., Martin, R. S., Nelson, J. P., Martin, D., and Morycz, R., 1985, EEG Sleep in elderly depressed, demented and healthy subjects, Biol. Psychiatry, 20:431.

Ron, M.A., Toone, B., Garralda, M. E., Lishman, W. A., 1979, Diagnostic accuracy in presenile dementia, Br. J. Psychiatry, 134:161.

Rowe, J. W., 1984, Physiologic changes of aging and their clinical impact, Psychosomatics, 25:6.

Schneck, M.K., Reisberg, B., and Feris, S. H., 1982, An overview of current concepts of Alzheimer's disease, Am. J. Psychiatry, 139:165.

Shraberg, D., 1978, The myth of pseudodementia: depression and the aging brain, Am. J. Psychiatry, 135:601.

Smith, J. S., and Kiloh, L. G., 1981, The investigation of dementia: results in 200 consecutive admissions, Lancet, 1:824.

Spar, J. E., and LaRue, A., 1983, Major depression in the elderly-DSM III criteria and the dexamethasone suppression test as predictors of treatment response. Am. J. Psychiatry, 140:844.

Stern, S. L., Rush, J. A., and Mendels, J., 1980, Toward a rational pharmacotherapy of depression, Am. J. Psychiatry, 137:545.

Straker, M., 1984, Depressive pseudodementia, Psychiatric Annals, 14:93.

Terry, R. D., and Katzman, R. K., 1983, Senile dementia of the Alzheimer type, Ann. Neurol., 14:497.

Ward, N. G., Rowlett, D. B., and Burke, P., 1978, Sodium amylobarbitone in the differential diagnosis of confusion, Am. J. Psychiatry, 135:75.

Wasylenki, D., 1980, Depression in the elderly, Can. Med. Assoc. J., 122:525.

Weingartner, H., Walter, K., Smallberg, S. A., Ebert, M. H., Gillin, J. C., Sitaram, N., 1981, Memory failures in progressive idiopathic dementia. J. Ab. Psychol., 90:181.

Weissman, M. M., 1970, The psychological treatment of depression: evidence for the efficacy of psychotherapy alone, in comparison with, and in combination with pharmacotherapy. Arch. Gen. Psychiatry, 36:1261.

Wells, C. E., 1981, A deluge of dementia, Psychosomatics, 22:837.

Wells, C. E., 1979, Pseudodementia, Am. J. Psychiatry, 136:895.

# THE EPIDEMIOLOGY OF THE CONCURRENCE OF DEPRESSION AND DEMENTIA

Barry Gurland and John Toner

Center for Geriatrics and Gerontology
Columbia University and
New York State Office of Mental Health

## INTRODUCTION

Depression and dementia are starkly contrasting conditions in their prognosis and response to treatment, and in their etiologies as presently understood. Therefore, when symptoms of these two conditions occur together, it raises questions about the clinical implications of the hybrid syndrome, and the circumstances that could lead to concurrence of the two conditions. This paper applies the epidemiological perspective to review findings of relevance to such questions.

### Definitions

Epidemiological methods rely heavily upon analysis of the relative frequencies (or distributions) of diseases and their associations among well described populations. The commonly used measures of frequency are prevalence and incidence. Prevalence is the frequency of a condition within a defined population observed over a given period of time or at a single point in time. Incidence is the frequency of new cases arising in a population during a given period of time, usually a year. Prevalence data on the concurrence of depression and dementia have a more direct bearing on the need for health services than do incidence data, but are less precise than incidence data for understanding the reasons for concurrence of the two conditions. Nevertheless, we will be referring primarily to prevalence data since these are more generally available.

A syndrome resembling the symptoms of dementia has been reported to occur among the elderly in cases diagnosed as primarily depressive disorder. The term pseudodementia was applied to this syndrome by Madden et al. (1952) and widely adopted by others, for example, in reviews by Kiloh (1961), Post (1975), Caine (1981), McAllister (1983), and Wells (1980). Pseudodementia has also been used to refer to other syndromes (Bulbena and Berrios, 1986), and conversely, the symptoms under discussion have been given other labels (such as depressive dementia) or subsumed under more inclusive categories, such as treatable or reversible dementia (Rabins, 1985). Any of these terms begs the question of the nature of this fluctuating intellectual impairment which is associated with some cases of depressive disorder. Since pseudodementia is still the most commonly understood term, we will adhere to this conventional usage for the most part.

THE FREQUENCY OF THE CONCURRENCE OF DEPRESSION AND DEMENTIA

## The Symptoms of Dementia Among Diagnosed Depressions

Madden et al. (1952) noted a prevalence rate for a dementia-like syndrome (disorientation and defects in recent memory, retention, calculation and judgment) of 10% among 300 patients with functional mental disorder starting after age 45 and admitted to the psychiatric unit of a general hospital. Kay et al. (1955) noted equivocal signs of cerebral disturbance such as mild memory defects or transient confusion and disorientation in around 10% of 175 affective disorders from consecutive admissions, aged 60 years old and over, to a mental hospital. In a series of elderly patients with diagnosed depression, Post (1984) described clinically evident "cerebral defects" in 10% and in 17% where psychological tests were applied.

## The Symptoms of Depression Among Diagnosed Dementias

Marsden (1972) reported depressive pseudodementia in 8 out of 106 (7.5%) patients admitted to a neurological hospital with a presumptive diagnosis of dementia. Nott and Fleminger (1975) studied 35 cases diagnosed as presenile dementia and followed to death or for a mean length of 10 years: twenty of these cases did not deteriorate in a way consistent with the diagnosis of dementia and 17 of these had a significant mood disturbance, predominantly depressed in 9 cases. Smith and Kiloh (1981) examined 200 patients (with an age range of 23 to 79 years) who had a provisional diagnosis of dementia and found that 10% had pseudodementia of which the most common cause was depression. Larson et al. (1985) evaluated 200 elderly outpatients who had been referred for suspected dementia: ten cases (5%) were primarily depressed with superimposed symptoms resembling dementia.

Rabins (1985) combined 8 studies comprising 630 cases of hospitalized patients who were given a diagnosis of dementia at some point but who were carefully evaluated for reversible dementia. Reversible conditions were found in 8% to 40% of cases, with a mean of 21%. Four percent were identified as being primarily cases of depression complicated by a syndrome resembling dementia.

Depression also occurs in cases correctly diagnosed as dementia. Larson et al. (1985) report that in their series there were 185 cases with a final diagnosis of dementia and 48 (26%) of these also met DSM III criteria for depression. Kral (1983) reviewed case material on 40 mental hospital patients (average age 78 years old) with Alzheimer's Disease and found depression in 15%.


REASONS FOR THE CONCURRENCE OF DEPRESSION AND DEMENTIA SYMPTOMS

## Concurrence by Chance

The first and simplest explanation of the concurrence of these two conditions would be that it occurs by chance alone. Gurland and Cross (1982), in a review of the prevalence of dementia, concluded that about 5% of the community residing elderly (65 years old and over) have a well established dementia; this rises to 20% or more after age 80. In nursing homes the prevalence of dementia can be as high as 50%. Therefore, depending on the settings and on the age groups from which the cases of depression are collected for study, one can expect a higher or lower proportion of cases to have concurrent dementia by pure chance.

Along the same lines, unless the dementia inhibits the development or expression of depression, cases of dementia will be depressed at least in proportion to the average rate of depression among the elderly population. Rates of depression appear to decrease in old age but are still substantial; for those over 65 years, the rate for all forms of clinical depression (including all subtypes) is in the region of 13% (Gurland et al., 1983), and for major depressions or endogenous depressions it is in the range of 1% to 3%. The ECA studies (Meyers et al., 1984) found that for all types of affective disorder in subjects 65 years and over, the prevalence rates in New Haven were 3.9%, in Baltimore 2.4% and in St. Louis 2.1%. Over the age of 80, when rates of dementia are rising, the rates of depression probably fall still further (at least for women), making chance concurrence less likely.

According to Smith and Kiloh (1981), pseudodementia predominantly occurs in middle age. In a study of patients of all ages with a provisional diagnosis of dementia, the prevalence rates of pseudodementia were respectively, 10% for those less than 45 years old, 13.6% for those between 45-64 years old, and 1.8% for those over 65 years old. Most of these pseudodementias were found to be due to depression. Wells (1979) reported 10 patients with a fully developed pseudodementia syndrome between the ages of 33 and 69 years. McAllister (1983) collated from several sources a series of pseudodementias with primary depression; their ages ranged between 22 and 85 years with a mean of 60.5 years of age. The age distribution of the frequency of pseudodementia appears in these data to parallel that of depression.

However, where depressions are taken as the base populations, the rates of pseudodementia may parallel those of dementia by rising with age. Cole and Hicking (1976) found the rate of minor organic signs rose with age in depressed patients 60 years old and over; 20% in the 60-69 age group, 45% in the 70-79 age group and 70% in the 80 plus age group.

The hypothesis that chance association accounts at least in part for the concurrence of depression and dementia poses a strong challenge to alternative explanations and is consistent with the observed age distributions of either condition viewed against the base population defined by the other condition.

Spurious Association Due to Selective Bias

In certain settings such as nursing homes, selective factors may lead to chance overlap of depression and dementia, or physicians with a special interest in geriatric depression may be referred a sample of patients with complications like concurrent dementia. However, it is difficult to estimate the effect on concurrence rates of selective factors unique to a particular series of patients. Some studies (e.g., Mindham et al., 1982) have introduced case-control comparisons (e.g., spouses, medically ill patients, etc.) to reduce the effects of bias in selection, but the controls also are subject to selective bias. Only clear and consistent findings on greater than chance concurrence of depression and dementia in a variety of samples will be convincing evidence.

On the other hand, pseudodementia may be selectively missing from some settings. Rabins et al. (1984) carried out a retrospective review of 136 outpatients evaluated for dementia in the Hopkins Hospital Psychogeriatric Clinic and found no reversible dementias; presumably these had been hospitalized.

Studies of representative samples of the community elderly are less liable to unintended biases of this nature, but exclude cases admitted to acute or long term care facilities. Among a random sample of community residing elderly (n=445), Gurland et al. (1983) noted a correlation between symptoms of depression and cognitive impairment that was in the low region (.10), although there were a number of cases of depression who had cognitive impairment and of dementia who had raised depression scores. Folstein et al. (1985) identified 44 subjects with possible or definite dementia among a representative sample of the community residing elderly; none of these was found to have a reversible dementia on the basis of a medical and mental examination and, for most cases (n = 36), a complete laboratory investigation.

Spurious Association Due to Misdiagnoses

A concurrence of depression and dementia may be apparent but not real when cases that are solely depressed are diagnosed as also having dementia or a dementia-like syndrome. This is often the result of a failure to distinguish between the symptoms of depression and those of cognitive impairment, or of overly broad criteria for dementia. Misclassification rates have been recently reviewed by Katzman et al. (1986) and show an overdiagnosis of dementia of between 10%-31% in four studies conducted between 1974 and 1981, in which diagnosis was checked by followup. However, in two studies reported in 1984 and 1985, the overdiagnosis dropped to less than 2%. Nevertheless, the misdiagnosis of dementia in cases that are later determined to be primarily a depression has been reported by Gurland et al. (1983), Garcia et al. (1981) and Rabins (1981), among others.

Katzman et al. (1986) attribute the recent improvement in the diagnosis of dementia to better methods of diagnosis, including the use of DSM III criteria. Others, particularly Wells (1980), have delineated certain features which may accompany the picture of cognitive impairment and point towards an underlying depression: exaggeration by patients of their impairments and the problems that ensue, uncooperativeness on testing (e.g. giving up too easily in attempts at answering questions in contrast with the true dementias who will invent answers or get as close as they can to the correct one), an onset which can be easily perceived because it is in sharp contrast to what is normal for that patient and comes on relatively quickly, rapid development of the clinical picture, a previous history of episodes of depression, raised anxiety and a sense of failure in relation to poor performance and islands of good memory or performance. Nott and Fleminger (1975) add that in pseudodementia there are not likely to be errors in language disturbance (perseveration and nominal dysphasia) or calculation; nor focal neurological signs such as apraxia, agnosia and dysgraphia; nor emotional lability. Ron et al. (1979) emphasized that a discrepancy in verbal-performance tests of the W.A.I.S. characterizes true dementia but not pseudodementia. Reding et al. (1985) found in a 3 year follow-up of depressed elderly patients referred to a dementia clinic that the following signs, among others, predicted a high risk of developing dementia: signs of cerebravascular, extrapyramidal or spinocerebellar disease; confusion on low doses of tricyclics. Rabins (1985) provides a logically ordered algorithmic battery of history, physical examination, psychiatric assessment and laboratory and special investigations for improving the accuracy of diagnosis of dementia; he insists that gradual progression and language disorder need be present for diagnosis of Alzheimer's Disease.

Cognitive symptoms of an acute confusional state (delirium) or other may complicate a depression and may be mistaken for dementia. This combination may present with a high frequency in medical settings where depression often accompanies the medical condition and acute confusional states are common as well. Correlations of depression and physical illness in the elderly are generally high (Gurland et al., 1983).

Cognitive impairment due to acute confusional state or other causes is frequent in the same medical settings that may have high rates of depression. Cognitive impairment has been detected by screening measures in 33% of patients (mean age of 55 years) in a general medical inpatient service (Knights and Folstein, 1977), 30% of patients with a mean age of 50.2 years in a neurology service (DePaulo and Folstein, 1978), and 25% in patients with a mean age of 63.4 years in a rehabilitation hospital (Garcia et al., 1984). Post (1984) asserts that confusional states present more commonly with paranoid or manic symptoms than with depressive symptoms, which are rare, but that confusional states may coincide with a depressive condition as a result of the medication prescribed for the depressive symptoms or of the often associated medical condition and its treatment.

Despite the encouraging trends in improving the diagnosis of dementia, it is still likely that misdiagnosis confounds estimates of the frequency of the concurrence of depression and the symptoms of dementia. Overall, the estimates are likely to be deflated by misdiagnosis. Fortunately, much of the data on pseudodementia comes from studies where diagnosis was carefully and expertly made, supported by special investigations and confirmed in some instances by follow-up and autopsy.

## Dementia Syndrome Resulting from Depression

A more interesting possibility than chance association between the two conditions is that there is a systematic concurrence of depression and the dementia syndrome and that it is because one condition increases the risk of the other occurring.

In cases where cognitive impairment is purely a result of depression, it should be expected not to progress, to disappear when the depression subsides and not to reemerge later as a full fledged dementia any more often than in the normal elderly population. Some cases of depression must by chance develop dementia at a later stage, the chances becoming greater the longer the follow-up. However, extrapolating from the estimates of Sluss et al. (1981), even if all subjects in a given series lived and were followed to age 85, only a minority (around a third) should by chance develop dementia.

Several of the earlier studies (Post, 1972; Madden et al., 1952) reported that during the course of depression, intellectual function may become impaired to a marked degree but return to a normal level spontaneously or when the mood state is relieved. Kay et al. (1955) found that the equivocal signs of cerebral disturbance which they noted in their series made no difference to patient outcome as determined by follow-up. Madden et al. (1952) noted that their 30 study patients with a dementia-like syndrome recovered with short-term therapy; however, there was no systematic follow-up to determine the eventual outcome of these patients.

Other and later investigators have reported a mixed outcome for pseudodementia. Rabins (1985) reviewed the scanty literature on the reversibility of dementia (Hutton, 1981; Smith and Kiloh, 1981; Fox et al., 1975; and Freemon, 1976) and concluded that, overall, about 50-60% of pseudodementias recover. Rabins (1981), in his personal series of 16 patients with coexistence of dementia and major depression, found that treatment for their depression led to improvement of cognitive function in 81% of cases, with most remaining well for 2 years. Similarly, Bul-

bena and Berrios (1986) report that the long-term outcome of the Fulbourn
Hospital sample of pseudodementias was mixed but not unlike results obtained by Murphy (1983) for elderly depressives.

However, Kral (1983) followed, for 4-18 years (average 8 years), 22
cases with a mean age of 76.5 years (ages ranged from 62-78 years) diagnosed as pseudodementia and, surprisingly, found that 20 developed
progressive dementia (confirmed by autopsy in 3 cases). Reding et al.
(1985) followed for 3 years 28 cases of depressive pseudodementia, of
whom 16 (57%) developed progressive dementia. Hutton (1981) noted that
in his series of 100 consecutive patients investigated for apparent
dementia, 8 did not have mental impairment and 18 had a functional
psychiatric disorder. There were 6 depressive pseudodementias; in a
follow-up of 4-11 months all of the depressive pseudodementias improved
on treatment, but 4 remained partially impaired. Cole and Hicking (1976)
studied 86 hospital admissions of depressed patients aged sixty years and
over and reported that minor organic signs (partial disorientation or
mild impairment of recent memory) predicted a poorer outcome. Davies et
al. (1978) found slightly unfavorable outcomes in elderly depressives
whose cognitive impairment was detectable in psychological and
psychophysiological tests.

A certain proportion of elderly depressives must by chance be in the
early subclinical stages of dementia; mood disturbance might then aggravate the intellectual difficulties and precipitate a pseudodementia.
In these instances the dementia symptoms would improve along with the
mood, but the dementia process would continue to deteriorate until it
surfaced again some time later regardless of mood. The odds of a chance
concurrence of depression and subclinical dementia are unknown because
there is so much inconsistency in the findings on early dementia in the
published studies. Estimates of the prevalence of early dementia are in
the range of 1-3 times the rates for established cases.

The evidence suggests that at least some cases which present with
the picture of pseudodementia are in fact in the early stages of a
progressive dementia; in some series these cases are a majority. Setting
aside methodological confounds such as selective bias and ambiguities
regarding diagnostic criteria, the evidence on outcome suggests that
pseudodementia is sometimes primarily a depression but often primarily a
dementia; in other cases chance association could account for the concurrence. Treatment of depression secondary to dementia with anticholinergic antidepressants does not appear to accelerate the dementing process
(Kral, 1983). The possibility that depression as such denotes a vulnerability to developing dementia needs further discussion.

Depression As a Precursor to Dementia

Roth (1955) and Post (1972) independently showed that cases of diagnosed depression do not develop dementia at any higher rate than the non-
depressed elderly population. Post (1972) reported the results from a 3
year follow-up of 92 elderly patients with depression: about two thirds
of the patients recovered completely, with or without relapses during the
3 year follow-up; in his opinion, this is quite comparable to recovery
rates published for younger patients. Moreover, only 6.5% of these
depressives developed dementia of "multi-infarct or senile" type, no
greater than would be expected for a population whose members were over
60 years old.

Tomlinson et al. (1968) and Roth (1980) found that brain changes in
depressives do not differ from those in other nondementing conditions
such as physical illness or paraphrenia. Yet, Jacoby et al. (1980, 1981)

reported that enlarged cerebral ventricles were found in 9 out of 10 of late onset depressions and none in early onset depressions; reduced brain tissue radiodensity also characterized the late onset depressives (Jacoby et al., 1983). The latter had a higher mortality rate in a 2 year follow-up, but this was not from dementia.

Mahendra (1985) notes that the earlier works (Nott and Fleminger, 1975; and Ron et al., 1979) emphasized that brain imaging techniques (at first the air encephalogram) showed abnormalities mainly in the true dements, but they did mention minor changes in the pseudodementias. Nott and Fleminger (1975) found almost as many cases with EEG abnormalities among the pseudodementias as in the true dementias.

Thus, both late onset depressions and pseudodementias may have a higher frequency of brain changes than other depressions in the elderly, but there is no evidence that these changes are characteristic of the progressive dementias.

## Depressive Reaction to Dementia

Some cases of depression will be superimposed on well established cases of dementia as reactions to the latter condition. Depression in fully established dementia is often fleeting and ill-defined but may fulfill DSM-III criteria for major depression in a substantial proportion of cases (Larson et al., 1985). In these types of cases, the dementia may improve but will tend not to recede with the depression (McAllister and Price, 1982; and Rabins, 1984).

High rates of such superimposed depressions could be expected if the rates were merely consistent with those observed for other types of disability (Gurland et al., 1983), especially in view of the greater disability imposed by dementia compared to most other disorders. A limit on the frequency of depression might be set by the inability of those with advanced intellectual deterioration to react normally or express their feelings, although it is not clear at what stage of dementia this actually occurs. Kral (1983) holds that in the later stages of Alzheimer's Disease the diagnosis of depression depends more on changes in the patient's behavior than on verbal complaints. Nevertheless, the depression might be not so much a reaction, but a direct effect of the brain change of dementia and thus independent of the patient's psychological awareness. This possibility is discussed below.

## Common Causes of the Two Conditions

The high rate of later development of dementia in some studies of pseudodementia might further be explained by a causal link between the two conditions. Either the depression is a psychological reaction to an incipient dementia, based on the person's awareness that his/her faculties are becoming impaired, or the two conditions arise out of a common biological process, possibly related to aging.

A specific biological association—as opposed to a non-specific psychological association—between depression and dementia should lead to differing rates of depression among sub-types of dementia. There is insufficient data to address this possibility, though there are claims that Parkinson's Disease has an especially high rate of both depression and dementia (Mayeux et al., 1981; Mindham et al., 1982). One estimate of the symptoms of depression in Parkinson's Disease has been as high as 90% (Mindham, 1970), though that study was conducted in a psychiatric hospital and, moreover, affective illnesses were of equal frequency in index (55 out of 89) and control (44 out of 89) groups. Mayeux et al. (1981)

found over 16% of their Parkinsonian patients to be moderately or severely depressed, with no such cases in spouses who were the controls.

Cognitive impairment has been reported to occur in around 20%-40% of Parkinsonian patients (Mayeux et al., 1981; Mindham et al., 1982), but opinion is divided as to whether the defects are those of dementia, and if so, whether this is of the Alzheimer type or a subcortical dementia (characterized by memory impairment, slowness of thought, apathy and depression and difficulty in manipulating knowledge, but no aphasia, apraxia or agnosia). Perry et al. (1983) have found that the cognitive impairments of Parkinson's Disease are associated with cortical cholinergic deficits but not with the neuropathological changes of Alzheimer's Disease.

The depression in Parkinson's Disease has been reported to be positively correlated with the level of cognitive impairment (Mayeux et al., 1981), but other relationships are less clear; it appears to be unrelated to the major subtypes of Parkinsonism (idiopathic, postencephaletic and arteriosclerotic) (Mindham et al., 1982). The depression seems often to coincide with the onset of Parkinsonism, but is not related to the severity of the Parkinsonian symptoms and may be relieved by antidepressives even when the Parkinsonian symptoms are not remittent. The depression may precede the Parkinsonian symptoms. Furthermore, equally disabled medically ill patients are not as depressed as Parkinsonian sufferers. Levodopa treatment is apparently not responsible for the depression in parkinsonian patients.

Mayeux et al. (1981) have reconciled these discrepancies in their observations that the depression of Parkinson's Disease is usually in the younger patient with a relatively slowly progressing illness; where it is not accompanied by a global dementia but rather by mild intellectual impairment, with impaired cognitive skills and inattention. The Alzheimer's type dementia occurs in the older patients with a rapidly progressive form of Parkinsonism. It may be that a reduction of norepinephrine and serotonin levels underlies some of the changes in Parkinson's Disease, dementia and depression.

Any theory on a common cause for the concurrent syndromes of depression and dementia must take into account differences in the features of the memory disturbance associated with the two conditions.

Caine (1981) studied 17 patients with depression and cognitive impairment and noted that many "cortically mediated" psychological functions commonly impaired in dementia were not affected, while attention, mental processing speed, spontaneous elaboration and analysis of detail were impaired. Gibson (1981) and Weingartner et al. (1982) suggest that memory is not disorganized in depression, but suppressed in proportion to the depression, especially for memory of unrelated events, which requires high and sustained effort and motivation. In dementia, the patient fails on even relatively easy memory tasks, despite the relationships between information and despite trying hard. Kral (1983) suggests that depression based on the brain changes of Alzheimer's Disease itself (as opposed to endogenous and reactive depression) is chronic with little variation in intensity and characterized by irritability, aggressiveness, paranoid ideation and nihilistic delusions. These depressions tend to be refractory to antidepressant treatment. Kral points to the possible role of the limbic system in serving both memory and mood.

Mahendra (1985) puts forward the view that if there is a neurobiological process common to dementia and depression which explains their relationships, whether positive or inverse, then it is complex (e.g., the role of monoamines or cholinergic activity). The process might favor depression at one extreme and dementia at the other, with some mixed conditions such as Parkinsonism between. He suggests that there might be a discrete entity involving a relatively benign and sometimes reversible type of dementia. In support of this concept, he points out that the dementia symptoms are often quite out of proportion to the level of depression (i.e., a progression of severity to the point of stuporous depression producing dementia no longer occurs with today's treatments); the depressive and dementing symptoms often pursue an independent course and concurrent depression tends to occur more commonly with the dementia of Parkinsonism, Huntington's Chorea and the slower senile types.

CLINICAL CONSIDERATIONS

In any event, pseudodementia or its synonyms and analogs occurs in a small but important minority of depressions (about 10%), and suspected cases of dementia (about 5%), and may account for as much as 20% of the reversible dementias. These figures underline the necessity and value of a full evaluation of depression in cases suspected of being demented. Depressive symptoms should be appropriately treated regardless of the presence of dementia or other cognitive impairment.

CONCLUSIONS

The various concepts and syndromes of relevance to a discussion of pseudodementia must be more clearly delineated in order to settle some of the inconsistencies in the findings of different studies. The concepts that are called upon as alternative explanations for the concurrence of depression and dementia have been reviewed in this paper. Some of these concepts are summarized below (together with suggestions for criteria) to define the clinical syndromes that reflect the concepts.

Depressive Pseudodementia

This concept implies that a primary depression presents with symptoms that have initially the clinical appearance but not the characteristic course of a progressive dementia. This concept excludes cases which are carelessly diagnosed as dementia because the typical symptoms of depression are overlooked or because symptoms such as subjective complaints of difficulty with memory or a syndrome of delirium (acute confusional state) are misinterpreted as indicating a dementia. Suggested criteria are: (a) fulfills criteria for a depressive disorder (except for tautological criteria such as ruling out an organic cause), (b) fulfills criteria for a dementia (except for tautological criteria such as ruling out depression), (c) the dementia ceases when the depression is relieved and (d) the criteria for dementia are not fulfilled during the subsequent 3 years except during episodes of depressive disorder or marked aggravation of depressive disorder.

Mahendra (1985) states that the criteria which underlie the concept that pseudodementia is caused by depression are that the symptoms of dementia are not progressive but improve with the depressive illness and that there is no causal relationship with brain disease. Bulbena and Berrios (1986) used the following precise but slightly broader criteria: the presence of cognitive impairment of the type seen in dementia, no relevant organic disorder and reversibility of the symptoms of dementia.

## Depression with Cognitive Impairment

This concept implies that a primary depression presents with the usual range of symptoms and that intellectual changes are only evident on very careful testing. Suggested criteria are: (a) fulfills criteria for a primary depressive disorder, (b) does not fulfill criteria for a dementia, (c) does not fulfill criteria for a dementia at any time in the next 3 years and (d) cognitive impairments, evident clinically or on testing, wax and wane with the depression.

Depressive pseudodementia does not include non-dementing conditions presenting as dementia for reasons other than a depressive precipitant (i.e., it excludes deliria, other treatable or reversible dementias, and other psychiatric causes).

## Dementia with Depression

The concept is that these cases are suffering from primary dementia and in addition have a depressive disorder. Suggested criteria are: (a) presently or within 3 years fulfills criteria for a dementia, (b) fulfills criteria for a depressive disorder and (c) the dementia symptoms precede and outlast the symptoms of depressive disorder or the dementia symptoms relapse without depression within 3 years.

It should be noted that in this concept and consistent with these criteria, the dementia may at the time of diagnosis be clinically evident or be subclinical.

There are also concepts covering cases that have a common biological process or occur together by chance, but these cannot be distinguished at present from the previous concepts by criteria that apply to the individual patient. These concepts can be examined by abstracting from data on large or special groups, and they will certainly be further clarified when markers of the two conditions are available.

It is tempting to add to these criteria the phenomenological indicators or predictors of depression or of dementia that have been mentioned in this paper; or to incorporate the evidence of special investigations such as brain imaging or evidence of specific neurotransmitter abnormalities. However, the usefulness of these indicators and predictors has not been well validated except insofar as they are already incorporated into criteria for depression and dementia separately. In the interim the consensual agreement on terms such as those listed above would resolve some of the apparent discrepancies in studies of pseudodementia and other conditions involving concurrence of depression and dementia and would clarify many of the issues that are raised.

REFERENCES

Arie, T., 1983, Pseudodementia, Br. Med. J., 286:277.
Bulbena, A., and Berrios, G.E., 1986, Pseudodementia: Facts and figures, Br. J. Psychiatry, 148:87.
Caine, E., 1981, Pseudodementia, Arch. Gen. Psychiatry, 38:1359.
Cole, M., and Hicking, T., 1976, Frequency and significance of minor organic signs in elderly depressives, Can. Psychiatr. Assoc. J., 21:7.
Cross, P., and Gurland, B., 1984, Age, period and cohort views of suicide rates of the elderly, in: "Suicide and the Life Cycle," C. Pfeffer, and J. Richman, The American Association of Suicidology, New York.
Davies, G., Hamilton, S., Hendrickson, D.E., Levy, R., and Post, F., 1978, Psychological test performance and sedation thresholds of

elderly dements, depressives and depressives with incipient brain change, Psychol. Med., 8:103.

DePaulo, J., and Folstein, M., 1978, Psychiatric disturbances in neurological patients: Detection, recognition, and course, Ann. Neurol., 4:225.

Folstein, M., Anthony, J.C., Parhad, I., Duffy, B., and Gruenberg, E.M., 1985, The meaning of cognitive impairment in the elderly, J. Am. Geriatr. Soc., 33:228.

Fox, J.H., Topel, J.L., and Huckman, M.S., 1975, Dementia in the elderly--A search for treatable illness, J. Gerontol., 30:557.

Freemon, F.R., 1976, Evaluation of patients with progressive intellectual deterioration, Arch. Neurol., 33:658.

Garcia, C., Reding, M., and Blass, J., 1981, Overdiagnosis of dementia, J. Am. Geriatr. Soc., 29:407.

Garcia, C., Tweedy, J., and Blass, J., 1984, Underdiagnosis of cognitive impairment in a rehabilitation setting, J. Am. Geriatr. Soc., 32:339.

Gibson, A., 1981, A further analysis of memory loss in dementia and depression in the elderly, Br. J. Clin. Psychol., 20:179.

Gurland, B., 1984, Public health aspects of Alzheimer's and related dementias, in: "Alzheimer's Disease and Related Dementias," W. Kelly, ed., Charles C. Thomas, New York.

Gurland, B., Copeland, J., Kuriansky, J., Kelleher, M., Sharpe, L., Dean, L.L., 1983, "The Mind and Mood of Aging," The Haworth Press, Inc., New York.

Gurland, B., and Cross, P., 1982, The epidemiology of psychopathology in old age: Some clinical implications, Psychiatr. Clin. of N. Am., 5:11.

Gurland, B., Golden, B., and Dean, L., 1980, Depression and dementia in the elderly of New York City, in: "Planning for the Elderly in New York City," New York Community Council of Greater New York.

Harrison, M.J.G., and Marsden, C.D., 1977, Progressive intellectual deterioration, Arch. Neurol., 34:199.

Hutton, J.T., 1981, Senility reconsidered, J. Am. Med. Assoc., 245:1025.

Jacoby, R.J., Dolan, R., Levy, R., and Baldy, R., 1983, Quantitative computed tomography in elderly depressed patients, Br. J. Psychiatry, 143:124.

Jacoby, R.J., Levy, R., and Bird, J.M., 1981, Computed tomography and the outcome of affective disorder: A follow-up study of elderly patients, Br. J. Psychiatry, 139:288.

Jacoby, R.J., Levy, R., and Dawson, J.M., 1980, Computed tomography in the elderly, 3. Affective disorders, Br. J. Psychiatry, 136:70.

Katzman, R., Lasker, B., and Bernstein, N., 1986, Accuracy of diagnosis and consequences of misdiagnosis of disorders causing dementia. Contract report prepared and submitted to U.S. Congress Office of Technology Assessment.

Kay, D.W.K., Roth, M., and Hopkins, B., 1955, Affective disorders in the senium, I, Their association with organic cerebral degeneration, J. Ment. Sci., 101:302.

Kiloh, L.G., 1961, Pseudodementia, Acta Psychiatr. Scand., 37:336.

Knights, E.B., and Folstein, M.F., 1977, Unsuspected emotional and cognitive disturbance in medical patients, Ann. Intern. Med., 87:723.

Kral, V., 1983, The relationship between senile dementia (Alzheimer Type) and depression, Can. J. Psychiatry, 28:304.

Larson, E., Reifler, B., Sumi, S., Canfield, C., and Chinn, N., 1985, Diagnostic evaluation of 200 elderly outpatients with suspected dementia, J. Gerontol., 40:536.

Madden, J.J., Luhan, J.A., Kaplan, L.A., and Manfredi, H.M., 1952, Nondementing psychoses in older persons, J. Am. Med. Assoc., 150:1567.

Mahendra, B., 1985, Depression and dementia: The multi-faceted relationship, Psychol. Med., 15:227.

Marsden, C.D., 1982, Basal ganglia disease, Lancet, ii:1141.

Marsden, C.D., and Harrison, M.J.G., 1972, Outcome of investigation of patients with presenile dementia, Br. Med. J., 2:249.

Mayeux, R., Stern, Y., Rosen, J., and Leventhal, J., 1981, Depression, intellectual impairment, and Parkinson's Disease, Neurology, 31:645.

McAllister, T.W., 1983, Pseudodementia, Am. J. Psychiatry, 140:528.

McAllister, T.W., and Price, T.R., 1982, Severe depressive pseudodementia with and without dementia, Am. J. Psychiatry, 139:626.

Mindham, R., 1970, Psychiatric symptoms in Parkinsonism, J. Neurol. Neurosurg. Psychiatry, 33:188.

Mindham, R., Ahmed, S., and Clough, C., 1982, A controlled study of dementia in Parkinson's Disease, J. Neurol. Neurosurg. Psychiatry, 45:969.

Murphy, E., 1983, The prognosis of depression in old age, Br. J. Psychiatry, 142:111.

Myers, J.K., Weissman, M.M., Tischler, G.L., Holzer, C.E. 3d, Leaf, P.J., Orvaschel, H., Anthony, J.C., Boyd, J.H., Burke, J.D. Jr., Kramer, M., et al., 1984, Six-month prevalence of psychiatric disorders in three communities 1980 to 1982, Arch. Gen. Psychiatry, 41:959.

Nott, P.N., and Fleminger, J.J., 1975, Presenile dementia: The difficulties of early diagnosis, Acta Psychiatr. Scand., 51:210.

Pearce, J., and Miller, E., 1973, "Clinical Aspects of Dementia," Baillere Tindall, London.

Perry, R., Tomlinson, B., Candy, J., Blessed, G., Foster, J., Bloxham, C., and Perry, E., 1983, Critical cholinergic deficit in mentally impaired parkinsonian patients, Lancet, ii:789.

Post, F., 1962, "The Significance of Affective Symptoms in Old Age," Oxford University Press, London.

Post, F., 1972, The management and nature of depressive illnesses in late life: A follow-through study, Br. J. Psychiatry, 212:393.

Post, F., 1975, Dementia, depression and pseudo-dementia, in: "Psychiatric Aspects of Neurological Disease," D.F. Benson and D. Blumer, eds., Grune and Stratton, New York.

Post, F., 1984, Affective psychoses, in: "Handbook of Studies on Psychiatry and Old Age," D.W. Kay, and G. Burrows, eds., Elsevier Science Publishers, Amsterdam and New York.

Rabins, P.V., 1981, The prevalence of reversible dementia in a psychiatric hospital, Hosp. Community Psychiatry, 32:490.

Rabins, P. V., 1985, The reversible dementias, in: "Recent Advances in Psychogeriatrics," T. Arie, ed., Churchill Livingstone, London.

Rabins, P.V., Merchant, A., and Nestadt, G., 1984, Criteria for diagnosing dementia caused by depression: Validation by 2 year follow-up, Br. J. Psychiatry, 144:488.

Reding, M., Haycox, J., and Blass, J., 1985, Depression in patients referred to a dementia clinic: A three year prospective study, Arch. Neurol., 42:894.

Reifler, B., Larson, E., and Hanley, R., 1982, Coexistence of cognitive impairment and depression in geriatric outpatients, Am. J. Psychiatry, 139:623.

Ron, M.A., Toone, B.K., Garralda, M.E., and Lishman, W.A., 1979, Diagnostic accuracy in presenile dementia, Br. J. Psychiatry, 134:161.

Roth, M., 1955, The natural history of mental disorders in old age, J. Ment. Sci., 101:281.

Roth, M., 1980, Senile dementia and its borderlands, in: "Psychopathology in the Aged," J. Cole and J. Barrett, eds., Raven Press, New York.

Sluss, T., Greenberg, E., and Kramer, M., 1981, The use of longitudinal studies in the investigation of risk factors for senile dementia-- Alzheimer Type, in: "The Epidemiology of Dementia," J. Mortimer and L. Schuman, eds., Oxford University Press, New York.

Smith, J.S., and Kiloh, L.G., 1981, The investigation of dementia: Results in 200 consecutive admissions, Lancet, i:824.

Tomlinson, B., Blessed, G., and Roth, M., 1968, Observations on the brains of non-demented old people, J. Neurol. Sci., 7:331.

Weingartner, H., Cohen, R., Bunney, W., Ebert, M., and Kaye, W., 1982, Memory-learning impairments in progressive dementia and depression, Am. J. Psychiatry, 139:135.

Wells, C.E., 1979, Pseudodementia, Am. J. Psychiatry, 136:895.

Wells, C.E., 1980, The differential diagnosis of psychiatric disorders in the elderly, in: "Psychopathology in the Aged," J. Cole and J. Barrett, Raven Press, New York.

# COGNITIVE FUNCTION AND BRAIN-ADRENAL AXIS ACTIVITY IN AGING, DEPRESSION AND DEMENTIA

Gregory F. Oxenkrug and Samuel Gershon

Department of Psychiatry
School of Medicine
Wayne State University
Detroit, Michigan

## INTRODUCTION

The brain-adrenal axis* represents one of the major adaptation mechanisms maintaining the body homeostatic balance (see Dilman, 1971). Since the 1960s it has become an object of increased attention to psychiatrists and has resulted in the avalanch of publications reviewed elsewhere (Stokes, 1987). This chapter reviews the findings of our research team as well as closely related literature in an attempt to offer a satisfactory explanation of the known facts and to suggest directions for further investigation.

The starting point of our studies was the understanding that brain-adrenal axis activation (initially viewed as a specific feature of, at least, a subgroup of depressions) is a non-specific phenomenon in regard to any pathological entity (Dilman, 1971; Dilman et al., 1979; Stokes et al., 1984). Brain-adrenal axis activation reflects rather, some brain-endocrine changes that might occur in the course of normal aging (see Dilman et al., 1979) and pathological conditions (depression, see Carroll et al., 1981; alcohol withdrawal, see Oxenkrug, 1978; primary degenerative dementia, see Raskind et al., 1982). Such an approach does not exclude the evaluation of brain-adrenal activity as an additional laboratory test (Carroll et al., 1981). Fever, in the same vein is a non-specific phenomenon for pneumonia or appendicitis but rather points to the presence of inflammation and might be useful for diagnostic and follow-up purposes.

Normal aging. There is ample experimental evidence of brain-adrenal activation in the course of normal aging (DeKosky et al., 1984; Landfield et al., 1978, 1981; Oxenkrug et al., 1983). Some hypotheses (see Dilman et al., 1979; Landfield, 1986) suggest that brain-adrenal activation is one of the main mechanisms of normal aging. This suggestion is in line with the findings that chronic exposure of the young animal to elevated levels of corticosteroids caused hippocampal morphological changes typical

---

*"Brain-adrenal" seems to be a more appropriate definition than hypothalamic-pituitary adrenal (at least in the context of the current review) since some other brain structures (hippocampus: McEwen et al., 1975; pineal: Wurtman & Altshule, 1959; Oxenkrug et al., 1984) might contribute to the regulation of adrenal activity.

of old animals (see Landfield, 1986); inhibited the sprouting of hippocampal noradrenergic neurons (DeKosky et al., 1984) and down regulated
hippocampal corticosterone receptors (Sapolsky & McEwan, 1986).

In contrast to abundant animal data, activation of the brain-adrenal
axis in <u>humans</u> has not been well established until recently. The routine
tool for the evaluation of brain-adrenal axis activity is dexamethasone
(DEX) suppression test; the failure of DEX (a synthetic glucocorticoid) to
suppress blood cortisol levels indicates an overactivation of brain-adrenal
axis. The use of 1 mg of DEX failed to find an age effect on post-DEX cortisol levels partly because 1 mg of DEX resulted in almost complete suppression of cortisol levels (mostly <1 microg/dl) (Tourigny-Rivard et al.,
1981). Recently, Rosenbaum et al. (1984) suggested that aging effect on
post 1 mg of DEX cortisol levels might be revealed with the use of radioimmunoassay but not competitive protein binding methods of plasma cortisol
determination. The use of 0.5 mg of DEX yields various degrees of cortisol
suppression (from <1 to 5 microg/dl) and allows for the establishment of a
positive correlation between plasma post-DEX cortisol levels and age in
normal volunteers (Oxenkrug et al., 1983). These results were in line with
the previously observed increase of post-prednisolone urine corticosteroid
levels in normal aged subjects (see Dilman et al., 1979). The other tool
for the evaluation of brain-adrenal axis activity is the determination of
24 h blood cortisol secretion. Positive correlation has been found in normal subjects between age and 24 h plasma cortisol levels (Halbreich et al.,
1985). According to Halbreich et al. (1985) each decade of age results in
0.65 microg/dl increase of 24 h plasma cortisol. The use of only one-point
(morning) plasma cortisol level fails to produce statistically significant
correlation between basal plasma cortisol levels and age (Oxenkrug et al.,
1983; Georgotas et al., 1986). However, linear regression analysis reveals
the contribution of basal (pre-DEX) morning plasma cortisol levels to age-
associated increase of post-DEX cortisol levels. The relationships between
age, pre- and post-DEX plasma cortisol levels was described by the following equation (Branconnier, Oxenkrug et al., 1984):

PostDEX cortisol = 0.12 (preDEX cortisol) + 0.04 (age) - 1.34     (I)

The highest post-DEX cortisol levels (4 to 5 microg/dl) were observed
among subjects older than 55 years suggesting that the use of one and the
same normal value (cut-off at the level of 4 to 6 microg/dl) is inappropriate for elderly population, at least, with the 0.5 mg of DEX test.
Theoretically, this equation might also be used for calculation of "age"
based on determination of pre- and post DEX cortisol levels:

"Age" = (PostDEX cortisol - 0.12 (preDEX cortisol) + 1.34):0.04   (II)

The calculated "age" might reflect some (but not all) age-associated
biological changes (mostly in brain-adrenal axis). Therefore, such a calculation might be used for the evaluation of the correspondence between
brain-adrenal axis activity and chronological age of the subject studied.

Therefore, both animal and human data suggest the progressive activation of brain-adrenal axis during the course of normal aging.

The memory changes are nearly universal in aging. Although no data
on the correlation between cognitive function and brain-adrenal axis activity during the course of the normal aging is available, one may suggest
the existence of such a correlation considering that age associates with
both brain-adrenal axis activation (Dilman et al., 1979; Oxenkrug et al.,
1983) and cognitive impairment (see Branconnier and De Witt, 1984).

<u>Cushing's and Down's Syndrome</u>.  Both syndromes are considered the

models of accelerated aging. Affective and cognitive changes in Cushing's syndrome were associated with the brain-adrenal overactivation (Starkman et al., 1986). We were particularly interested in evaluating the brain-adrenal activity in Down's syndrome patients since age-associated brain morphological changes (plaques, tangles) (Ball and Nuttall, 1979) as well as early development of dementia (Thase et al., 1984) similar to senile dementia of Alzheimer's type (primary degenerative dementia, DSM-111) were observed in this genetic disorder as early as in the third decade of life (see Wishnievski, this volume).

Post-DEX plasma cortisol levels were below 4 microg/dl in two out of six patients (Oxenkrug et al., 1987a). The limited number of observations did not allow us to conclude (according to Carroll's criteria) whether non-suppressors were more frequent among Down's syndrome patients. However, post-DEX plasma cortisol level calculated according to equation #I was identical to the obtained cortisol level only in one patient, 26 years old. In the rest of the patients calculated postDEX levels were higher than obtained ones and the differences between calculated and obtained cortisol levels positively correlated (r=0.73, p<0.05) with the age of the subjects.

In the same vein, calculated "age" (equation #II) was almost identical with the chronological age of the patient in the second decade of life. However, patients of the third to sixth decade of chronological age revealed the persistent increase of their calculated "age". The calculated "ages" of patients in the fifth and sixth decades were above the limits of the equation (82 years). In fact, if the same equation was based on the data obtained from normal subjects up to 200 years old, the calculated "age" of these Down's syndrome patients would be around 180 years.

Therefore, brain-adrenal activation was observed in both normal aging and in Down's syndrome. The striking difference between these two conditions is a dramatically accelerated development of brain-adrenal activation and cognitive impairment in Down's syndrome. The direct assessment of such a correlation has so far been done in primary degenerative dementia and major depressive disorder.

Primary degenerative dementia. Brain-adrenal overactivation in dementia has been observed by several research teams (Coppen et al., 1983; Spar and Gerner, 1982; Raskind et al., 1982). Further studies reported brain-adrenal overactivation in severe (but not mild) forms of primary degenerative dementia (Jenike and Albert, 1984; Pomara, Oxenkrug et al., 1984). It is noteworthy that both studies came to a similar conclusion on the correlation between cognitive impairment and brain-adrenal activation despite the fact that severity of dementia was assessed by two different methods: Dementia Scale (Jenike and Albert, 1984) and Memory and Information Test of Roth and Hopkins (1953) (Pomara, Oxenkrug et al., 1984). Recently, we observed a positive correlation between post-DEX plasma cortisol levels and Global Deterioration Scores (GDS) (Reisberg et al., 1982) in primary degenerative dementia (Oxenkrug et al., 1987b). However, the correlation between GDS scores and post-DEX cortisol levels in the primary degenerative dementia was not observed by Georgotas et al. (1986). The possible reasons for the descrepancy between their data and our results are the wider range of GDS scores in our patients than in the Georgotas et al. study and the use of different modifications of the DEX test. The 0.5 mg DEX method apparently is a more sensitive tool for the evaluation of brain-adrenal axis disfunction than the 1 mg of DEX test since it results in a wider range of post-DEX cortisol values.

A positive correlation between cognitive impairment and brain-adrenal overactivation observed in primary degenerative dementia provides an additional indirect support for the suggestion that brain-adrenal overactivation might contribute to cognitive impairment in normal aging, Down's syndrome and primary degenerative dementia.

Depression. Overactivation of brain-adrenal axis is generally acknowledged in, at least, a subgroup of depressed patients. Cognitive impairment, a clinical feature of depression, (McAllister, 1981; Weingartner et al., 1981) has been shown to be more pronounced in DEX test non-suppressors (Brown and Shuey, 1980; Reus, 1982) and to correlate with free urinary cortisol (Rubinov et al., 1984) and post-0.5 mg DEX cortisol levels (Siegel et al., 1987) in depressed patients. The possible correlation between cognitive impairment and brain-adrenal activation was substantiated recently by finding of the association of memory deficit and nonsuppression to 1 mg of DEX with radioimmunoassay of plasma cortisol in depressed patients (Winokur et al., 1987).

It is noteworthy that correlations between cognitive function and brain-adrenal axis activity in depressed patients were observed by several authors despite the different methods used for the evaluation of both cognitive function and brain-adrenal axis activity (Brown and Shuey, 1980; Rubinov et al., 1984; Reus, 1982). However, our observation of correlation between GDS scores and post-DEX cortisol levels in elderly depressed patients (Siegel et al., 1987) is at variance with Georgotas et al. (1986). Since the number of observations and the average GDS scores in our study were very similar to that of Georgotas et al., the possible reason for the discrepancy might be the use of 0.5 mg of DEX in our study versus 1 mg of DEX in the Georgotas et al. (1986) study.

Therefore, literature and our data produced the repeated observations of a positive correlation between brain-adrenal activation and cognitive impairment in depressed patients.

It is feasible that interaction of age and depression effects on brain-adrenal axis (Stangl et al., 1986) might result in higher degree of brain-adrenal axis activation (Alexopolus et al., 1984; Davis et al., 1984; Greden et al., 1986; Nelson et al., 1984) and more severe cognitive impairment (Rubinov et al., 1984; Seigel et al., 1987) in elderly depressed subjects. The degree of cognitive impairment in elderly depressed patients might be, indeed, indistinquishible from that in primary degenerative dementia (see Siegel and Gershon, this volume).

Comments. The review of the available data suggests that brain-adrenal activation correlates with cognitive impairment in, at least, a subgroup of depressives, as well as in primary degenerative dementia, Down's syndrome and in normal aging. One might suggest that cognitive impairment and brain-adrenal axis activation may be independently triggered by one and the same mechanisms and, therefore, the correlation between cognitive function and brain-adrenal activity is just an epiphenomen. The alternative suggestion might be that the observed correlation reflects the cause-effect relationships between brain-adrenal axis activation and cognition. Such a hypothesis is in line with the experimental data which suggests that brain-adrenal axis activation might impair cognition through cortisol effect on glucocorticoid receptors (Sapolsky & McEwen, 1986) and adrenergic neurons (DeKosky et al., 1984) in hippocampus—the structure intimately involved in memory processes (Hyman et al., 1985). Since normal aging and, at least, some subtypes of depression, dementias and Down's syndrome associate with both brain-adrenal axis overactivation and cognitive impairment, one might argue that brain-adrenal axis overactivation contributes to the development of cognitive impairment in these conditions. (The lack of data does not allow us to consider different subtypes of dementia or depression.)

The positive correlation between brain-adrenal axis activation and cognitive impairment also implies that the degree of brain-adrenal axis activation might, at least partly, determine the degree of cognitive impairment. Some literature and our data discussed in this review are in line with such a suggestion, since in the course of normal aging brain-adrenal axis activation and cognitive impairment are minimal in the young subjects and become prominent only in the aged population. In the case of Down's syndrome, both cognitive impairment and brain-adrenal axis activation are dramatically accelerated. Primary degenerative dementia might be considered as some what in the middle between normal aging and Down's syndrome.

The mechanisms and natural course of brain-adrenal axis dysfunction (and cognitive impairment) in depression might be different from the other reviewed conditions. Aging associated changes in brain-adrenal activity and cognition are expected to be irreversible and genetically predetermined. The same arguments might be applied to Down's syndrome and primary degenerative dementia. Recent studies suggest that both disorders might have the genetic defects related to chromosome 21. Depression-associated changes on the contrary in general are reversible and may be associated with the defect of chromosome 11. It is noteworthy that both brain-adrenal axis activation and cognitive impairment are stat rather than trait-related features of depression. (This does not exclude the possibility of irreversible brain changes caused by prolonged brain-adrenal axis activation in depression --Kral et al., 1983).

In conclusion, we suggest that age-associated activation of brain-adrenal axis might affect the potential demented patients at an earlier time of life and might contribute to development of cognitive impairment. Such a suggestion is in line with the hypothesis that activation and acceleration of the normal "machinery" of brain aging might contribute to the manifestations of dementia (see Landfield, 1986). The results of further investigations of the mechanisms of brain-adrenal activation in primary degenerative dementia might be used therefore for the development of methods of identification of populations-at-risk and for rational biological treatments of dementia.

ACKNOWLEDGEMENT

Supported by NIMH grant MH 40924 01A1 (G.O.)

REFERENCES

Alexopulos, G.S., Young, R.C., Kocsis, J.H., Brockner, N., Butler, T.A., Stokes, P.E., 1984, Dexamethasone suppression test in geriatric depression. Biol. Psychiat., 19:1567-1571.

Ball, M.J., and Nuttall, K., 1979, Neurofibrially tangles, granulova-cuolar degeneration neuron loss in Down's syndrome: Comparison with Alzheimer dementia. Ann. Neurol.., 7:462.

Branconnier, R., DeWitt, D., 1983, The early detection of incipient alzheimer's disease: some methodological considerations on computed diagnostics, in: "Alzheimer's Disease: The Standard Reference," B. Reisberg, ed., Free Press, New York.

Branconnier, T., Oxenkrug, G.F., McIntyre, I.M., Pomara, N., Stanley, M., Harto-Truax, N.E., Gershon, S., 1984, Prediction of serum cortisol response to dexamethasone in normal volunteers: a multivariate approach. Psychopharmacology, 84:274-275.

Brown, W.A., And Shuey, I., 1980, Response to dexamethasone and subtype of depression. Arch. Gen. Psychiat., 37:747-751.

Carroll, B., Feinberg, M., Greden, J., 1981, A specific laboratory test for the diagnosis of melacholia. Arch. Gen. Psychiat., 38:15-22.

Coppen, A., Abou-Saleh, M., Milln, P., 1983, Dexamethasone suppression text in depression and other psychiatric illness. Br. J.

text in depression and other psychiatric illness. **Br. J. Psychiat.**, 142:498-504.

Davis, K.L., B.M., Mathe, A.A., Mohs, R.C., Rothpearl, A.B., Levy, M.I., Corman, L.K., Berger, P., 1984, Age and the Dexamethasone suppression test in depression, **Am. J. Psychiat.**, 141:872-874.

DeKosky, S.T., Sohoff, S.W., Cotman, C.W., 1984, Elevated corticosterone levels, a possible cause of reduced axon sprouting in aged animals, **Neuroendocrinology**, 38:33-38.

Dilman, V.M., 1971, Age-associated elevation of hypothalamic threshold of feedback control and its role in development, aging and disease, **Lancet.**, i:1211-1216.

Dilman, V.M., Lapin, I.P., and Oxenkrug, G., 1979, Serotonin and aging, **in:** "Serotonin in Health and Diseases," W. Essman, ed., Spectrum Press, N.Y., London.

Georgotas, A., McCue, R.E., Kim, O.M., Hapworth, W.,E., Reisberg, B., Stoll, P.M.S.E., Fanelli, C., and Stokes, P.E., 1986, Dexamethasone suppression in dementia, depression and normal aging, **Am J. Psychiat.**, 143:452-456.

Greden, J.F., Fiegel, P., Haskett, R., 1986, Age effects in serial hypothalamic-pituitary-adrenal monitoring, **Psychoendocr.**, 11:195-204.

Halbreich, U., Asnis, G.M., Zumoff, B., and Nathan, R.S., 1985, The effect of age and sex on cortisol secretion in depressives and normals, **Psychiat. Res.**, 13:141-148.

Hyman, B.T., Hoesenvan, G.W., Damasio, A.R., and Barnes, C.L., 1984, Alzheimer's disease: Cell-specific pathology isolates the hippocampal formation, **Sci.**, 225:1168-1170.

Jenike, M.A., and Albert, M.S., 1984, The dexamethasone suppression test in patients with presenile and senile dementia of the Alzheimer's type, **J. Amer. Geriat. Soc.**, 32:441-443.

Kral, V.A., 1978, The relationship between senile dementia (Alzheimer type) and depression, **Can. J. Psychiat.**, 28:304-396.

Landfield, P.W., 1986, Preventive approaches to normal brain aging and Alzheimer's disease, **in:** "Treatment development strategies for Alzheimer's disease," T. Crook, R. Bartus, S. Ferris and S. Gershon, eds., Mark Powley Ass.

Landfield, P.W., 1978, Hippocampal aging and adrenocorticoids: Quantitative correlation, **Science,** 202:1098-1102.

Landfield, P.W., Baskin, R.K., and Pitler, T.A., 1981, Brain aging correlates: retardation by hormonal-pharmacological treatments, **Sci.**, 214:581-584.

McAllister, T.W., 1984a, Overview: Pseudodementia, **Am. J. Psychiat.**, 140:528-533.

McEwen, B.S., Gerlach, J.L., Micco, D.J., 1975, Putative glucocorticoid receptors in hippocampus and other regions of the rat brain, **in:** "The Hippocampus," R.L. Isaacson and K.H. Pribram, eds., New York, Plenum Press.

Nelson, W.H., Orr, W.W., Shane, S.R., and Stevenson, J.M., 1984, Hypothalamic-pituitary-adrenal axis activity and age in major depression, **J. Clin. Psychiat.**, 3:120-122.

Oxenkrug, G.F., 1978, Dexamethasone test in alcoholics, **Lancet,** i:195.

Oxenkrug, G.F., Balon, R., Hoksema, R., 1987a, Cortisol response to dexamethasone in Down's syndrome (Submitted).

Oxenkrug, G.F., Gurevich, D., Siegel, B., 1987b, Cognitive impairment and cortisol response to dexamethasone in primary degenerative dementia (submitted).

Oxenkrug, G.F., McIntyre, I.M., and Gershon, S., 1984b, Effect of pinalectomy and aging on the serum corticosterone circadian rhythm in rats, **J. Pineal. Res.**, 1:181-185.

Oxenkrug, G.F., Mcintyre, I.M., Stanley, M., Gershon, S., 1984a, Dexamethasone suppression test: Experimental model and effect of age, Biol. Psych., 19:413-416.

Pomara, N., Oxenkrug, G.F., McIntyre, I.M., Block, R., Stanley, M., and Gershon, S., 1984, Dexamethasone suppression test in primary degenerative dementia, Biol. Psychiat., 19:1481-1487.

Raskind, M.A., Reskind, E.R., Halter, J.B., Jimmerson, D.C., 1984, Noradrenaline and MHPG levels in CSFG and plasma in Alzheimer's disease, Arch. Gen. Psychiat., 41:343-346.

Reisberg, B., Ferrris, S., DeLeon, M.J., and Crook, T., 1982, The global deterioration scale for the assessment of primary degenerative dementia, Am. J. Psychiat., 189:1136-1139.

Reus, V.I., 1982, Pituitary-adrenal disinhibition as the independent variable in the assessment of behavioral symptoms, Biol Psychiat., 17:317-326.

Rosenbaum, A.H., Schatzberg, A.F., Mclaughlin, R.A., Snyder, K., Jiang, N.S., Gestrup, D., Rothschild, A.J., Kliman, B., 1984, The dexamethasone suppression test in normal control subjects: Comparison of two assays and effect of age, Am J. Psychiat., 141:1550-1554.

Roth, M. and Hopkins, B., 1953, Psychological test performance in patients over 60: Senile psychosis and affective disorders of old age, J. Ment. Sci., 99:439-450.

Rubinow, D.R., Post, R.M., Savard, R., and Gold, P,W., 1984, Cortisol Hypersecretion and cognitive impairment in depression, Arch. Gen. Psychiatr., 41:279-288.

Sapolsky, R.M., and McEwen, B.S., 19876, Stress, glucocorticoids, and their role in degenerative changes in the aging hippocampus, in: "Treatment Development Strategies for Alzheimer's disease," T. Crook, R. Bartus, S. Ferris and S. Gershon, eds., Mark Powley Association.

Siegel, B., Gurevich, D., and Oxenkrug, G.F., 1987, Cognitive impairment and cortisol resistance to dexamethasone suppression test distinguish dementia from depression? Am. J. Psychiat., 139:238-240.

Spar, J.E., Gerner, R., 1982, Does the dexamethasone suppression test distinguish dementia from depression. Am. J. Psychiat., 139: 238-240.

Stangl, D., Pfohl, B., Zimmerman, M., Coryell, W., and Corenthal, C., 1986, The relationship between age and post-dexamethasone cortisol: A test of three hypotheses, J. Affect. Dis., 11:185-197.

Starkman, M.N., Schteingart, D.E., and Schork, M.A., 1986, Cushing's syndrome after treatment: Changes in cortisol and ACTH levels and amelioration of the depressive symptoms, Psychiat. Res., 19:177-188.

Stokes, P., 1987, DST update: The hypothalamic-pituitary-adrenocortical axis and affective illness, Biol. Psychiat., 22:245-248.

Stokes, P., Stoll, P.M., Koslow, S.H., Mass, F.M., Swann, A.C., and Robins, E., 1984, Pretreatment hypothalamic-pituitary-adrenocortical function in depressed patients and comparison groups: A multicenter study, Arch. Gen. Psychiat., 41:257-267.

Thase, M., Tigner, R., Smeltzer, D., and Liss, L., 1984, Age-related neuropsychological deficits in Down's syndrome, Biol. Psychiat., 19:571-586.

Tourigny-Rivard, M.D., Raskind, M., and Rivard, D., 1981, The dexamethasone suppression test in an elderly population, Biol. Psychiat., 16:1177-1184.

Weingartner, H., Cohen, R.M., Murphy, D.L., Martello, J., and Gerdt, C., 1981, Cognitive processes in depression, Arch. Gen. Psychiat., 38:42-47.

Winokur, G., Black, D.W., and Nasrallah, A., 1987, DST nonsuppressor

Status:  Relationship to specific aspects of the depressive
     syndrome, Biol. Psychiat., 22:360-368.

Wurtman, R.J., Altschule, M.O., 1959, Effect of pinealectomy and of
     bovine pineal extract in rats, Am. J. Physiol., 197:108-111.

# FROM FAMILY STUDIES TO MOLECULAR HYPOTHESIS IN ALZHEIMER'S DEMENTIA

Marcia L. Morris and Leonard L. Heston

University of Minnesota
Minneapolis, Minnesota

## INTRODUCTION

That dementia of the Alzheimer's type (DAT) runs in families is clear from modern family studies. With minor differences, explainable by variation in severity of DAT in the probands selected, these studies have discovered the same basic recurrence rates among relatives of affected probands. At equal ages, these rates of DAT recurrence are significantly higher than those of the general population. This data forms one basic set of facts upon which causal hypotheses must depend.

A second set of data defines associations between DAT and Down's syndrome (DS). These associations permit important focusing of etiologic thinking at the molecular level.

## FAMILY STUDIES

The results of five recent family studies based on probands with DAT can be seen in Figure 1. Note first in Figure 1, that the five lines depicting cumulative risk to relatives are reasonably close to parallel which permits concluding that the several studies found about the same rate of recurrent illness. However, the ages at which the risk begins to be increased over the general population differs considerably among the studies. This age is represented on Figure 1 by the origin on the X-axis for each line.

This difference in age of increased risk can be explained by the observation that age of probands will have a major influence on age of secondary cases. A general finding applicable to all studies is that secondary cases in families are older at onset of illness by 5 to 10 years than the probands through whom the family was located. Moreover, it is rare that a secondary case is younger than the proband for the family. In the Heston series, for example, only 9 secondary cases among 87 had onsets of illness while younger than the family's proband (Heston et al., 1981). This occurs no doubt because probands are highly selected for relatively severe, dramatic illnesses. Therefore, they would tend also to have earlier onset of illness.

Each of these studies have special features that impinge on the ages of probands and thus of secondary cases. Åkesson (Åkesson, 1969) studied probands who were over age 65 at the onset of DAT, were located in nursing homes, and were severely ill. In order to become a proband, a nursing home resident had to be constantly disoriented. Thus one would expect most of Åkesson's secondary cases to be 65 or older and, on average, older than those found in studies starting with younger probands. Second, because these probands were severely ill, their families would have higher risks than families located through probands of the same age with more moderate illnesses.

Probands in Larsson's study (Larsson et al., 1963) were also over age 65, but were not selected for relative severity. Therefore, few secondary cases with onset before 65 would be expected and the risk to relatives would be fairly small. This is indeed what is reported and shown in Figure 1.

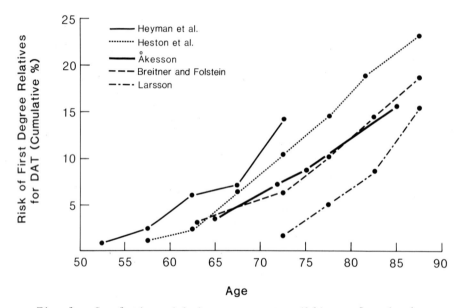

Fig. 1. Cumulative risk in percents to siblings of probands with DAT or presumed DAT as found in five modern family studies.

Heston's probands (Heston et al., 1981) were all ages, but younger probands were oversampled to a small extent. Breitner and Folstein's (1984) sampling design potentially included all ages but older probands were over-represented. These two studies report very similar results.

Probands located by Heyman were all under age 65 (Heyman et al., 1983). It would be expected, therefore, that relatives of these probands would have a relatively high risk of DAT, and that secondary cases would be younger at onset. The data confirms this expectation as shown in Figure 1.

Figure 1 not only summarizes the major findings from these family studies, but it also points to a consistency among the studies and to an agreement with expectations based on a multifactorial disease to which genetic factors make an etiologic contribution. It appears that these studies are recognizing the same phenomona, which is surely a genetic component in DAT. Until more sophisticated hypotheses are developed, there seems no need to go on repeating the same experiment.

## DAT AND DOWN'S SYNDROME

Several associations link DAT with Down's Syndrome (DS). The neuropathology found in DAT is also found in persons affected with DS who live at least to early adulthood. Of DS cases coming to autopsy after age 45, 100% have been found to exhibit the characteristic neuropathology of DAT (Malamud, 1972). Although dementia in retardates is difficult to demonstrate, cross-sectional studies strongly suggest that a large proportion of DS persons experience a decline in mental functioning with age consistent with phenotypic DAT (Thase, 1982; Haxby, 1985). In addition, DS and DAT brains appear identical under the electron microscope and exhibit similar patterns of change in neurotransmitters and enzymes, especially choline acetyl transferase, cholinesterase, and superoxide dismutas-1.

Weinreb (1985) has reported that a clinic population of DAT cases exhibited dermatoglyphic patterns (fingerprint, palm and sole) which deviated from normal in directions consistently found in DS. Moreover, DAT is the only disorder, including a variety of neurologic, psychiatric, and retarded control conditions, in which like deviations have been observed. The only other group in which the similarities are significant are the parents of DS cases, especially their mothers.

In addition, the rate of new onset seizures in DAT is reported to be about 10% higher than the general age population, and between 5% and 15% higher in older DS patients (Morris, 1985; Hauser, 1984; Tangye, 1979). Other research has shown that similar chromosomal aberrations occur in DS and DAT cells treated with bleomycin, a chemical that produces x-ray like damage to DNA. This is ascribed to defective DNA repair mechanisms shared by DS and DAT (Lijima et al., 1984; Hirsch et al., 1982)

## SYNTHESIS

Available data concerning the overlapping pathological traits of DAT and DS point not to a shared disease mechanism that results from a defective gene(s) or product(s), but to pathologic results caused by increased amounts of essentially normal products of genes located on a small area of chromosome 21. This interpretation is predicated on acceptance of a near 100% incidence of phenotypic DAT in DS, and that the pathophysiology leading to dementia is the same in the two conditions. We regard this as the most parsimonious interpretion of the available evidence.

In 96% of cases, DS is caused by a trisomy of chromosome 21, while most remaining cases result when a small segment of 21 becomes 'trisomic' due to a translocation. It is known that virtually all of the phenotypic traits commonly associated with DS can be caused by trisomy of only the 21q22 area of chromosome 21.

To date, three genetic loci have been mapped to this distal region of the long arm of chromosome 21. They are the superoxide dismutase-1 enzyme (SOD-1) (Epstein et al., 1982), the phosphoribosylglycinamide synthetase enzyme (GARS) (Wiranowsha-Stewart and Stewart, 1977), and the interferon receptor complex (AVG-for "anti-viral gene") (Feaster et al., 1977). For all three loci, DS cells produce more gene product than normal disomic cells.

An analogous excess of gene product has been found in DAT in the case of SOD-1. Theinhaus (1985) assayed SOD-1 activity in cultured skin fibroblasts derived from cases of DAT and DS, and normal control. He confirmed Feaster's previous finding of increased SOD-1 activity in DS cells and also showed that the SOD-1 activity was significantly increased in the DAT case. Increased SOD-1 activity has also been demonstrated in brains from DAT cases (Scott, 1986).

A like excess of AVG gene product has been sought but not consistently demonstrated. Mowshowitz (1983), using cultured fibroblasts from three familial DAT cases, found a wide variation in interferon sensitivity that fell within the ranges noted in controls. Further studies using greater numbers, a non-fibroblast or neuronal test system, and controls more closely matched for age could be helpful since Tan (1975) has shown that the concentration of interferon needed to induce the AVG gene is decreased in fibroblast lines derived from persons over age 64 compared to those under age 30.

A conclusive demonstration of increased product from the inducible AVG gene would go toward explaining the observed secondary phenotypic traits common to DS and DAT. Increased levels of interferon receptor protein produced at the AVG locus results in increased sensitivity of cells to interferon (Epstein and Epstein, 1980). Lin (1980) has shown that interferon inhibits epidermal growth factor, and thus may play a role in the dermatoglyphic patterns shared by DAT and DS. Interferon can also induce amyloidogenic proteins, and amyloid deposition is an important element in the pathological plaques and tangles of DAT and DS (Maury et al., 1983). The AVG gene product in excess has been implicated in nondisjunction. It is known to secondarily be antimitogenic in lymphocytes, increase the frequency of abortive mitoses, and interfere with cytokinesis (Pfeffer et al., 1980; Maroun, 1980; Gajdusek, 1985).

Unfortunately, we know of no study that has measured the activity of GARS in DAT cases.

MOLECULAR HYPOTHESIS

Excess gene product in DS is attributable to excess chromosomal DNA. An excess of gene product in DAT which would account for the observed phenotypic similarities between DAT and DS, could be produced in three known ways: the critical sequence of DNA must either be (1) selectively increased relative to the remainder of the genome, thus making more DNA available for transcription; or (2) a normal disomic complement of DNA must be transcribed at a proportionately increased rate; or (3) the mRNA product of the transcription of the critical sequence must be more stable or translated at a proportionately increased rate.

Theinhaus (1985) and Feaster et al. (1977) considered only the first possibility and assumed increased SOD-1 activity was due to undiscovered excess chromosome 21 material. Schweber has also proposed a "unitary genetic hypothesis" suggesting that a small segment of chromosome 21 is tripled in DAT by an unknown mechanism. She also noted that the excess chromosomal material should be discoverable in DAT.

We regard this hypothesis as unlikely. Exceptionally careful studies, including those by Matsuyama and Jarvik, have explored this hypothesis since the 1960's without positive result (Matsuyama, 1981; Frohlander and

Adolfson, 1985). Further, in an attempt to measure variation in DNA content, Cook-Deegan (1983) used uncultured lymphocytes taken freshly from familial DAT cases, their unaffected though "at rusk" relatives, and unrelated controls. (Previous studies had used cultured cells which allowed several opportunities for artifacts to be introduced). Cook-Deegan found no correlations between DNA concentrations and the presence or absence of DAT.

If a selective increase of DNA is ruled out, we are left with increased transcription or translation of a subset of genes present in the 21q22 area of chromosome 21. While these concepts have been virtually ignored, Sajdel-Sulkowka et al. (1983) noted that mRNA species recovered from DAT brains were translationally less active than their control counterparts. She had isolated functionally active mRNA species to explore protein synthesis at the molecular level, and to follow up on existing information concerning DNA and RNA in brains of persons affected with senile DAT which indirectly sugggested a protein synthesis deficit. While this data does not alone provide a definitive basis on which to rule out increased translation of one or a few specific mRNA species as primary pathologic event in DAT, it adds support to our carefully considered decision to choose increased transcription as the point at which to encourage research efforts.

To help focus this research, we hypothesize that a DNA enhancer sequence inserts into a critical area of at least one of the chromosome 21 homologs of DAT victims. This sequence acts in cis to increase the efficiency of transcription from a small subset of genes on the 21q22 area independent of 3' or 5' orientation to the affected genes. Such an enhancer could account for the observed increases in normal enzyme activity, could be influenced by age or neuronal tissue specific factors, and could account for the genetic observations of the family studies. Such a sequence, when stably incorporated but have an apparently sporadic appearance when recombination events brought inducible promoters of the relevant genes.

Since their discovery in the small DNA tumor virus, SB40, enhancer elements have become increasingly well-known. Some of the best studied enhancers reside within the long terminal repeat sequences (LTR's) of the retroviruses (RNA tumor viruses). They have also been found within the genomes of the polyoma, papilloma, BK and AIDS viruses, as well as the human immunoglobin genes (Hamer and Khoury, 1983; Mercola et al., 1985).

It is known that various sequences contained in LTR's can activate cellular proto-oncogenies following proviral integration. There is increasing evidence that enhancer sequences occur naturally within the human genome and are influenced by cell and tissue specific factors. They can inflate transcription if diverse genes relatively independent of position and orientation to the gene, can act over fairly large genomic distances, and are known to move about the fluid genome through genomic recombination. In mature neurons which do not undergo mitosis, recombination, like proviral integration, can take place during DNA repair (Johnson, 1982).

As Epstein (1983) has observed, previous attempts to consolidate molecular mechanisms which lead to the etiology of the pathologies of both DS and DAT into a single unifying entity have led to hypotheses that were largely untestable. However, molecular genetic techniques now exist, and additional methodologies are rapidly evolving that make this hypothesis testable.

Sadjel-Sulkoska's studies are useful as a start because a test of an hypothesis of increased transcription of a particular subset of genes would be to demonstrate an increased amount of mRNA species from those genes. These studies, which found an overall decreased amount of total mRNA species from the postmortem brains of severely demented senile DAT victims, in conjunction with the decreased protein synthesis intuitively expected from brains severely encumbered with dead and dying neurons, unfortunately cannot be considered a definitive test for this hypothesis for several reasons. First, as Sadjel-Sulkoska noted, unusual postmortem processing of mRNA may occur that would affect both the recovery and translational activity of the brain mRNA from DAT cases. In addition, it seems unlikely that the sensitivity of the method would detect increased levels of mRNA from only a tiny fraction of the genome in generally decreased pool.

Moreover, all of the brains were from severely affected SDAT cases. The experimental design allows for the possibility that what is being measured are secondary or late stage effects upon transcription or translation or, both, rather than a critical primary pathological event. This reservation is supported by Comar et al. (1981), whose preliminary studies using L-(IIC) methionine incorporation kinetics shown a decline in protein synthesis as dementia progresses. The in vivo incorporation of methionine into protein of mildly demented patients was 58% of normal compared to 30% in severely demented patients. It is also notable that interferon depresses synthesis of mRNA and DNA (Sen. 1984).

More direct manipulation of the DNA sequence itself is needed and recent work done by Hasse (Hasse et al., 1985) has advanced applicable methods further. He has used cDNA and cloning techniques to identify a single gene whose expression was increased in the brains of mice, and he has accomplished preferential hybridization of a cloned DNA probe to both murine brain cells and neuritic plaques of DAT victims. This research has also confirmed Finch's (Finch, 1985) critical prediction that brain mRNA species would demonstrate a remarkable postmortem stability that would invite the aggressive use of molecular genetic technology.

Additional techniques are being employed, and studies are currently underway in affiliated laboratories that will form the basis of critical tests of this hypothesis. Using an SOD-1 gene probe and samples being collected from DAT affected families, preliminary tests can begin to search for restriction length polymorphism in these families with an eye toward eventual fine mapping of the SOD-1 and AVG gene areas of chromosome 21 and discovery of the presence or absence of genetic insertions in this area.

If in fact nature has graciously provided an elegant key to greater understanding of the entire human genome through the concurrence of DAT and DS, it behooves all to use our creative resources to utilize the opportunity.

REFERENCES

Akesson, H.O., 1969, A population study of senile, and arteriosclerotic psychoses, Human Heredity, 19: 546-66.
Breitner, J.C.S., and Folstein, M.F., 1984, Familial Alzheimer's Dementia: a prevalent disorder with specific clinic features, Psychological Medicine, 14: 63-80.
Comar, D., 1981, Regional brain uptake and metabolism of 11C-methionine in dementia, "Proceedings of the Third World Congress of Biological Psychiatry," Stockholm, Abstract S63.
Cook-Deegan, R.M., 1983, Implications of Normal Lymphocyte DNA content in familial Alzheimer's Disease, American Journal of Medical Genetics, 15: 511-513.
Epstein, C.J., Epstein, L.B., Weil, J., Cox, D.R., 1982, Trisomy 21, Mechanism and Model, Ann. NY, Acad. Sci., 396: 107-118.

Epstein, C.J., 1983, Down's syndrome and Alzheimer's disease: Implications and Approaches, in: Banbury report 15, "Biological Aspects of Alzheimer's Disease," Robert Katzman, ed., Cold Spring Harbor.

Epstein, C.J., Epstein, L.B., 1980, T-lymphocyte function and sensitivity to interferon in trisomy 21, Cell Immunol., 51: 303-318.

Fester, W., Kwok, L., Epstein, C., 1977, Dosage effects for superoxide-1 in nucleated cells aneuploid for chromosome 21, Am J. Hum. Gen., 29: 563-570.

Finch, C., 1985, Alzheimer's Disease: A biologist's perspective, Science, 230: 47130.

Frohlander, N., Adolfson, R., 1985, Human Heredity, 35: 25-29.

Gajdusek, D.C., 1985, Hypothesis: Interference withi axonal transpoort of neurofilament as a common pathogenatic mechanism in certain disease of the central nervous siystem, New England Journal of Medicine, 11: 714-719.

Hamer, D.H., and Khoury, G., 1983, Enhancers and eucaryotic gene expression, in: "Current Communications in Molecular Biology," Y. Gluzman and T. Shenk, eds., Cold Spring Harbor.

Hauser, W.A., Morris, M.L., Jacobs, M.P., Heston, L.L., Anderson, V.E., 1984, Unprovoked sizures in patients with Alzheimer's disease, Epilepsia, 25: 658.

Haxby, J.V., 1985, Clinical and neuropsychological studies of dementia in Down's syndrome, in: "Moderator, Alzheimer's disease and Down's syndrome: New insights," N.R. Cutler, ed., Ann. Intern. Med., 103: 566-578.

Heston, L.L., Mastri, A.R., Anderson, V.E, White, J., 1981, Dementia of the Alzheimer's type: Clinical genetics, natural history, and associated conditions, Arch. Gen. Psychiatryi, 38: 1085-1090.

Heyman, A., Wilkinson, W.E, Hurwitz, B.H., Schmechel, D., Sigmon, A.H., Weinberg, T., Helms, M.J., Swift, M., 1983, Alzheimer's disease: Genetic aspects and associated clinical disorder, Annals of Neurology, 14: 507-515.

Hirsch, B., Heston, L.L., Cervenka, V., 1982, DNA repair in Alzheimer's disease, Am. J. of Human Genetics, 34: 434.

Lijima, K., Morimotor, K., Koizumi, A., Higurashi, M., Hirayama, M., 1984, Bleomycin-ilnduced chromosomal aberrations and sister chromatid exchanges in Down's syndrome cultures, Human Genetics, 66: ;57-61.

Johnson, R.T., 1982, "Viral infections of the Nervous System," Raven Press, New York.

Larsson, T., Sjogren, T.M., Jacobson, G., 1963, Senile dementia, ACTA Psychiat Scand., 39: 1-259.

Lin, S., Ts'o Po, M., Hollenberg, 1980, The effects of interferon on epidermal growth factor action, Biochem. Biophys. Res. Comm., 96: 168-174.

Malamud, N., 1979, "Aging and the Brain," C.M., Gaits, ed., Plenum Press, New York.

Maroun, L.E., 1980, interferon action and chromosome 21 trisomy, J. Theor. Biol., 86: 603-606.

Matsuyama S., 1981, Report of the White House Conference on Aging, January 15 and 16.

Maury, C.P., Enholm, E., Teppo, A.M., 1983, Is interferon an "inducer" of serum amyloid?, N. Engl. J. Med., 309: 1060-1061.

Mercola, M., Goverman, J., Mirell, C., Calame, K., 1985, Immunoglobulin heavy chain enhancer requires one or more tissue-specific factors, Science, 227: 266-270.

Morris, M.L., 1985, Unprovoked seizures and myoclonus in patients with Alzheimer's disease, J. Mn. Acad. Sci., 51:2: 8-10.

Mowshowitz, S.L., Dawson, G.J., Elizan, T.S., 1983, Antiviral response of fibroblasts from familial Alzheimer's disease and Down's syndrome to human interferon-alpha, J. Neural Transmission, 57: 121-126.

Pfeffer, L.M., Wang, E., Tamm, I., 1980, Interferon effects on micro-
    filament organization, cellular fibroconnection distribution, and cell
    motility in human fibroblasts, J. Cell Biol., 85: 9-17.
Sadjel-Sulkowska, E.M., Coughlin, J.F., 1983, In vitro protein synthesis
    by messenger RNA from the Alzheimer's disease brain, in: "Biological
    Aspects of Alzheimer's Disease," Katzman, R., ed., Banbury Report 15,
    Cold Spring Harbor, New York.
Scott, M., 1986, personal communication.
Sen., G.C., 1984, Biochemical pathways in interferon-action, Pharmac. Ther.
    24: 235-257.
Tangye, S.R., 1979, The EEG and the incidence of epilepsy in Down's
    syndrome, J. Ment. Defic., Res., 23: 17-24.
Thase, M.E., Liss, L., Smeltzer, D., Maloon, J., 1982, Clinical evaluation
    of dementia in Down's syndrome: A preliminary report, J. Ment. Defic.
    Res., 26: 239-244.
Thienhaus, O.J., Cliffe, C., Zemlan, F.P., Bosmann, H.B., 1985, Superoxide
    dismutase in fibroblasts: Possible chromosome 21 abnormality in
    Alzheimer's disease, in: Presentation-13th Ann. Meet. of Amer. Psych.
    Assoc.," Dallas, Texas.
Weinreb, H.J., 1985, Fingerprint patterns in Alzheimer's disease, 1985,
    Archives of Neurology, 42: 50-54.
Wietgrefe, S., Zupancic, M., Hasse, A., 1985, Cloning of gene whose express-
    ion is increased in scrapie and in senile plaques in human brain,
    Science, 230: 1171-1179.
Wiranowska-Stewart, W.E., 1977, The role of human chromosome 21 in sensit-
    ivity to interferons, J. Gen. Virol., 37: 629-633.

SCRAPIE PRIONS, AMYLOID PLAQUES, AND A POSSIBLE LINK WITH

ALZHEIMER'S DISEASE

Michael P. McKinley and Stanley B. Prusiner

Departments of Neurology and of Biochemistry and Biophysics
University of California
San Francisco, California 94143

INTRODUCTION

Scrapie and Creutzfeldt-Jacob disease (CJD) are caused by prions which are different from both viruses and viroids. Prions have a protein required for infectivity, but no nucleic acid has been found within them. Prion proteins and a cellular homologue are encoded by a cellular gene and not by a nucleic acid within the infectious prion particle. A cellular homologue of the prion protein has been identified. The role of this homologue in metabolism is unknown. Prion proteins aggregate into rod-shaped particles that are histochemically and ultrastructurally identical to amyloid. Extracellular collections of prion proteins form amyloid plaques in scrapie- and CJD-infected brains. Within the plaques, amyloid filaments are composed in part of prion proteins. Elucidating the molecular difference between the prion protein and its cellular homologue may be important in understanding the chemical structure and replication of prions.

PRION DISEASE OF ANIMALS AND HUMANS

In developing models for the study of degenerative neurologic diseases, we have focused our attention on the study of scrapie, a degenerative neurologic disorder of sheep and goats. Scrapie occurs after a prolonged incubation period and is readily transmissible to laboratory rodents. The disease is characterized by progressive neurologic dysfunction caused by degeneration of the CNS. Neuropathologic changes include proliferation of glial cells, vacuolation of neurons and deposition of extracellular amyloid in the form of placque.

Three degenerative human diseases similar to scrapie have been described: kuru, CJD and Gerstmann-Strassler syndrome (GSS). All three of these disorders are transmissible to experimental animals. Kuru presents as a cerebellar ataxia (Gajdusek, 1977). Kuru appears to have been transmitted during ritualistic cannibalism amongst New Guinea natives. CJD occurs at a rate of one per million population throughout the world. It is a dementing disorder much like Alzheimer's disease (AD), but in addition, myoclonus is frequently seen. GSS presents much like kuru as a cerebellar ataxia (Masters et al., 1981). Later, dementia becomes a prominent symptom of GSS prior to death. GSS is very rare and is apparently inherited as an autosomal dominant trait. In all three of these human diseases, as well as scrapie, the host remains afebrile, and there is no inflammatory response despite an overwhelming and fatal CNS "slow infection."

## IMPROVED BIOASSAY FOR PRION PURIFICATION

The development of effective purification protocols of the infectious particles causing scrapie is leading to an understanding of their chemical structure (Prusiner et al., 1981; Prusiner et al., 1982a; Prusiner et al., 1983; Prusiner et al., 1984). Numerous attempts have been made to purify the scrapie agent over the past three decades (Mould et al., 1965; Hunter, 1972; Millson et al., 1976; Siakotos et al., 1976; Brown et al., 1978; Diringer et al., 1983; Marsh et al., 1984). Few advances in this area of investigation were made until a relatively rapid and economical bioassay was developed (Prusiner et al., 1980; Prusiner et al., 1982b). This bioassay based on incubation times was a seminal advance in studies on the chemical and physical properties of the scrapie agent. Over a period spanning nearly a decade, our investigations of the molecular properties of the scrapie agent have been oriented toward developing effective procedures for purification. Our studies first determined the sedimentation properties of the scrapie agent in fixed angle rotors and sucrose gradients (Prusiner et al., 1977; Prusiner et al., 1978a; Prusiner et al., 1978b), then extended those findings and demonstrated the efficacy of nuclease and protease digestions as well as sodium dodecyl sarcosinate gel electrophoresis in the development of purification protocols (Prusiner et al., 1980a; Prusiner et al., 1980b). Once a 100-fold purification was achieved, convincing evidence was obtained demonstrating that a protein is required for infectivity (Prusiner et al., 1981; McKinley et al., 1981).

## PRIONS ARE NOVEL INFECTIOUS PATHOGENS

Progress in purification of the scrapie agent allowed us to establish that a protein molecule is required for infectivity. No dependence of infectivity upon a nucleic acid has been demonstrated. Based upon these observations, the term prion was suggested in order to distinguish this class of novel infectious pathogens from viruses and viroids (Prusiner, 1982). Prions are defined as "small proteinaceous infectious particles that resist inactivation by procedures which modify nucleic acids." This is an operational definition; it does not prejudge the chemical composition of the scrapie except to state that is does contain a protein.

Some investigators have misinterpreted the term prion. They have used prion to signify infectious proteins (Manuelidis et al., 1985; Carp et al., 1985) or even as a synonym for scrapie-associated fibrils (Multhaup et al., 1985). This misuse of the term prion has led to confusion and is inappropriate.

## SCRAPIE PRIONS CONTAIN A SIALOGLYCOPROTEIN

In our search for a scrapie-specific protein, discontinuous sucrose gradients in vertical rotors were substituted for gel electrophoresis (Prusiner et al., 1982a), resulting in the first identification of a macromolecule which appears to be a component of the scrapie prion (Bolton et al., 1982; McKinley et al., 1983; Prusiner et al., 1983; Prusiner et al., 1984; Bolton et al., 1984). Many lines of evidence indicate that PrP 27-30 is both required for and inseparable from infectivity. This molecule is a sialoglycoprotein designated PrP 27-30 (Bolton et al., 1985). The development of a large-scale purification protocol has allowed us to determine the N-terminal sequence of PrP 27-30 and to raise antibodies against it (Prusiner et al., 1984; Bendheim et al., 1984; Bendheim et al.,

1985). Other investigators using purification steps similar to those developed by us have apparently demonstrated the presence of this protein in their preparations (Diringer et al., 1983).

Many lines of evidence indicate that PrP 27-30 is both required for and inseparable from scrapie infectivity (Prusiner et al., 1983; McKinley et al., 1983; Prusiner et al., 1984; Bolton et al., 1984). First, PrP 27-30 and scrapie prions copurify; PrP 27-30 is the most abundant macromolecules in purified preparations of prions. Second, PrP 27-30 concentration is proportional to prion titer. Third, procedures that denature, hydrolyze or selectively modify PrP 27-30 also diminish prion titer; The molecular properties of PrP 27-30 mirror those of the infectious prion. Fourth, recent studies with inbred strains of mice indicate that the cellular gene encoding PrP 27-30 is linked to a gene which controls the length of the scrapie incubation times (Carlson et al., 1986).

SEARCH FOR A PRION GENOME

The size of the smallest infectious unit remains controversial, largely because of the extreme heterogeneity and apparent hydrophobicity of the scrapie prion (Prusiner, 1982; Diringer and Kimberlin, 1983; Prusiner, 1984; Rohwer, 1984). Early studies suggested a molecular weight of 60,000 to 150,000 (Alper et al., 1966). While an alternate interpretation of that data has been proposed (Rohwer, 1984), there is no firm evidence to suggest that these molecular weight calculations are incorrect. In fact, sucrose gradient sedimentation, molecular sieve chromatography and membrane filtration studies all suggest that a significant portion of the infectious particles may be considerably smaller that the smallest known viruses (Prusiner, 1982; Rohwer, 1984). However, the propensity of the scrapie agent to aggregate makes molecular weight determinations subject to artifact.

Some investigators have identified a 4.3 S RNA in density gradient fractions from scrapie-infected brain which appears to be absent in uninfected brains based on fingerprinting studies (German et al., 1985; Dees et al., 1985). We have failed to identify a similar molecule in our purified preparations of scrapie prions (K. Gilles, D. Riesner and S.B. Prusiner, unpublished data). Other investigators have repeatedly suggested that the scrapie agent is the first example of a filamentous animal virus (Rohwer, 1984; Merz et al., 1984). Our studies show that the molecular properties of scrapie prions with respect to nucleic acids are antithetical to those of the filamentous bacteriophage M13 and the rod-shaped plant viruses, tobacco mosaic virus and potato X virus (McKinley et al., 1986; C.G. Bellinger-Kawahara, T.O. Diener and S.B. Prusiner, in preparation).

CELLULAR GENE ENCODES PRION PROTEINS

A cDNA encoding PrP 27-30 has been used as a probe to show that the gene for PrP is found in healthy uninfected hamsters (Oesch et al., 1985). From the cloning of cDNAs and genomic DNA encoding PrP, a primary sequence for the prion protein has been deduced. When limited proteinase K digestion is used during purification of prions, the N-terminal -67 amino acids of the scrapie protein designated PrP 33-35Sc are removed and PrP 27-30 is generated (Oesch et al., 1985). Whether or not the C-terminus is slightly truncated during this digestion remains to be established. The primary sequence of the prion protein is unique and is clearly different from that of known proteins.

The cloned PrP cDNA has been used to search for a complementary nucleic acid within purified preparations of prions (Oesch et al., 1985). To date, we have failed to identify either a PrP-related DNA or RNA molecule in these preparations. Assuming PrP is a component of the infectious scrapie particle, our observations demonstrate that scrapie prions are not typical viruses. As noted, we still cannot eliminate the possibility of a small. nongenomic nucleic acid which lies highly protected within the prion core.

PrP-related candidate genes have been detected by hybridization on Southern blots in scrapie and CJD susceptible hosts such as sheep, goats, mice, rats, cats and humans (Oesch et al., 1985; Westaway and Prusiner, 1986). In addition, PrP-related sequences have been found in the DNA of Drosophila, nematodes and yeast (Westaway and Prusiner, 1986). The widespread presence of the PrP gene amongst eukaryotes suggests that its cellular product (PrPc) may have an important role in normal metabolism.

CELLULAR AND SCRAPIE PRION PROTEIN ISOFORMS

Molecular cloning studies led to the discovery of PrP 33-35C, the cellular isoform of the prion protein. This protein can be distinguished from PrP 33-35c, by its sensitivity to proteases and its inability to polymerize into amyloid filaments (Table 1) (Oesch et al., 1985;Meyer et al., 1986). The role of PrP 33-35C in cellular metabolism is unknown. The scrapie prion protein,Prp 33-35c, accumulates to high levels in infected brains and forms amyloid filaments. Proteolytic digestion converts PrP 33-35c to PrP 27-30 which is relatively resistant to further digestion (Oesch et al., 1985). PrP 33-35C appears to be an integral membrane protein, while PrP 33-35Sc is an amphiphatic protein displaying characteristics of both an integral membrane protein and a filamentous protein (Meyer et al., 1986). How the accumulation of PrP 33-35Sc disrupts cellular metabolism and central nervous system (CNS) function is unknown. PrP mRNA levels remain constant during scrapie infection. Only a single 2.1 kb mRNA has been detected in hamsters by norther blotting (Oesch et al., 1985). Similar results from scrapie-infected mouse brain poly (A+) have been reported by other investigators (Chesebro et al., 1985). In situ hybridization has shown that PrP mRNA within brain is largely confined to neurons (Kretzschmar et al., 1986). The same mRNA is found at lower levels in organs outside the CNS (Oesch et al., 1985).

Table 1. Cellular and scrapie prion protein isoforms

| Properties | PrP 33-35C | PrP 33-35Sc |
|---|---|---|
| Uninfected brain | Present | Absent |
| Scrapie brain | Level unchanged | Accumulates |
| Concentration* | <1 ug/g | 10 ug/g |
| Purified prions molecules/ID | Absent | 10 |
| Genetic origin | One cellular gene | One cellular gene |
| mRNA | 2.1 kb | 2.1 kb |
| Localization | | |
| Intracellular | Membrane-bound | Membrane-bound |
| Extracellular | None | Amyloid filaments with plaques |
| Detergent extraction | Soluble | Amyloid rods formed |
| Protease digestion | Degraded | Converted to PrP 27-30^ |

*Expressed as microgram of prion protein per gram of brain tissue.
^PrP 27-30 is derived from PrP 33-35SC during proteinase K digestion in the absence or presence of detergent.

Whether or not prions contain macromolecules other than PrP 33-35Sc remains to be established. The apparent biologic properties of prions argue in favor of a small nucleic acid, but there is no physical or biochemical evidence for such a molecule (Prusiner, 1982; Prusiner, 1984). How proins replicate is unknown. Understanding the chemical differences between PrP 33-35c and PrP 33-35Sc will be important in unraveling the mechanism of prion biosynthesis.

The discovery of PrP 33-35C explains one of the most interesting, yet perplexing, features of scrapie. This slow infection progresses in the absence of any detectable immune response (McFarlin et al., 19873; Kasper et al., 1981). Since PrP 33-35C and PrP 33-35Sc share epitopes, PrP 33-35C probably renders the host tolerant to PrP 33-35Sc (Oesch et al., 1985).

## ULTRASTRUCTURAL MORPHOLOGY OF PRION AGGREGATES

Many investigators have used the electron microscope to search for a scrapie-specific particle. Spheres, rods, fibrils and tubules have been described in scrapie, kuru and CJD-infected brain tissue (David-Ferreira et al., 1968; Field, et al., 1969; Bignami and Parry, 1971; Lampert et al., 1971; Narang, 1974; Baringer and Prusiner 1978; Vernon et al., 1979). Notable amongst the early studies are reports of rod-shaped particles in sheep, rat and mouse scrapie brain measuring 15 to 26 nm in diameter and 60 to 75 nm in length (Narang, 1974). Studies with ruthenium red and lanthanum nitrate suggested that the rod-shaped particles possessed polysaccharides on their surface; these findings are of special interest since PrP 27-30 has been shown to be a sialoglycoprotein (Bolton et al., 1985).

In purified fractions prepared from scrapie-infected brains, rod-shaped particles were found measuring 10 to 20 nm in diameter and 100 to 200 nm in length (Figure 1) (Chesebro et al., 1985). Although no unit morphologic structure could be identified, most of the rods exhibited a relatively uniform diameter and appeared as flattened cylinders. In the fractions containing rods, one major protein (PrP 27-30) and 10  ID  units of prions per ml were also found (Table 2). The high degree of purity of our preparations demonstrated by radiolabeling and SDS polyacrylamide gel electrophoresis indicated that the rods are composed of PrP 27-30 molecules. Since PrP 27-30 had already been shown to be required for and inseparable from infectivity (McKinley et al., 1983), we concluded that the rods must be a form of the prion (Prusiner et al., 1983). Recent immunoelectron microscopic studies using antibodies raised against PrP 27-30 have confirmed that the rods are composed in part of PrP 27-30 molecules (Barry et al., 1985).

Table 2.  Prion rods contain PrP 27-30 molecules

1.  Fractions with high prion titers contain one protein, PrP 27-30, by sodium dodecyl sulfate polyacrylamide gel electrophoresis and rods by electron microscopy (Prusiner et al., 1982a; Prusiner et al., 1983).

2.  Gas phase sequencing of the prion rods give the same N-terminal sequence as found for PrP 27-30 (Prusiner et al., 1984).

3.  Antibodies raised against PrP 27-30 or synthetic peptides corresponding to portions of the PrP 27-30 sequence decorate the prion rods (Barry et al., 1985).

4.  Boiling purified fractions in sodium dodecyl sulfate causes the rods to disappear, PrP 27-30 to become protease-sensitive and the prion titer to diminish (Prusiner et al., 1983; Kretzschmar et al., 1986).

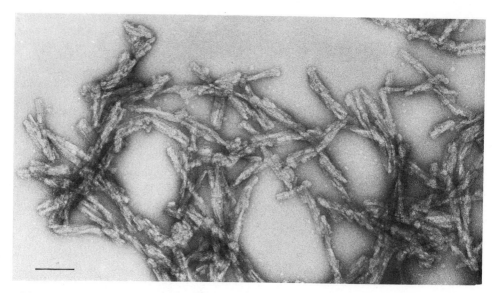

Fig. 1. Ultrastructure of Prion Rods Isolated From Sucrose Gradients.
Electron micrograph of negatively stained scrapie prion rods in
fractions from discontinuous sucrose gradients. Scrapie prion
titer was >109.5 $ID_{50}$ units/ml. Bar = 100 nm.

POLYMORPHIC FORMS OF PRIONS

Several experimental approaches indicate that the prion rods are not
the smallest infectious unit. First, no elongated structures similar to
prion rods could be identified in 10% homogenates of scrapie-infected
hamster brains. Second, microsomal fractions contained no rods associated
with prion infectivity. Third, detergent extraction of microsomal membranes
isolated from scrapie-infected hamster brains was accompanied by the
formation of prion rods (Figure 2). Thus, the prion rods in our purified
fractions result from the detergent extractions used during purification.
Sonication of the prion rods reduced their mean length to 60 nm and
generated many spherical particles without altering infectivity titers
(McKinley edt al., 1986). Sedimentation of these sonicated fractions into
sucrose gradients resulted in a distribution of particles ranging from small
spheres at the top (8 nm diameter) to relatively undisrupted rods at the
bottom. Prion infectivity was associated with each fraction such that the
relationship between protein concentration and prion titer remained constant
throughout the gradient. These studies demonstrated that elongated
structures were not necessary for scrapie infectivity. In contrast,
fragmentation of M13 filamentous bacteriophage by brief sonication reduced
infectivity significantly.

Spherical particles have been found within postsynaptic evaginations of
the brains of scrapie-infected sheep and mice as well as CJD-infected humans
and chimpanzees (David-Ferreira et al., 1968; Bignami and Parry, 1971;
Lampert et al., 1971; Baringer and Prusiner, 1978); these particles measured
23 to 35 nm in diameter. Since sonication fragmented prion rods and
generated spheres measuring 10 to 30 nm in diameter (McKinley et al., 1986),
the question arises as to whether or not the spherical particles observed in
brain tissue are related to the spheres generated by sonication of the prion
rods.

It seems doubtful whether electron microscopic studies to date have
been able to demonstrate the smallest infectious unit or fundamental
particle of the scrapie prion; certainly, the morphology of the unit

structure has not been identified. The extreme morphologic heterogeneity of the rods is inconsistent with the recently advanced hypothesis that prions are filamentous viruses (Merz et al., 1984).

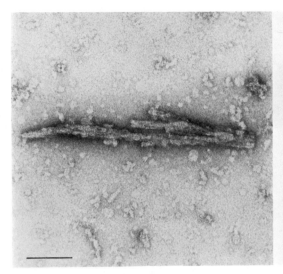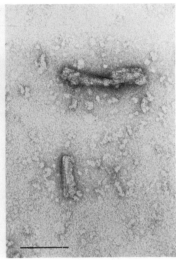

Fig. 2.    Detergent Solubilization of Scrapie-Infected Brain Microsomes Produces Prion Rods. Both panels depict rods formed after addition of Sarkosyl to a concentration of 2% (w/v). All specimens were negatively stained with uranyl formate. Bars = 100 nm.


PRION RODS AND FILAMENTS ARE AMYLOID

The ultrastructure of the prion rods is indistinguishable from many purified amyloids (Prusiner et al., 1983). Histochemical studies with Congo red dye have extended this analogy in purified preparations of prions (Prusiner et al., 1983) as well as in scrapie-infected brains where amyloid plaques have been shown to stain with antibodies of PrP 27-30 (Bolton et al., 1985; DeArmond et al., 1985). Amyloid plaques have also been found in three transmissible disorders similar to scrapie and CJD: kuru and GSS of humans as well as chronic wasting disease of mule deer and elk (Klatzo et al., 1959; Hunter, 1972; Bahmanyar et al., 1985). Recent studies have shown that PrP antisera stain amyloid plaques in human CJD and GSS brains as well as rodent brains with experimental CJD (Kitamoto et al., 1986). These findings raise the possibility that Prion-like molecules might play a causative role in the pathogenesis of nontransmissible disorders such as Alzheimer's disease (Prusiner, 1984). Amyloid proteins are prevalent in Alzheimer's disease, but for many decades these proteins have been considered a consequence rather that a possible cause of the disease.

Immunocytochemical studies with antibodies to PrP 27-30 have shown that filaments measuring approximately 16 nm in diameter and up to 1,500 nm in length within amyloid placques of scrapie-infected hamster brain composed in part of prion proteins (DeArmond et al., 1985). The antibodies to PrP 27-30 did not react with neurofilaments, glial filaments, microtubules and microfilaments in brain tissue. The prion amyloid filaments have a relatively uniform diameter, rarely show narrowings and possess all the morphologic features of amyloid. Except for their length, they appear to be identical unltrstructurally to the rods which are found in purified fractions of prions.

Abnormal structures, labeled scrapie-associated fibrils, were distinguished from other filamentous structures in extracts of scrapie-infected rodent brains by their characteristic and well defined morphology (Merz et al., 1981). Published electron micrographs show 2 or 4 subfilaments wound into two types of helical fibrils of 300 to 800 nm in length exhibiting a regular periodicity. Type I fibrils contain 2 subfilaments, measure 12 to 16 nm in diameter and exhibit a perioditicy of 40 to 60 nm; type II contain 4 subfilaments, measure 27 to 34 nm in diameter and exhibit a periodicity of 80 to 110 nm. Based on their extensive ultrastructural characteristics, the unique fibrils have been reported repeatedly to be different from amyloid (Merz et al., 1981; Merz et al., 1983). Attempts to stain the fibrils with Congo red dye have yielded negative results (Merz et al., 1981; Merz et al., 1983; Merz et al., 1984); however, even a positive result would have been uninterpretable because of impurities in the extracts.

No particles with the ultrastructural morphology of scrapie-associated fibrils have been found either in thin sections of scrapie-infected brain or in purified preparations of scrapie prions. Some investigators have used the scrapie-associated fibrils (Diringer et al., 1983a; Kimberlin, 1984) to describe the rod-shaped particles found in purified preparations of prions (Prusiner et al., 1982a; Prusiner et al., 1983). Renaming the prion rods is both confusing and misleading (Multhaup et al., 1985). It suggests that scrapie-associated fibrils as originally described are amyloid (Somerville, 1985) and that they are found in purified fractions of prions (Diringer et al., 1983a); neither statement is true. Some investigators have suggested that scrapie-associated fibrils are filamentous animal viruses (Chesebro et al., 1985) while others claim that they are pathologic products of infection (Multhaup et al., 1985). We believe the term scrapie-associated fibrils should be reserved for those abnormal structures meeting the morphologic criteria set forth in originally defining the fibrils (Merz, et al., 1981). With respect to the prion rods, considerable data indicates that they are neither filamentous viruses or pathologic products of infection.

THE PRION HYPOTHESIS

New knowledge about the molecular structure of scrapie prions is beginning to accumulate rapidly. If prions were typical viruses, then they should contain a genomic nucleic acid which encodes PrP 27-30. They do not! To explain the apparent biological diversity of prions, a small, nongenomic nucleic acid which does not encode PrP 27-30 has been proposed; however, ther continues to be no chemical or physical evidence to indicate the existence of such a nucleic acid. Alternatively, prions may be devoid of nucleic acid. Information for the synthesis of new prion proteins is encoded within the host genome. A cloned PrP cDNA as well as antibodies to the protein provide new tools with which to extend our investigation of the chemical structure of prions.

Once it is determined whether or not prions contain other macro-molecules besides glycoproteins, chemical studies to determine the molecular mechanisms by which prions reproduce and cause disease should become possible. Indeed, efforts to purify and characterize the infectious particles causing scrapie and CJD have yielded important new information about the structure and biology of prions

ACKNOWLEDGEMENTS

Important contributions from Drs. R. Barry, C. Bellinger-Kawahara, J. Bockman, D. Bolton, S. DeArmond, D. Kingsbury, R. Meyer, M. Scott, D. Stites and D. Westaway are gratefully acknowledged. Collaborative studies with Drs. R. Aebersold, J. Cleaver, T. Diener, W. Hadlow, L. Hood, S. Kent, B.

Oesch and C. Weissmann have been important to the progress of these studies. The authors thank K. Bowman, M. Braunfeld, P. Cochran, D. Groth and L. Pierce for technical assistance as well as M. Canevari, F. Elvin, L. Gallagher and J. Sleath for editorial and administrative assistance. This work was supported by research grants from the National Institutes of Health (AG02132 and NS14069) as well as by gifts from R.J. Reynolds Industries, Inc. and the Sherman Fairchild Foundation.

REFERENCES

Alper, T., Haig, D.A., and Clarke, M.C., 1966, The exceptionally small size of the scrapie agent, Biochem. Biophys. Res. Commun., 22:278.

Bahmanyar, W., Williams, E.S., Johnson, F.B., Young, S., and Gajdusek, 1985, Amyloid plaques in spongiform encephalopathy of mule deer, J. comp. Pathol., 95:1.

Baringer, J.R., and Prusinger, S.B., 1978, Experimental scrapie in mice – ultrastructural observations, Ann. Neurol., 4:205.

Barry, R.A., McKinley, M.P., Bendheim, P.E., Lewis, G.K., DeArmond, S.J., and Prusinger, S.B., 1985, Antibodies to the scrapie protein decorate prion rods, J. Immunol., 135:603.

Bendheim, P.E., Barry, R.A., DeArmond, S.J., Stites, D.P., and Prusiner, S.B., 1984, Antibodies to a scrapie prion protein, Nature, 310:418.

Bignami, A., And Parry, H.A., 1971, Aggregations of 35-nanometer particles associated with neuronal cytopathic changes in natural scrapie, Science, 171:389.

Bolton, D.C., Meyer, R.K., and Prusiner, S.B., 1985, Scrapie PrP 27-30 is a sialoglycoprotein, J. Viro., 53:596.

Bolton, D.C., McKinley, M.P., and Prusiner, S.B., 1984, Molecular characteristics of the major scrapie prion protein, Biochemistry, 23:5898.

Bolton, D.C., Mckinley, M.P., and prusiner, S.B. 1982, Identification of a protein that purifies with the scrapie prion, Science, 218:1309.

Brown, P., Green, E.M., Gajdusek, D.C., 1978, Effect of different gradient solutions on the buoyant density of scrapie infectivity, Pro, Soc. Exp. Bio. Med., 158:513.

Carlson, G.A., Goodman, P., Kingsbury, D.T., and Prusiner, S.B., 1986, Scrapie incubation time and prion protein genes are linked, Clin, Res., (in press).

Carp, R.I., Merz, P.A., Moretz, R.C., Somerville, R.A., Callahan, S.M., and Wisniewski, H.M., 1985, Biological particles of scrapie: an unconventional slow virus, in: "Subviral Pathogens of Plants and Animals: Viroids and Prions," K. Maramorosch and J.J. McKelvey, Jr., eds., Academic Press, Orlando.

Chesebro, B., Race, R., Wehrly, K., Nishio, J., Bloom, M., Lechner, S., Berstrom, S., Robbins, K., Mayer, L., Keith, J.M., Garon, C., and Hasse, A., 1985, Identification of scrapie prion protein-specific mRNA in scrapie-infected and uninfected brain, Nature, 315:331.

David-Ferriera, J.I., David Ferriera, K.L., Gibbs, C.J., Morris, J.A., 1968, Scrapie mice: ultrastructural observations in the cerebral cortex, Proc, Soc. Exp. Biol. Med., 127:313.

DeArmond, S.J., McKinley, M.P., Barry, R.A., Braunfeld, M.B., McColloch, J.R., and S.B., Prusiner, 1985, Identification of prion amyloid filaments in scrapie-infected brain, Cell, 41:221

Dees, C., McMillan, B.C., Wade, W.F., German, T.L., and Marsh, F.F., 1985, infected hamster brain, J. Virol., 55:126.

Diringer, H., Hilmert, H., Simon, D., Werner, E., and Ehlers, B., 1983a, Towards purification of the scrapie agent, Eur. J. Biochem., 134:555.

Diringer, H., Gelderblom, H., Hilmert, H., Ozel, M., Edelbluth, C., and Kimberlin, R.H., 1983b, Scrapie infectivity, fibrils and low molecular weight protein, Nature, 306:476.

Diringer, H., and Kimberlin, R.H., 1983, Infectious scrapie agent is apparently not as small as recent claims suggest, Biosci. Rep., 3:563.

Field, E.J., Matthew, J.D., and Raine, C.S., Electron microscopic observations on the cerebellar cortex in kuru, J. Neurol. Sci., 8:209.

Gajdusek, D.C., Unconventional viruses and the origin and disappearance of kuru, Science, 197:943.

German, T.L., McMillan, B.C., Castle, B.E., Dees, C., Wade, W.F., and Marsh R.F., 1985, Comparison of RNA from health and scrapie-infected hamster brain, J. Gen. Virol., 55:126.

Hunter, G.D., 1972, Scrapie: A prototype slow infection, j. Infect. Dis., 125:427.

Kasper, K.C., Bowman, K., Stites D.P., and Prusiner, S.B., 1981, Toward development of assays for scrapie-specific antibodies, in: "Hamster Immune Responses in infectious and Oncologic Diseases," J.W. Streilein, D.A. Hart, J. Stein-Streilein, S.R. Duncan and R.E. Billingham, eds., Plenum Press, New York.

Kimberlin, R.H., 1984, Scrapie: The disease and the infectious agent, Trends in Neuroscience, 7:312.

Kitamoto, T., Tateishi, J., Tashima, T., Takeshita, I., Barry, R.A., DeArmond, S.J., and Prusiner, S.B., 1986, Amyloid plaques in Creutzfeld-Jacob disease stain with prion protein antibodies, Ann. Neuro., (in press).

Klatzo, I., Gajdusek, D.C., and Zigas, V., 1959, Pathology of kuru, Lab. Invest., 8:799.

Kretzschmar, H.A., Prusiner, S.B., Stowring, L.W., and DeArmond, S.J., 1986, Scrapie prion proteins are synthesized in neurons, Am. J. Pathol., 122:1.

Lampert, P.W., Gajdusek, D.C., Gibbs, C.J., 1971, Experimental Spongiform encephalopathy (Creutzfeldt-Jakob disease) in chimpanzees, J. Neuropathol. Exp. Neurol., 30:20.

Manuelidis, L., Valley, S., Manuelidis, E.E., 1985, Specific proteins associated with Creutzfeldt-Jakob disease and scrapie share antigenic and carbohydrate determinants, Proc. Natl. Acad. Sci. USA, 82:4263.

Marsh, R.F., Dees, C., Castle, B.E., Wade, W.F., and German, T.L., Purification of the scrapie agent by density gradient centrifugation, J. Gen. Virol., 65:415.

Master, C.L., Gajdusek, D.C., and Gibbs, C.J., 1981, Creutzfeldt-Jakob disease virus isolations from the Gerstmann-Straussler syndrome, Brain, 104:559.

McFarlin, D.E., Raff, M.C., Simpson, E., Nehlsen, S., 1971, Scrapie in immunologically deficient mice, Nature, 233:336.

Mckinley, M.P., Bolton, D.C., Prusiner, S.B., 1983, A protease - resistant protein is structural component of the scrapie prion, Cell, 35:57.

McKinley, M.P., Masiarz, F.R., and Prusiner, S.B., 1981, Reversible chemical modification of the scrapie agent, Science, 214:1259.

McKinley, M.P., Braunfeld, M.B., Bellinger, C.G., and Prusiner, S.B., 1986, J. Infect. Dis., (in press).

Mertz, P.A., Wisniewski, H.M., Somerville, R.A., Bobin, S.A., Masters, C.L., and Iqbal, K., 1983, Ultrastructural morphology of amyloid fibrils from neuritic and amyloid plaques, Acta Neuropathol. (Berl.), 60:113.

Mertz, P.A., Rohwer, R.J., Kascsak, R., Wisniewski, H.M., Somerville, R.A., Gibbs, C.J., and Gajdusek, D.C, 1984. Infection-specific article from the unconventional slow virus diseases, Science, 225:437.

Mertz, P.A., Somerville, R.A., Wisniewski, H.M., and K. Iqbal, 1981, Abnormal fibrils from scrapie-infected brain, Acta. Neuropathol. Berl.), 54:63.

Meyer, R.K., McKinley, M.P., Bowman, K.A. Barry, R.A., and Prusiner, S.B., 1986, Separation and properties of cellular and scrapie prion proteins, Proc. Natl. Acad. Sci. USA, (in press).

Millson, G.C., Hunter, G.D., Kimberlin, R.H., 1976, The physico-chemical nature of the scrapie agent, in: "Slow Virus Diseases of Animals and Man," R.H. Kimberlin, ed., American Elsevier, New York.

Mould, D.L., Smith, W., and Dawson, A.M., 1965, Centrifugation studies on the infectivities of cellular fractions derived from mouse brain infected with scrapie ('Suffolk strain'), J. Gen. Microbiol., 40:71.

Multhaup, G., Diringer, H., Hilmert, H., Prinz, H., Heukeshoven, J., and Beyreuther, K., 1985, The protein component of scrapie-associate fibrils is a glycosylated low molecular weight protein, EMBO J., 4:1495.

Narang, H.K., 1974, An electron microscopic study of natural scrapie sheep brain: Further observations on virus-like particles and paramyxovirus-like tubules, Acta neuropathol. (Berl.), 28:317.

Oesch, B., Westaway, D., Walchli, M., McKinley, M.P., Kent, S.B.H., Aebersold, R., Barry, R.A., Tempst, P., Teplow, D.B., Hood, L.E., Prusiner, S.B., and Weissmann, C., 1985, A cellular gene encodes scrapie PrP 27-30 protein, Cell, 40:735.

Prusiner, S.B., 1984, Some speculations about prions, amyloid and Alzheimer's disease, N. Engl. J. Med., 31:661.

Prusiner, S.B., Cochran, S.P., Groth, D.F., Downey, D.E., Bowman, K.A., and Martinez, H.M., 1982b, Measurement of the scrapie agent using a incubation time interval assay, Ann. Neurol., 11:353.

Prusiner, S.B., Groth, D.F., Cochran, S.P., Masiarz, F.R., McKinley, M.P., and Martinez, H.M., 1980b, Molecular properties, partial purification and assay by incubation period measurements of the hamster scrapie agent, biochemistry, 1:4883.

Prusiner, S.B., Groth, D.F., Bolton, D.C., Kent, S.B., and Hood, L.E., 1984, Purification and structural studies of a major scrapie prion protein, Cell, 38:127.

Prusiner, S.B., McKinley, M.P., Groth, D.F., Bowman, K.A., Mock, N.I., Cochran, S.P., and Masiarz, F.R., 1981, Scrapie agent contains a hydrophobic protein, Proc. Natl. Acad, Sci. USA, 78:6675.

Prusiner, S.B., 1982, Novel proteinaceous infectious particles cause scrapie, Science, 216:136.

Prusiner, S.B., Groth, D.F., Bildstein, C., Masiarz, F.R., 1980a, Gel electrophoresis and glass permeation chromatography of the hamster scrapie agent after enzymic digestion and detergent extraction, Biochemistry, 19:4892.

Prusiner, S.B., McKinley, M.P., Bowman, K.A., Bolton, D.C., Bendheim, P.E., Groth, D.F., Glenner, G.G., 1983, Scrapie prions aggregate to for amyloid-like birefringent rods, Cell, 35:349.

Prusiner, S.B., Groth, D.F., Bilstein, C., Masiarz, F.R., McKinley, M.P., and Cochran, S.P., 1980, Electrophoretic properties of the scrapie agent in agarose gels, Proc. Natl. Acad. Sci. USA, 77:2984.

Prusiner, S.B., Hadlow, W.J., Garfin, D.E., Cochran, S.P., Baringer, J.R., Race, R.E., and Eklund, C.M., 1978b, Partial purification and evidence 10 for multiple molecular forms of the scrapie agent, Biochemistry, 17:4993.

Prusiner, S.B., Hadlow, W.J., Eklund, C.M., Race, R.E., Cochran, S.P., Sedimentation characteristics of the scrapie agent from murine spleen and brain, Biochemistry, 17:4987.

Prusiner, S.B., Bolton, D.C., Groth, D.F., Bowman, K.A., Cochran, S.P., 1978a, and McKinley, M.P., 1982 a, Further purification and characterization of scrapie prions, Biochemistry, 21:6942.

Prusiner, S.B., 1984, Prions - novel infectious pathogens, in: "Advances in virus Research," M.A. Lauffer and K. Maramorosch, eds., Academic Press, New York.

Prusiner, S.B., Hadlow, W.J., Eklund, C.M., Race, R.E., 1977, Sedimentation properties of the scrapie agent, Proc. Natl. Acad. Sci. USA, 74:4656.

Rohwer, R.G., 1984, Scrapie infectious agent is virus-like in size and susceptibility to inactivation, Nature, 308:58.

Siakotos, A.N., Gajdusek, D.C., Gibbs, C.J., Traub, R.D., and Bucana, C., 1976, Partial purification of the scrapie agent from mouse brain by pressure disruption and zonal centrifugation in sucrose-sodium chloride gradients, Virology, 70:230.

Somerville, R.A, 1985, Ultrastructural links between scrapie and Alzheimer's disease, Lancet, 1:504.

Vernon, M.L., Horta-Barbosa, L., Fuccillo, D.A., Sever, J.L., Baringer, J.R. and Birnbaum, G., 1979, Virus-like particles and nucleoprotein-type filaments in brain tissue from two patients with Creutzfeldt-Jakob disease, Lancet, 1:964.

Westaway, D., Prusiner, S.B., 1986, Conservation of the cellular gene encoding the scrapie prion protein PrP 27-30, Nucleic acids res., (in press).

ALZHEIMER'S DISEASE, DOWN SYNDROME, AND PARKINSON'S DISEASE:

SELECTED PATHOLOGIC FEATURES

Henry M. Wisniewski, Paul E. Bendheim and David C. Bolton

New York State Office of Mental Retardation and
Developmental Disabilities, Institute for Basic Research
in Developmental Disabilities, Staten Island, NY 10314

INTRODUCTION

Alzheimer's disease (AD), Parkinson's disease (PD) and Down syndrome
(DS) are distinct nosological entities. They are distinguishable
clinically and pathologically, with the exception that the brain from a
DS individual over the age of 35-40 years shows pathological changes
that cannot be distinguished from those found in AD patients' brains
(Malamud, 1966; Heston, 1977; Liss et al., 1980; Wisniewski K., et al.,
1985). This is true whether or not the DS patient had a clinically
recognized dementia during life. Dementia defines the clinical
symptomatology of AD, so the incidence of dementia in this disease is
100%. In the DS population over the age of 40 years the incidence of
dementia is uncertain, but appears to be at least 15-30% (Wisniewski K.
et al., 1985; Oliver and Holland, 1986) and in PD the incidence of
dementia is reported in the literature to be anywhere from 20-90%
(Lieberman et al., 1979; Huber et al., 1986). Shared neuropathologic
features suggest that a common mechanism may be responsible for select
aspects of the neurodegenerative changes seen in these three disorders.
This is not to imply that they share etiologies, but rather that several
diverse factors may act separately to produce similar clinical and
pathological features. This review will concentrate on these shared
morphological features in Alzheimer's disease, Parkinson's disease, and
Down syndrome.

ALZHEIMER'S DISEASE

The microscopic pathology of AD is characterized by the abundant
occurrence of neuritic (senile) plaques, neurofibrillary tangles (NFT),
granulovacuolar degeneration of neurons and congophilic angiopathy.
Plaques and tangles are found in characteristic locations throughout the
brains of AD victims, but they also occur in reduced numbers and in a
more topographically restricted distribution in the brains of normal
aged persons. Autosomal dominant cases of AD, although uncommon,
usually have an earlier onset, more rapid progression, and denser
accumulation of amyloid and NFT (Feldman et al., 1963; Nee et al.,
1983). This suggests that the mechanisms responsible for the formation
of plaques and tangles may have relevance beyond AD and that
understanding these mechanisms might contribute to a broader discussion
of normal and aged neuronal function, dysfunction and cell death.

Separately, plaques and tangles can be found in diseases other than AD. However, the only conditions in which these two lesions occur together in abundance are AD and Down syndrome (Malamud, 1966; Heston, 1977; Liss et al., 1985, Wisniewski K. et al., 1985). The brains of DS individuals over the age of 40 years uniformly show AD neuropathology irrespective of the presence or absence of clinical dementia. Amyloid plaques are also a conspicuous feature of the transmissible spongiform encephalopathies (Masters et al., 1981, Bendheim et al., 1984). These include Creutzfeldt-Jakob disease, Gerstmann-Straussler syndrome and kuru of humans and scrapie in animals. Tangle formation is seen in post-encephalitic Parkinson's disease, the Parkinsonism-dementia complex of the Chamorro natives on Guam, certain viral infections, tuberous sclerosis, Hallervorden-Spatz disease, dementia pugilistica, and several other neurologic disorders. The above lists should serve to emphasize that plaques and particularly tangles are not markers of specific etiologic processes, but rather that they are the final pathological products of abnormal mechanisms which can be triggered in various ways.

Neuritic (senile) plaques are classified as (1) immature, (2) mature, and (3) amyloid, compact or "burned out" (Wisniewski, H. et al., 1986). This nomenclature conceptualizes the hypothesis that the various forms of these plaques are a reflection of stages in their evolution. It seems probable that at a molecular level the constituent proteins are present in related, but different forms depending on the age of the plaque. Immature or young plaques have amyloid fibrils that are diffuse and not yet compacted into a central core. The fibrils are found dispersed among microglia, and other reactive cells. Microglia may play a role in the processing of the amyloid proteins or their precursors. Mature plaques have a central core of amyloid surrounded by astrocytes, microglia and neuronal processes (neurites) in various stages of degeneration and regeneration. The amyloid plaque consists of a dense, amyloid core with very few or no surrounding abnormal neurites.

Neurofibrillary tangles are fibrous structures located within the cytoplasm of neurons and their processes. They consist primarily of paired helical filaments (PHF). Tangles, as noted above, are present excessively in AD brain, but are found also in other conditions (Wisniewski, K., et al., 1979). Tomlinson et al. (1970) correlated the density of tangles in brain tissue with the degree of dementia noted during life in Alzheimer's disease patients.

PHF are paired pathological fibrils in which each filament measures 10-12 nm in diameter and is helically wound around its partner (Kidd, 1963; Terry, 1963; Wisniewski, H., et al., 1984; Wischik et al., 1985). The total PHF diameter is therefore 20-24 nm and has repeating nodes at 80 nm intervals. Negative stain electron microscopic studies using ultrathin sections have revealed that each 10-12 nm PHF is constructed from four protofilaments. Bundles of straight filaments, 10-20 nm in diameter, can coexist with PHF within tangles (Yagashita et al., 1981; Yoshimura et al., 1984). Antibodies specific for PHF also stain these straight filaments suggesting that they may share amino acid sequences (Rasool and Selkoe, 1985; Perry et al., 1986).

The morphological characteristics of PHF differ from those of normal neurofilaments and neurotubules. NFTs, like neuritic plaque amyloid, demonstrate affinity for congo red stain and show green-red birefringence in polarized light. Additionally, X-ray diffraction studies of PHF and extraneuronal amyloid fibers isolated from AD brain demonstrated evidence of a β-pleated sheet type of protein conformation (Kirschner et al., 1986). Normal neurofilaments do not have these amyloid properties. Recently it was shown that a constituent of PHF is the microtubule associated protein, tau (Brion et al., 1985; Grundke-Iqbal et al., 1986a; Kosik et al., 1986; Nukina and Ihara, 1986; Wood et al., 1986). It appears that tau protein is abnormally phosphorylated in PHF (Grundke-Iqbal et al., 1986b; Ihara et al., 1986). Whether or not this abnormal phosphorylation is responsible for the formation of PHF from tau, and perhaps other proteins, is not known.

A prominent feature of PHF is their relative resistance to solubilization. This can be considered an "in vitro" correlate to their natural resistance to degradation within the brain. Whether this accumulation is secondary to a failure of normal degradation mechanisms or is an intrinsic property of PHF themselves is not known. Their resistance to solubilization can be used as an argument that it is an intrinsic property of the filament. PHF are relatively unaffected by proteases, denaturing detergents, reducing agents, urea, chaotropic chemicals, and 0.2N HCl (Goni et al., 1984; Yen and Kress, 1983). Solubilization of PHF was achieved using sonication and heating in the presence of SDS and β-mercaptoethanol (Iqbal et al., 1984).

PHF appear to be distinct morphologically from the amyloid fibrils found in both the plaques and vascular walls of AD brains (Merz et al., 1983). Amino acid sequencing of an AD vascular amyloid protein demonstrated that this protein did not share homology with other known amyloid proteins (Glenner and Wong, 1984). Later, similar amino acid composition and N-terminal sequences for plaque amyloid and a subunit protein of PHF (Masters et al., 1985) were reported. This led to the suggestion that PHF, plaque amyloid and cerebrovascular amyloid in AD contain deposits of the same protein (Kidd et al., 1985; Masters et al., 1985). Other workers using biochemical and immunocytochemical methods could not confirm these data (Grundke-Iqbal et al., 1986a; Selkoe et al., 1986).

Immunohistochemical studies have demonstrated that some antisera to microtubules and neurofilaments identify antigenic sites on NFTs. The 145 KDa and 200 KDa neurofilament polypeptides, but not the 68 KDa neurofilament protein, have been shown to share epitopes with PHF (Anderton et al., 1982; Perry et al., 1986). The microtubule associated protein, tau, shares antigenic sites with PHF and, as noted above, an abnormally phosphorylated form of tau appears to be a constituent of PHF. MAP-2 (microtubule-associated protein-2) also shares epitopes with NFT (Kosik et al., 1984; Perry et al., 1985). Although the exact relationships between these normal neuronal proteins and NFT is not completely elucidated, it appears now that normal cytoskeletal proteins or abnormal variants of these proteins are intimately associated with, and probably actually constitute, a significant portion of PHF. Whether this occurs as a consequence of deranged transcriptional, translational, post-translational, or other regulatory processes, is not known.

AD has not been transmitted to any experimental animal (Goudsmit et al., 1980) and the amyloid plaques in AD are not identified by an antisera that stains amyloid plaques in scrapie and the other transmissible spongiform encephalopathies (Roberts et al., 1986). The major proteins of the agents causing scrapie and Creutzfeldt-Jakob disease (CJD) are derived from host cellular proteins (Oesch et al., 1985; Bassler et al., 1986; Liao et al., 1986), but the gene encoding the human CJD amyloid protein is on chromosome 20, not on chromosome 21 (Liao et al., 1986). These data argue against the suggestion that AD could be caused by a transmissible agent similar to the agents of scrapie and CJD (Prusiner, 1984). However, that all well characterized amyloid proteins, including the cerebrovascular and plaque amyloid of AD

(Robakis et al., 1987), are derived from normal protein precursors suggests that similar abnormalities in protein metabolism might explain amyloid formation in AD, scrapie, and CJD (Wisniewski et al., 1986).

DOWN SYNDROME

Down syndrome (DS) has an estimated incidence of 1-1.3 per 1000 live births. Among the host of abnormalities which may be seen as an expression of the chromosomal disorder (trisomy 21) underlying this syndrome, only mental retardation is seen in all DS individuals (Ropper and Williams, 1980). Increasingly, DS individuals are living into middle age and in this population a striking incidence of clinical and pathological Alzheimer's disease has been documented (Malamud, 1966; Liss et al., 1980; Wisniewski K. et al., 1985; Oliver and Holland, 1986). The true incidence of clinical AD dementia in the older DS population is not known, but appears to be 15-30%, perhaps higher (Scott et al., 1983; Wisniewski, K. et al., 1985). Virtually 100% of brains examined from DS patients over the age of 40 years satisfy current pathological criteria for AD (Malamud, 1966; Heston, 1977; Liss et al., 1980; Wisniewski, K. et al., 1985). Why a greater percentage of these individuals are not demented during life is not known.

The microscopic examination of the brains of older DS individuals reveals senile plaques and neurofibrillary tangles in a pattern indistinguishable from the pattern seen in a non-DS patient's brain with AD. Plaques have been noted even in the second decade in some DS cases. Malamud studied 35 brains from subjects with DS over the age of 40 years and found AD pathology in all. A morphometric study of 100 DS brains was reported by K. Wisniewski and colleagues. AD pathology was present in 49 of 49 brains from patients above 30 years of age, while 7 of 50 brains from cases below 30 years satisfied neuropathological criteria for AD. In the frontal cortex and hippocampus the mean number of plaques increased markedly in the 31-40 years old brains, but a similar rise in tangle concentration was not observed until 51-60 years. We could find no evidence in the literature for such a primacy of plaques over neurons with neurofibrillary changes in the brains of aging and/or dementing persons without DS. Recent studies from our and other laboratories have demonstrated that a gene on chromosome 21 encodes the precursor of the amyloid protein which accumulates in blood vessel walls and neuritic plaques. The discovery of the amyloid gene on chromosome 21 appears to provide evidence, for the first time, for a gene dose effect on neuritic plaque formation and for a direct genetic link between DS and AD (Robakis et al., submitted). Thirteen of 49 patients older than 30 years (27%) had been diagnosed as demented and these brains contained more than twenty plaques or plaques and tangles per $1.5 \times 10^{6}$ um$^{2}$ of cerebral cortex. These authors suggested that in DS patients, as is the case in non-DS AD patients, a correlation exists between clinical dementia, the number of plaques and tangles, and age. However, the DS people appear to better tolerate the increased number of plaques and tangles than do non-DS aged people.

The accumulation of AD changes in the brains of DS individuals occurs in the setting of a brain already abnormal, in contradistinction to the non-DS AD patient. Brains of DS subjects are below normal in weight (Wisniewski, K. et al., 1985), appear grossly smaller by radiological and pathological examination (Wisniewski, K. et al., 1982), and contain a reduced number of neurons (Ross et al., 1984). This reduction in neurons is most pronounced in the granular layers of the visual cortex (Takashima et al., 1981). Other changes also are evident microscopically. Dendritic spines and average dendritic length are reduced and this dendritic atrophy has been proposed as a major contributing factor to the mental retardation seen in DS (Becker et al., 1986).

Abnormalities of the nucleus basalis of Meynert (nbM) have been noted in AD brains (Whitehouse et al., 1981; Arendt et al., 1983). Neurons in this nucleus provide a major cholinergic input via their projections to the neocortex. That a cholinergic deficit may be responsible for some AD symptoms is strengthened by reports of therapeutic efficacy by a potent central acting anticholinesterase drug (Summers et al., 1986). The number of neurons in the nbM was reduced in brain sections from five DS patients, varying in age from 16 to 56 years, as compared to controls (Casanova et al., 1985). However, whether low nbM neuron counts reflect developmental nbM hypoplasia in DS or a progressive loss of nbM in neurons such as occurs in AD is uncertain.

There have been limited biochemical comparisons made between the plaques, tangles and their constituent macromolecules from DS brains with AD and non-DS AD. The cerebrovascular amyloid protein from one adult case of DS was isolated, purified and analyzed by amino acid sequencing (Glenner and Wong, 1984). It was shown to share sequence homology with a protein isolated and sequenced from AD cerebrovascular amyloid. Subsequently, the amyloid core protein in AD and DS were partially characterized (Masters et al., 1985). Amino acid compositions, molecular masses, and N-terminal sequences of this protein were found to be nearly identical to the cerebrovascular amyloid protein of AD and DS (Glenner and Wong, 1984). It has been suggested that a genetic defect in AD, by analogy with DS, could be localized on human chromosome 21 (Heston, 1977; Glenner and Wong, 1984). A cDNA probe generated from the N-terminal sequence of AD cerebrovascular amyloid hybridizes to chromosome 21 and would appear to confirm this prediction (Robakis et al., 1987). As indicated above amyloid plaque deposits are found at early ages in DS and the gene for this amyloid protein maps to chromosome 21. There may be a causal relationship between the gene dosage effect seen in trisomy 21 and Alzheimer neuropathology.

PARKINSON'S DISEASE

Dementia is now recognized to occur in a significant percentage of PD patients. Estimates of the incidence of dementia in PD range from 20 to 90% (Lieberman et al., 1979; Huber et al., 1986). A long-standing debate has centered upon the question of whether the dementia seen in patients with PD is an integral feature of the disease, the expression of concomitant AD or represents another disorder (Hakim and Mathieson, 1979; Lieberman et al., 1979; Boller et al., 1980; Mayeux, 1982; Perry et al., 1985; Huber et al., 1986; Whitehouse, 1986). PD is an age-associated disorder and it is not surprising that some patients also develop AD neuropathology with or without cognitive deficiency. Even so, the incidence of dementia in PD is greater than one would predict if dementia was not an integral part of PD, or if PD did not predispose to the development of dementia.

The essential pathologic changes in the brains of PD patients are the degeneration of pigmented nerve cells in the substantia nigra, locus coeruleus, and dorsal nucleus of the vagus, and the occurrence of Lewy bodies (Forno and Alvord, 1971). Lewy bodies are eosinophilic inclusions found in neurons and their processes, primarily in the substantia nigra, but also in the dorsal motor nucleus of the vagus. Lewy bodies, examined by electron microscopy, consist of filaments compacted into cores of variable density (Duffy and Tennyson, 1965).

The systemic administration of the neurotoxin MPTP (1-methyl-4-phenyl-1,2,3,6-tetrahydropyridine) accurately reproduced the pathological changes of PD in squirrel monkeys (Forno et al., 1986).

Relevant to a discussion of shared pathological features between AD, and PD is the subset of PD patients with the postencephalitic form of the disease. The virus responsible for postencephalitic PD has not been identified. Most cases followed the pandemic of encephalitis lethargica which occurred in 1916-1927. This disease is an example of a neurodegenerative disorder developing, in some cases after many years, as a sequel to a viral infection. Brains from these patients contain Lewy bodies and a decreased number of striatal neurons, but they also show accumulation of neurofibrillary tangles (Forno and Alvord, 1971). Neurofibrillary tangles found in neurons in postencephalitic PD and studied by tilt-stage electron microscopy were demonstrated to be composed of paired helical filaments (Wisniewski, H. et al., 1976). These tangles closely resemble the tangles of AD and DS. The frequency of dementia in a large series of patients was 26% in the postencephalitic group versus 29% in the idiopathic group (Mortilla and Rinne, 1976). Cell loss in the nbM was not found in three cases of postencephalitic PD examined in a separate study (Whitehouse et al., 1983). A potential animal model for postencephalitic PD now exists with the report of a relatively specific infection of the basal ganglia by murine coronavirus (Fishman et al., 1985). This virus, MHV-A59, causes infected animals to assume a hunched posture and exhibit difficulty in motility, signs resembling certain PD features. Neurofibrillary tangles were not observed in the brains of these experimental animals.

The pathologic basis for the dementia in idiopathic PD is uncertain (Hakim and Mathieson, 1979; Boller et al., 1980; Perry et al., 1985; Chui et al., 1986; Whitehouse, 1986). The association with AD lesions (plaques and tangles) in the cortex is inconsistent. In two series, each containing only a small number of cases, investigators were unable to detect an increased number of plaques and tangles in the hippocampi of demented versus nondemented PD patients (Mann and Yates, 1983; Ball, 1984). AD lesions, in the quantity required to make the diagnosis of AD, do not appear to be necessary for the dementia of PD. Neuronal loss occurs in the locus ceruleus and nbM in both conditions, but these findings are again inconsistent.


PROSPECTIVE

Intraneuronal filamentous inclusions are a pathological characteristic of AD and PD (Goldman and Yen, 1986). Appel (1981) postulated that AD and PD might each result from the lack of a disorder specific neurotropic hormone. Gajdusek (1985) theorized that interference with axonal transport of neurofilaments might be the common pathogenetic mechanism in AD, PD, and the spongiform encephalopathies. Significant progress has been made in characterizing the pathological structures of AD. The demonstration that an AD amyloid protein is encoded on chromosome 21 represents an exciting, if preliminary, confirmation of a prediction based on neuropathologic observations in AD and DS. The precise etiologies of AD and PD certainly differ, but certain shared neuropathologic features indicate that abnormal molecular mechanisms may be shared. Further application of the tools of molecular biology promises to increase our understanding of these pathologic features, the mechanisms responsible for their production, and the etiologies of the diseases themselves.

ACKNOWLEDGMENT

Supported in part by NIH grant AGO–4220.

REFERENCES

Anderton, B.H., Breinburg, D., Downes, M.J., Green, P.J., Tomlinson,
    B.E., Ulrich, J., Wood, J.N., and Kahn, J., 1982, Monoclonal
    antibodies show that neurofibrillary tangles and neurofilaments
    share antigenic determinants, Nature, 298:84.
Appel, S.H., 1981, A unifying hypothesis for the cause of amyotrophic
    lateral sclerosis, parkinsonism, and Alzheimer disease, Ann.
    Neurol., 10:499.
Arendt, T., Bigl, V., Arendt, A., and Tennstedt, A., 1983, Loss of
    neurons in the nucleus basalis of Meynert in Alzheimer's disease,
    paralysis agitans, and Korsakoff's disease, Acta Neuropathol.,
    (Berl), 61:101.
Ball, M.J., 1984, The morphological basis of dementia in Parkinson's
    disease, Can. J. Neurol. Sci., 11:180.
Bassler, K., Oesch, B., Scott, M., Westaway, D., Walchli, M., Groth,
    D.F., McKinley, M.P., Prusiner, S.B., and Weissmann, C., 1986,
    Scrapie and cellular PrP isoforms are encoded by the same
    chromosomal gene, Cell, 46:417.
Becker, L.E., Armstrong, D.L., and Chan, F., 1986, Dendritic atrophy in
    children with Down's syndrome, Ann. Neurol., 20:520.
Bendheim, P.E., Barry, R.A., DeArmand, S.J., Stites, D.P., and
    Prusiner, S.B., 1984, Antibodies to a scrapie prion protein,
    Nature, 310:418.
Boller, F., Mizutani, T., Roessmann, U., and Gambetti, P., 1980,
    Parkinson disease, dementia, and Alzheimer disease: clinico-
    pathological correlations, Ann. Neurol., 7:329.
Brion, J.P., von den Bosch de Aguilar, P., and Flament-Durand, J., 1985,
    Senile dementia of the Alzheimer type: morphological and
    immunocytochemical studies, in: "Senile Dementia of Alzheimer
    Type, Adv. Appl. Neurol. Sci., Vol. II," W. Gispen and J. Traser,
    eds., Springer, Berlin.
Casanova, M.F., Walker, L.C., Whitehouse, P.J., and Price, D.L., 1985,
    Abnormalities of the nucleus basalis in Down's syndrome, Ann.
    Neurol., 18:310.
Chui, H.C., Mortimer, J.A., Slager, U., Zarrow, C., Bondareff, W., and
    Webster, D.D., 1986, Pathologic correlates of dementia in
    Parkinson's disease, Arch. Neurol. 43:991.
Duffy, P.E., and Tennyson, V.M., 1965, Phase and electron microscopic
    observations of Lewy bodies and melanin granules in the substantia
    nigra and locus ceruleus in Parkinson's disease, J. Neuropath.
    Exp. Neurol., 24:398.
Feldman, R.G., Chandler, K.A., Levy, L.L., and Glaser, G.H., 1963,
    Familial Alzheimer's disease, Neurology, 13:811.
Fishman, P.S., Gass, J.S., Swoveland, P.T., Lavi, E., Highkin, M.K., and
    Weiss, S.R., 1985, Infection of the basal ganglia by a murine
    coronavirus, Science, 229:877.
Forno, L.S., and Alvord, E.C., 1971, The pathology of Parkinsonism, in:
    "Recent Advances in Parkinson's Disease," F.H.K. McDowell and
    C.H. Markham, eds., F.A. Davis, Philadelphia.
Forno, L.S., Langston, J.W., DeLanney, L.E., Irwin, I., and Ricaurte,
    G.A., 1986, Locus ceruleus lesions and eosinophilic inclusions in
    MPTP-treated monkeys, Ann. Neurol., 20:449.
Gajdusek, D.C., 1985, Hypothesis: interference with axonal transport of
    neurofilament as a common pathogenetic mechanism in certain

diseases of the central nervous system, New Engl. J. Med., 312:714.

Glenner, G.G., and Wong, C.W., 1984, Alzheimer's disease and Down's syndrome: sharing of a unique cerebrovascular amyloid fibril protein, Biochim. Biophys. Res. Commun., 122:1131.

Goldman, J.E., and Yen, S.-H., 1986, Cytoskeletal protein abnormalities in neurodegenerative diseases, Ann. Neurol., 19:209.

Goni, F., Pons-Estel, B., Alvarez, F., Gorevic, P., and Frangione, B., 1984, Alzheimer's disease: isolation and purification of neurofibillary tangles, in: "Proceedings IVth International Symposium on Amyloidosis," G.G. Glenner, ed., Plenum Press, New York.

Goudsmit, J., Murrow, C.H., Asher, D.M., Yanagihara, R.T., Masters, C.L., Gibbs, Jr., C.J., and Gajdusek, D.C., 1980, Evidence for and against the transmissibility of Alzheimer's disease, Neurology, 30:945.

Grundke-Iqbal, I., Iqbal, K., Quinlan, M., Tung, Y.-C., Zaidi, M.S., and Wisniewski, H.M., 1986a, Microtubule-associated protein tau: a component of Alzheimer paired helical filaments, J. Biol. Chem., 261:6084.

Grundke-Iqbal, I., Iqbal, K., Tung, Y.-C., Quinlan, M., Wisniewski, H.M., and Binder, L.I., 1986b, Abnormal phosphorylation of the microtubule-associated protain tau in Alzheimer cytoskeletal pathology, Proc. Natl. Acad. Sci., USA, 83:4913.

Hakin, A.M., and Mathieson, G., 1979, Dementia in Parkinson disease: a neuropathologic study, Neurology, 29:1209.

Heston, L.L., 1977, Alzheimer's disease, trisomy 21, and myeloproliferative disorders: associations suggesting a genetic diathesis, Science, 196:322.

Huber, S.J., Shuttleworth, E.C., and Paulson, G.W., 1986, Dementia in Parkinson's disease, Arch. Neurol., 43:987.

Ihara, Y., Nukina, N., Miura, R., and Ogawara, M., 1986, Phosphorylated tau protein is integrated into paired helical filaments in Alzheimer's disease, J. Biochem., 99:1807.

Iqbal, K., Zaidi, T., Thompson, C.H., Merz, P.A., and Wisniewski, H.M., 1984, Alzheimer paired helical filaments: bulk isolation, solubility and protein composition, Acta Neuropathol. (Berl), 62:167.

Kidd, M., 1963, Paired helical filaments in electron microscopy of Alzheimer's disease, Nature, 197:192.

Kidd, M., Allsop, D., and Camdon, M., 1985, Senile plaque amyloid, paired helical filaments and cerebrovascular amyloid in Alzheimer's disease are all deposits of the same protein, Lancet, 1:278.

Kirschner, D.A., Abraham, C., and Selkoe, D.J., 1986, X-ray diffraction from intraneuronal paired helical filaments and extraneuronal amyloid fibers in Alzheimer disease indicates cross-B conformation, Proc. Natl. Acad. Sci., USA, 83:503.

Kosik, K.S., Duffy, L.K., Dowling, M.M., Abraham, C., McCluskey, A., and Selkoe, D.J., 1984, Microtubule-associated protein 2: monoclonal antibodies demonstrate the selective incorporation of certain epitopes into Alzheimer neurofibrillary tangles, Proc. Natl. Acad. Sci. USA, 81:7941.

Kosik, K.S., Joachim, C.L., and Selkoe, D.J., 1986, The microtubular associated protein, tau, is a major antigenic component of paired helical filaments in Alzheimer's disease, Proc. Natl. Acad. Sci., USA 83:4044.

Liao, Y.-C.J., Lebo, R.V., Clawson, G.A., and Smuckler, E.A., 1986, Human prion protein cDNA: molecular cloning, chromosomal mapping, and biological implications, Science, 233:364.

Lieberman, A., Dziatolowski, M., Kupersmith, M., Serby, M., Goodgold, A., Korein, J., and Goldstein, M., 1979, Dementia in Parkinson disease, Ann. Neurol., 6:335.

Liss, L., Shim, C., Thase, M., Smeltzer, D., Maloon, J., and Couri, D.,
    1980, The relationship between Down's syndrome (DS) and dementia
    Alzheimer type (DAT), J. Neuropath. Exp. Neurol., 39:371.

Malamud, N., 1966, The neuropathology of mental retardation, in:
    "Prevention and Treatment of Mental Retardation," I. Philips, ed.,
    Basics Books, New York.

Mann, D.M.A., and Yates, P.O., 1983, Pathological basis for
    neurotransmitter changes in Parkinson's disease, Neuropathol.
    Appl. Neurobiol., 9:3.

Martilla, R.J., and Rinne, U.K., 1976, Dementia in Parkinson's disease,
    Acta Neurol. Scand., 54:431.

Masters, C.L., Gajdusek, D.C., and Gibbs, Jr., C.J., 1981, Creutzfeldt-
    Jakob disease virus isolations from the Gerstmann-Straussler
    syndrome, Brain, 104:559.

Masters, C.L., Multhaup, G., Simms, G., Pottigiesser, J., Martins, R.N.,
    and Beyreuther, K., 1985, Neuronal origin of a cerebral amyloid:
    neurofibrillary tangles of Alzheimer's disease contain the same
    protein as the amyloid of plaque cores and blood vessels, EMBO J.,
    4:2757.

Masters, C.L., Simms, G., Weinman, N.A., Multhaup, G., McDonald, B.L.,
    and Beyreuther, K., 1985, Amyloid core protein in Alzheimer's
    disease and Down syndrome, Proc. Natl. Acad. Sci., USA, 82:4245.

Mayeux, R., 1982, Depression and dementia in Parkinson's disease, in:
    "Movement Disorders," C.D. Marsden and S. Fahn, eds., Butterworth,
    London.

Merz, P.A., Wisniewski, H.M., Somerville, R.A., Bobin, S.A.,
    Masters, C.L., and Iqbal, K., 1983, Ultrastructural morphology of
    amyloid fibrils from neuritic and amyloid plaques, Acta
    Neuropathol. (Berl), 60:113.

Nee, L.E., Polinsky, R.J., Eldridge, R., Weingartner, H., Smallberg, S.,
    and Ebert, M., 1983, A family with histologically confirmed
    Alzheimer's disease, Ann. Neurol., 40:203.

Nukina, N., and Ihara, Y., 1986, One of the antigenic determinants of
    paired helical filaments is related to tau protein, J. Biochem.,
    99:1541.

Oesch, B., Westaway, D., Walchli, M., McKinley, M.P., Kent, S.B.H.,
    Aebersold, R., Barry, R.A., Tempst, P., Teplow, P.B., Hood, L.,
    Prusiner, S.B., and Weissmann, C., 1985, A cellular gene encodes
    scrapie PrP 27-30 protein, Cell 40:735.

Oliver, C., and Holland, A.J., 1986, Down's syndrome and Alzheimer's
    disease: a review, Psychol. Med., 16:307.

Perry, E.K., Curtis, M., Pick, D.J., Candy, J.M., Atack, J.R., Bloxham,
    C.A., Blessed, G., Fairbaira, A., Tomlinsin, B.A., and Perry,
    R.H., 1985, Cholinergic correlates of cognitive impairment in
    Parkinson's disease: comparisons with Alzheimer's disease,
    J. Neurol. Neurosurg. Psych., 48:413.

Perry, G., Rizzuto, N., Autilio-Gambetti, L., and Gambetti, P., 1985,
    Alzheimer's paired helical filaments contain cytoskeletal
    components, Proc. Natl. Acad. Sci. USA, 82:3916.

Perry, G., Selkoe, D.J., Block, B.R., Stewart, D., Autilio-Gambetti, L.,
    and Gambetti, P., 1986, Electron microscopic localization of
    Alzheimer neurofibrillary tangle components recognized by an
    antiserum to paired helical filaments, J. Neuropath. Exp. Neurol.,
    45:161.

Prusiner, S.B., 1984, Some speculations about prions, amyloid and
    Alzheimer's disease, New Engl. J. Med., 310:661.

Rasool, C.G., and Selkoe, D.J., 1985, Sharing of specific antigens by
    degenerating neurons in Pick's disease and Alzheimer's disease,
    New Engl. J. Med., 312:700.

Robakis, N.K., Wisniewski, H.M., Jenkins, E.C., Devine-Gage, E.A., Houck,
    G.E., Yao, X-L., Ramakrishna, R., Wolfe, G., Silverman, W.P., and
    Brown, W.T., Chromosome 21q21 sublocalization of the gene encoding

the B-amyloid peptide present in vessels and neuritic (senile) plaques of people with Alzheimer disease and Down syndrome, (submitted).

Robakis, N.K., Wolfe, G., Ramakrishna, N., and Wisniewski, H.M., 1987, Isolation of a cDNA clone encoding the Alzheimer disease and Downs syndrome amyloid paptide, in: "Neurochemistry of Aging," Banbury Report, Cold Spring Harbor Laboratory, New York, in press.

Roberts, G.W., Lofthouse, R., Brown, R., Crow, T.J., Barry, R.A., and Prusiner, S.B., 1986, Prion-protein immunoreactivity in human transmissible dementias, New Engl. J. Med., 315:1231.

Ropper, A.H., and Williams, R.S., 1980, Relationship between plaques, tangles, and dementia in Down's syndrome, Neurology, 30:639.

Ross, M.H., Galaburda, A.M., Kemper, T.L., 1984, Down's syndrome: is there a decreased population of neurons?, Neurology, 34:909.

Scott, B.S., Becker, L.E., and Petit, T.L., 1983, Neurobiology of Down's syndrome, Prog. Neurobiol., 21:199.

Selkoe, D.J., Abraham, C.R., Podlisny, M.B., and Duffy, L.K., 1986, Isolation of low-molecular-weight proteins from amyloid plaque fibers in Alzheimer's disease, J. Neurochem., 146:1820.

Selkoe, D.J., Ihara, Y., and Salazar, F.J., 1982, Alzheimer's disease: insolubility of partially purified helical filaments in sodium dodecyl sulfate and urea, Science, 215:1243.

Summers, W.K., Majorski, L.V., Marsh, G.M., Tachiki, K., and Kling, A., 1986, Oral tetrahydroaminoacridine in long-term treatment of senile dementia, Alzheimer type, New Engl. J. Med., 315:1241.

Takashima, S., Becker, L.E., Armstrong, D.L., and Chan, F., 1981, Abnormal neuronal development in the visual cortex of the human fetus and infant with Down's syndrome. A quantitative and qualitative study, Brain Res., 225:1.

Terry, R.D., 1963, The fine structure of neurofibrillary tangles in Alzheimer's disease, J. Neuropath. Exp. Neurol., 22:629.

Tomlinson, B.E., Blessed, G., and Roth, M., 1970, Observations on the brains of demented old people, J. Neurol. Sci., 11:205.

Whitehouse, P.J., 1986, The concept of subcortical and cortical dementia: another look, Ann. Neurol., 19:1.

Whitehouse, P.J., Hedreen, J.C., White, C.L., and Price, D.L., 1983, Basal forebrain neurons in the dementia of Parkinson disease. Ann. Neurol., 13:243.

Whitehouse, P.J., Price, D.L., Clark, A.W., Coyle, J.T., and DeLong, M.R., 1981, Alzheimer disease: evidence for selective loss of cholinergic neurons in the nucleus basalis, Ann. Neurol., 10:122.

Wischik, C.M., Crowther, R.S., Stewart, M., and Roth, M., 1985, Subunit structure of paired helical filaments in Alzheimer's disease, J. Cell Biol., 100:1905.

Wisniewski, H.M., Clinical, pathological and biomedical aspects of Alzheimer's disease, 1986, in: "Alzheimer's and Parkinson's Disease," A. Fisher, I. Hanin and C. Lachman, eds., Plenum Press, New York.

Wisniewski, H.M., Iqbal, K., Grundke-Iqbal, I., Rubenstein, R., Wen, G.Y., Merz, P.A., Kascsak, R., and Kristensson, K., 1986, Amyloid in Alzheimer's disease and unconventional viral infections, International Symposium on Dementia and Amyloid (Tokyo), "Neuropathology" Supplement 3, pp. 87–94.

Wisniewski, H.M., Merz, P.A., and Iqbal, K., 1984, Ultrastructure of paired helical filaments of Alzheimer's neurofibrillary tangle, J. Neuropath. Exp. Neurol., 43:643.

Wisniewski, H.M., Narang, H.K., and Terry, R.D., 1976, Neurofibrillary tangles of paired helical filaments, J. Neurol. Sci., 27:173.

Wisniewski, K.E., French, J.H., Rosen, J.F., Kozlowski, P.B., Tenner, M., and Wisniewski, H.M., 1982, Basal ganglia calcification in Down's syndrome - another manifestation of premature aging. Ann. N.Y. Acad. Sci., 396:179.

Wisniewski, K., Jervis, G.A., Moretz, R.C., and Wisniewski, H.M., 1979, Alzheimer neurofibrillary tangles in diseases other than senile and presenile dementia, Ann. Neurol., 5:288.

Wisniewski, K.E., Wisniewski, H.M., and Wen, G.Y., 1985, Occurrence of neuropathological changes and dementia of Alzheimer's disease in Down's syndrome, Ann. Neurol., 17:278.

Wood, J.G., Mirra, S.S., Pollock, N.J., and Binder, L.I., 1986, Neurofibrillary tangles of Alzheimer's disease share antigenic determinants with the axonal microtubule-associated protein tau, Proc. Natl. Acad. Sci. USA,, 83:4040.

Yagashita, S., Itoh, T., Nau, W., and Amano, N., 1981, Reappraisal of the fine structure of Alzheimer's neurofibrillary tangles, Acta Neuropathol., (Berl) 54:239.

Yen, S.-H., and Kress, Y., 1983, The effect of chemical reagents or proteases on the ultrastructure of paired helical filaments, in: "Banbury Report 15: Biological Aspects of Alzheimer's Disease," R. Katzman, ed., Cold Spring Harbor Laboratory, New York.

Yoshimura, N., 1984, Evidence that paired helical filaments originate from neurofilaments, Clin. Neuropathol., 3:22.

# NEUROTRANSMITTERS IN THE AGEING BRAIN AND DEMENTIA

D.M. Bowen and A.N. Davison

Department of Neurochemistry
Institute of Neurology
London, U.K. WC1 3BG

Cognitive processes especially short-term memory are primarily impaired in normal ageing and more dramatically so in dementing diseases.  Other psychological effects are also evident.  There is with age a general decay in sensorimotor processing including visual, auditory, somatosensory, gustatory and olfactory systems (Flicker et al, 1985) but in dementia these modalities are not enhanced.  The control of behaviour is largely mediated within the brain by the limbic system (amygdala, hippocampus, septum, mamillary bodies of the hypothalamus and their connecting fibres).  The frontal and parietal lobes of the neocortex (association areas) are more concerned with higher functions of thought and perception. The temporal lobe contains large areas of association cortex and is involved with memory of visual tasks and learning of auditory patterns.  More subtle higher functions connected with movement and speech are also controlled by the cortex.  There is generally loss of weight in the ageing brain and in non-vascular dementia atrophy may be pronounced.  Selective loss or shrinkage also occurs.  Biochemical methods have been used to identify the neurotransmitter systems and metabolic pathways affected.

## Neurotransmitters and higher mental functions

Since communication between neurons is mediated at the synapse by the release of low molecular-weight excitatory and inhibitory neurotransmitters, measurement of the ability of brain tissue to synthesize such transmitters and their absolute concentration in CNS tissue together with assessment of their receptor concentration may give a clue to selective defects in their metabolism.  This is particularly relevant, for modification of the sensitive mechanism of synaptic transmission can result in altered brain function as happens in psychiatric or neurological disorder as a result of changes in neurotransmitter or receptor concentration.

Function within the CNS depends on neuronal interaction in which different chemical transmitters may participate.  For example dopaminergic pathways in the basal ganglia are of especial importance in controlling movement and loss of neurons from the substantia nigra and the projections to the striatum is associated with the tremor of Parkinson's disease.  Cell counts in the substantia nigra, where this dopaminergic tract originates, suggest that, despite cell loss, decrease in tyrosine hydroxylase activity is largely due to decreased activity of residual cells. In Huntington's disease impaired GABAergic neuronal activity in the striatum, is associated with chorea, but the dementia seen in this condition is likely to be due to changes in the cortex rather than the subcortex where there is no loss of nucleus basalis cells.

Of the different centrally acting neurotransmitters it has long been considered that acetylcholine is particularly involved in learning mechanisms (Deutsch, 1971). However the design of some of the early experimental lesioning procedures has been criticised. More persuasive are pharmacological studies on young men treated with the anticholinergic agent scopolamine who show cognitive and memory defects comparable to those seen in the elderly (Drachman and Leavitt, 1974). While the cholinergic muscarinic antagonist, arecholine, has been found to increase serial learning in normal human subjects (Baker et al., 1971). In addition; physostigmine given to young normal subjects significantly enhances storage of information into long-term memory and improves recall. Since physostigmine acts as an inhibitor of CNS cholinesterase, this again implicates acetylcholine in memory mechanisms. Finally, lesioning of the cholinergic nucleus basalis area in the rat results in impaired cognitive function which can be partially restored by cholinergic ventral forebrain grafts (Fine et al, 1985).

Long term memory

It has been argued that long term memory traces relate to structural or permanent molecular changes at the synaptic level (Hebb, 1949). This concept receives support from the finding after very brief periods of intense activity of persistent increases in postsynaptic potentials within cortical and hippocampal pathways. The amplitude of the long term potential correlates with the speed of complex maze learning by rats (Lynch and Baudry, 1984). Peptide and biogenic amines may be later implicated through action on receptors and control of second messengers to regulate genetic expression of glycoprotein for it is associated with memory traces lasting for more than one day (Goelet et al, 1986).

Cholinergic neurones and acetylcholine

Cholinergic nerve cells synthesize, store and release acetylcholine (ACh). The enzyme protein is synthesized in the neuronal perikaryon, together with the hydrolase AChE, ACh is transported down the axon to the nerve terminals. In the presynaptic terminal ACh is formed and stored within synaptic vesicles. Released acetylcholine interacts with the predominantly muscarinic (M1) receptor on the postsynaptic neuronal surface. There is a feed back control mechanism on the presynaptic terminals where muscarinic (M2) autoreceptors are predominantly located. The radioactively labelled ligand quinuclidinyl benzilate has been widely used to quantitate total muscarinic binding sites. Receptor subtypes can be classified on the basis of high and low affinity pirenzepine binding (M1 and M2 respectively) and further subdivided using high and low affinity for agonists (Birdsall et al, 1978). Muscarinic receptors are coupled to guanine nucleotide binding regulatory proteins (G proteins). Later stages in receptor mediated signal transduction involve the phosphoinositols and protein kinase C system.

## Nicotine receptors

Nicotinic receptors have been assayed using labelled α-bungaro-toxin but some studies show that the distribution of binding sites differ from that using nicotine as specific ligand (Clarke et al., 1985). Using tritiated nicotine Flynn and Mash (1986) have studied the receptor characteristics in human cerebral cortex. Since supersensitivity has been demonstrated on iontophoretic application of nicotine to nucleus basalis lesioned rats it is likely that the nicotine receptors have a postsynaptic localisation. Autoradiographic localisation shows a high density in cortical layer 1V (Whitehouse et al, 1985) indicating that these sites may process thalamocortical sensory information.

## Acetylcholine metabolism

In-vitro studies indicate that radioactive ACh is derived from acetyl-coenzyme A and radioactive choline through the action of choline acetyltransferase (ChAT), an enzyme present in excess in the presynaptic terminal. On depolarization of the neuron, release of ACh is dependent on calcium ions and inhibited by magnesium ions. Choline, once taken up by the nerve terminal, serves as a critical substrate for biosynthesis of the neurotransmitter, acetyl-CoA and ChAT may also have a rate-limited role in ACh synthesis (Tucek, 1985). Choline is derived from the blood and to a lesser extent from breakdown of phosphatidylcholine within the nerve cell. Although low affinity transport of choline may contribute to uptake, a sodium-dependent high affinity choline uptake system (Kuhar and Murrin, 1978) is primarily involved. This system is uniquely localized to cholinergic neurons and their nerve terminals.

## Distribution of the cholinergic system

An axonal tract originates from the septal region and forms cholinergic synapses with hippocampal neurons. It also appears that arousal projections that pass to the neocortex from the midbrain reticular formation, hypothalamus, striatum and septum are predominantly cholinergic. Cholinergic interneurons in the striatum interact with nigrostriatal dopaminergic projections (McGeer et al., 1971). In the cortex dopaminergic projections augment cortical ACh release rather than inhibit as occurs in the striatum (Lloyd, 1978).

The regional activity of ChAT gives an indication of the density of cholinergic nerves within the CNS. Thus ChAT activity is highest within the striatum and caudate nucleus of the basal ganglia and relatively low within the frontal cortex. In the primate there are widely disseminated cholinergic cortical projections from the basal forebrain (Walker et al 1985).

## Changes in transmitter synthesizing enzyme in the ageing brain

Well recognised physiological changes are found in the elderly. Besides decreased motor activity there are altered sleep patterns, mood flattening and declining mental activity. As a result it may be anticipated that there would be parallel changes in the ability of the brain to synthesize the relevant neurotransmitters. Some of the behavioural changes can be explained by a decrease in catecholamine synthesis in various brain regions, although there is an increase in monoamine oxidase activity with age. In the human brain, Bertler (1961) and Carlsson and Winblad (1976) found a significant decline in the dopamine content of the caudate nucleus and putamen in the elderly (over 70 years old). Rossor and Iversen (1986) found steady loss of noradrenalin in the cingulate cortex (60-100 years). Increased concentrations occur with age of the principal dopamine metabolite, homovanillic acid (HVA), and the serotonin metabolite, 5-hydroxyindoleacetic acid, in the CSF (Winblad et al., 1978). Presynaptic markers (5-hydroxytryptamine uptake and impripramine binding) show little alteration with age although indices of postsynaptic 5-hydroxytryptamine receptors show a reduction in the cortex (Allen et al, 1983). These changes in neurotransmitter concentration may be due to nerve cell loss. Thus reduction in concentration of noradrenalin could be the result of diminished neuronal population in the locus coeruleus, 5-hydroxytryptamine to neuronal loss in the raphe nucleus. There is a small decline in GABA content of intrinsic neurons in the frontal cortex (Rossor and Iversen, 1986). Other neurotransmitter concentrations do not alter markedly with age. No age-related alterations was found in the ability of fresh neocortical tissue to synthesise and release ACh (Sims et al, 1983). Indeed there is relative preservation of ascending projections from basal forebrain and brain stem.

In contrast, there is some evidence that ChAT activity slowly declines with increasing age except in the caudate nucleus and the frontal cortex. The loss of ChAT activity is especially marked in the hippocampus (Perry et al., 1977) and in the caudate nucleus (Allen et al., 1983). From the age of 60 years onwards, there is a slow decline in muscarinic cholinergic receptor binding in the human frontal cortex (White et al., 1977) and throughout life loss of cortical nicotine binding sites (Flynn and Mash, 1986).

Alzheimer's disease

This condition is typified by an acquired progressive decline in memory with global cognitive impairment. Details of the clinical definition and diagnosis for Alzheimer's disease (AD) have been summarized (McKhann et al., 1984). Atrophy especially of the cerebral cortex is common with ventricular dilation. Areas of the limbic system such as the hippocampus and amygdala seem to be particularly affected (Ball., 1982). Neuritic plaques and tangles with loss of neurons occurs in these regions. The cortex particularly the temporal, parietal and frontal lobes are also similarly affected. Other areas such as the motor cortex, sensory regions and primary visual areas show less pathology (Pearson et al., 1985). Excessive loss of cholinergic neurons from the nucleus basalis of Meynert (Price et al., 1982) and other nuclei in the basal forebrain have been related to neuritic plaque formation in the cortex (Kitt et al., 1984; Mann, Yates & Marcyniuk 1985). Similarly loss or damage to neurons in the raphe nucleus may lead to reduction in cortical serotonergic innervation (Ishii 1966). For the concentration of serotonin and its receptors appear to be reduced in the temporal cortex of AD patients (Bowen et al., 1983). In the locus coeruleus diminished neuronal populations could, it is thought, affect noradrenergic terminals within the neocortex (Tomlinson, Irving & Blessed, 1981) and account for reduced noradrenalin levels in the temporal cortex (Francis et al., 1985).

The cholinergic hypothesis

In 1965 Pope and his colleagues published preliminary histochemical data to suggest a loss of AChE in the frontal cortex of AD patients. Defects in the activity of ChAT were first noted by Bowen and his colleagues (Bowen et al., 1976) and the loss of the synthetic enzyme found to relate to the degree of neuropathological damage. At about the same time Davies & Maloney (1976) and Perry et al., (1977) showed significant reduction in ChAT activity particularly in the hippocampus, amygdaloid and mamillary body in the brain of AD patients.

Later Wilcock et al, (1982) demonstrated that loss of ChAT related to the severity of the dementia and the numbers of neurofibrillary tangles in the cortex. Reductions have been found in other markers of cholinergic activity - AChE (particularly the G4 form, Perry 1986) activity and the concentration of presynaptic muscarinic M1 cortical autoreceptors are for example decreased although overall muscarinic receptor concentration is little affected (Bowen and Davison, 1986). For example in the hippocampus significant reduction in M1 high affinity pirenzepine binding and high affinity carbachol binding have been reported (table 1). There is about 75% loss of ChAT and half the AChE activity of the hippocampus.

Since ChAT is not rate controlling in formation of acetylcholine, it was essential to demonstrate its altered synthesis in fresh tissue from Alzheimer's patients. Fresh biopsy tissue from 'presenile cases of dementia' assessed by histopathology were used in a collaborative study (Neary et al, 1986). Tissue prisms were prepared and incubated with radioactive glucose in medium containing low and high potassium concentrations. Thus the ability of the nervous tissue to respond to stimulation could be measured (Sims et al, 1983). The formation of acetylcholine under stimulating and resting conditions was found to be reduced in AD as was the uptake of choline by the diseased prisms (Fig. 1). Reduced synthesis of ACh was significantly correlated with premortem cognitive impairment (Francis et al, 1985). Since there is comparable reduction in sodium dependent high energy choline uptake (table 2), ACh synthesis and ChAT activity in fresh neocortical tissue it is likely that these changes are due to loss of presynaptic terminals from afferent fibres projecting from the nucleus basalis of Meynert (Whitehouse et al, 1982). The cholinergic hypothesis has several shortcomings: most patients with clinical AD but absent histological features have no evidence of cholinergic denervation; some overlap between ChAT activities in control and AD subjects has also been noted (Palmer et al, 1986). Finally the hypothesis also fails to account for the typical intrinsic changes in the cortex (e.g. tangle formation).


Biochemical changes in cortical neurons

The reports of reduced blood flow to the cortex and the hypometabolism of glucose especially in the parietal, temporal and frontal cortices (Foster et al, 1984) in AD suggest that this part of the CNS is affected. Loss of large neurons has been found in the cortex. Tangles are found in the pyramidal cells of layers III and V. The clustering of tangles and laminar distribution support the concept that affected regions are interconnected by well defined possibly glutamergic pathways along which the disease process may extend. Pearson and his colleagues (1985) raise the possibility that olfactory tracts may be initially involved and that the disease may spread from the subcortex by corticofugal or petal fibres and transcortically by corticocortical association fibres. The amygdala, which receives a direct projection from the olfactory tract, also has direct cholinergic innervation from the basal nucleus of Meynert. ChAT activity in the amygdala is significantly reduced to only 33% of control in cortical ChAT-deficient AD subjects (Rossor et al, 1982;

Table 1.  Receptor Binding in Hippocampus

| Possible Localisation | Pirenzepine affinity M₁ high | M₂ low | Agonist (carbachol) affinity high | low | N-Methyl scopolamine Total muscarinic |
|---|---|---|---|---|---|
| | | | — mainly postsynaptic — | | |
| Normal | 209 ± 38 (9) | 191 ± 34 | 265 ± 17 | 286 ± 48 | 551 ± 65 |
| Alzheimer's disease | 166 ± 32*(6) | 155 ± 31 | 225 ± 42* | 239 ± 78 | 465 ± 111 |
| Parkinson's with dementia Disease | 210 ± 50 (4) | 190 ± 41 | 264 ± 58 | 291 ± 53 | 555 ± 108 |
| without dementia | 196 ± 64 (6) | 231 ± 59 | 304 ± 69 | 352 ± 61* | 656 ± 123 |

(fmol/mg protein mean ± SD)

(Data from Smith et al, 1987, J. Neurochem. in press)

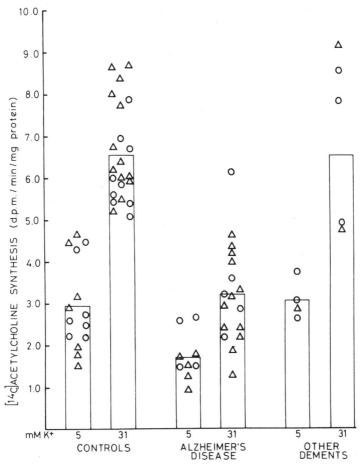

Fig. 1. [$^{14}$C]Acetylcholine synthesis measured in the presence of either 5 mM K$^+$ or 31 mM K$^+$ in samples of temporal neocortex (Δ) and frontal neocortex (O) from neurosurgical controls, patients with histologically confirmed Alzheimer's disease and other demented patients. Samples from patients with Alzheimer's disease were significantly different (p<0.01; Wilcoxon rank test) from control samples measured under the same conditions.

(reproduced with permission from Sims et al., 1983 and the Journal of Neurochemistry).

Palmer et al, 1986). The reduction is the same in the cortical ChAT-spared subjects (Palmer et al, 1986) who had been clinically demented, with AD histopathology. This suggests that cholinergic denervation occurs early in the amygdala. The disease process could then spread to the cortex along the direct connections between the amygdala and cortex, with the degeneration of the basal nucleus of Meynert being a secondary phenomenon.

Although the amygdala is involved in memory, loss of its cholinergic innervation seems unlikely to be a prerequisite for the syndrome of dementia since amygdaloid ChAT activity is not reduced in undiagnosed dementia (Palmer et al, 1986). Thus deficits in other neurotransmitters may underlie clinical dementia. Although postmortem studies suggest that ascending serotonergic and noradrenergic (corticopetal) projections are affected in AD, examination of these neurons in biopsy samples failed to show any relationships with the severity of dementia (Palmer et al, 1987). It has been proposed that loss of excitatory amino acid-releasing neurons should be considered as an alternative neurotransmitter basis of dementia and that 2-amino-4-sulphobutyric acid is one of a group of sulphur-containing compounds that have some characteristics of such neurotransmitters (Bowen and Davison 1986, Procter and Bowen 1987). Brattstrom et al, (1987) have argued that individuals with Down's syndrome may be protected against arteriosclerosis due to the increased expression of the gene for cystathionine-B-synthase located on chromosome 21. The authors speculated that a similar explanation might also account for the low prevalence of arteriosclerosis said to occur in AD. The gene loci for familial AD, amyloid-B-protein and cystathionine-B-synthase are all now known to be located on the long arm of chromosome 21. The synthase locus, at 21q2.1$\rightarrow$ 21q22.1 is however thought to be distal to the putative location of the AD and amyloid protein loci at 21q11.2$\rightarrow$ 21q2.1 (see Kraus et al, 1986; St George-Hyslop et al, 1987). Altered synthase activity has nevertheless been implicated, albeit indirectly, in AD as one substrate of the enzyme (homocysteine) is also the likely precursor of 2-amino-4-sulphobutyric acid (Fig. 2). Free serine (one synthase substrate) has been determined by high performance liquid chromatography (HPLC) in neocortex from diagnostic craniotomies of patients with presenile dementia and controls (Neary et al, 1986). Serine and a small HPLC peak (retention time of methionine, precursor of homocysteine, Fig. 2) are elevated in AD consistent with decreased synthase activity. The possibility that cystathionine co-eluted with methionine is under study but these data (as well as that of Tarbit et al, 1980) suggests that at least one gene on the long arm of chromosome 21 may be underexpressed in sporadic AD (table 3).


Neuropeptides

The concentration of many neuropeptides does not undergo change in AD. Even the amounts of vasoactive intestinal polypeptide (VIP) do not alter in the cortex despite the report of co-existence of VIP and ChAT in cortical neurons (Emson and Lindvall, 1986). In contrast somatostatin levels are consistently lowered (Rossor and Iversen, 1986). The loss of the peptide is greatest in the temporal cortex but this change is not so marked in elderly patients (in comparison with age matched controls) and is not a conspicious feature of biopsy samples of the frontal or temporal lobe. There is some evidence, however, that an early loss of somatostatin occurs from the parietal lobe (see Francis et al, 1987). An interesting possibility is that neuropeptides may function as trophic factors (Jones and Hendry, 1986). The concentration of corticotropin-releasing factor (CRF)-like

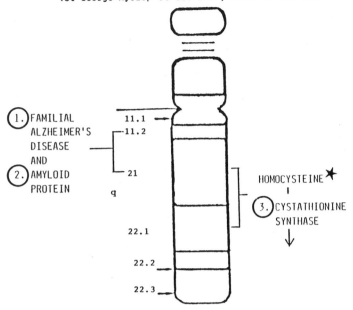

THREE GENE LOCI ON CHROMOSOME 21
(St George-Hyslop et al. 1987; Kraus et al. 1986)

1. FAMILIAL ALZHEIMER'S DISEASE AND
2. AMYLOID PROTEIN

11.1
11.2
21
22.1
22.2
22.3
q

HOMOCYSTEINE ✱
|
3. CYSTATHIONINE SYNTHASE
↓

✱LIKELY PRECURSOR ALSO OF 2-AMINO-4-SULPHOBUTYRIC ACID,
PROPOSED AS A NEUROTRANSMITTER OF CORTICOCORTICAL ASSOCIATION
FIBRES AND TO BE DECREASED IN ALZHEIMER'S DISEASE (Procter and Bowen, 1987).

Fig.2.   Underexpression of cystathionine-B-synthase may occur in
Alzheimer's disease (in the remaining cells) and 2-amino-
4-sulphobutyric acid is also cytotoxic.
(see May and Grey, 1985)

Table 2.   Choline Uptake of samples from demented patients and
neurosurgical controls compared with values for other
presynaptic cholinergic markers in the same demented
patients.

| | Choline uptake (in 31 mM K+) (pmol/min/mg protein) | [$^{14}$C]Acetylcholine synthesis (31 mM K+) (dpm/min/mg protein) | ChAT activity (pmol/min/mg protein) |
|---|---|---|---|
| Controls | 3.04 ± 0.33 (6) | 6.6 ± 1.2 (22) | 86 ± 21 (11) |
| Alzheimer's disease | 1.72 ± 0.58 (6)[a] | 3.9 ± 1.2 (6)[a] | 37 ± 25 (6) |
| Other demented patients | 2.71,2.73 | 4.9,8.5 | 70,74 |

Values are expressed as mean ± SD with number of samples in parentheses
where appropriate.   [a]$p < 0.01$ compared with control (Wilcoxon rank test).

(after Sims et al, 1983)

Table 3. Underexpression of a chromosome 21 gene in Alzheimer's disease?

| Synthase indices? | Alzheimer's Disease (n=10) | Other Dements (A) (n=6) | Controls (B) (n=31) |
|---|---|---|---|
| Serine | $13.20 \pm 8.11^{a}$ | $6.80 \pm 3.53$ | $8.41 \pm 3.80$ |
| Methionine? | $1.07 \pm 0.57^{b}$ | $0.58 \pm 0.27$ | $0.67 \pm 0.22$ |

Values are means ± S.D. For each amino acid Kruskal-Wallis ANOVA revealed significant differences ($p<0.05$) in ranks between groups. Individual group means were compared by the Mann-Whitney U-test, [a]$p<0.05$ from both A and B: [b]$p<0.05$ from B.

(after Bowen et al, 1987)

Table 4. Indications for Replacement Therapy

| Neurotransmitter | Evidence of: | | | |
|---|---|---|---|---|
| | Major role in cognition | Loss early in disease | Compensation for loss | Receptor loss* |
| Acetylcholine | + | + | − | − |
| Serotonin | − | + | + | + |
| Noradrenaline | − | + | + | − |
| Somatostatin | − | − | − | + |
| Glutamate | − | − | − | + |
| Dopamine | − | − | − | − |
| GABA | − | − | − | − |
| Corticocortical cells | +? | +? | ? | +? |

*Severely affected cases post-mortem.

(After Bowen, 1987)

immunoreactivity is reduced in the occipital, frontal and temporal but not cingulate cortex of Alzheimer's patients (De Souza et al. 1986). Conversely there is up-regulation of CRF receptor binding in the same cortical areas. This is consistent with the concept that CRF acts as a neurotransmitter in normal cortical function. The peptide is localised in intrinsic neurons in layers 2 and 3 with terminals in layers 1 and 4 of the neocortex. A sub-population of brain stem cholinergic neurons containing CRF project to the forebrain where it may exert a neuromodulatory function on the cholinergic system.

## Conclusion

The aetiology of AD is still uncertain. Reduction in ACh synthesis in fresh Alzheimer tissue obtained ante-mortem correlates with cognitive impairment (Francis et al., 1985). These changes and reductions in ChAT activity and choline uptake are probably due to loss of cholinergic presynaptic terminals originating from shrunk or lost cells in the basal forebrain. Similarly decreased serotonin and noradrenalin concentrations in the neocortex may relate to defective projections from subcortical nuclei. Post-mortem data suggests that cortical nerve cells utilising excitatory amino acid transmitters may also be affected in AD but it is not known if this is the site of primary damage. Although a pure cholinergic basis for Alzheimer's disease would seem to be unlikely, evidence accumulated in recent years continues to be consistent with the cholinergic alterations making an important contribution to this disorder (Table 4, Sims and Bowen 1987).

## References

Allen, S.J., Benton, J.S., Goodhardt, M.J., Haan, E.A., Sims, N.R., Smith, C.C.T., Spillane, J.A., Bowen, D.M., and Davison, A.N., 1983, Biochemical evidence of selective nerve cell changes in the normal ageing human and rat brain, J. Neurochem., 41:256.

Baker, R.W., 1971, Structure and activity of muscarinic stimulants, Nature, 230:439.

Ball, M.J., 1982, Limbic predilection in Alzheimer dementia: Is reactivated herpesvirus involved?, Canad. J. Neurol. Sci., 9:303.

Bertler, A., 1961, Occurrence and localization of catecholamines in the human brain, Acta Physiol. Scand., 51:97.

Birdsall, N.J.M., Hulme, E.C., Kromer, W., Peck, B.S., Stockton, J.M., and Zigmond, M.J., 1986, Two drug binding sites on muscarinic receptors, in: "New Concepts in Alzheimer's Disease," M. Briley, A. Kato, M. Weber, ed., Macmillan Press, Hampshire.

Bowen, D.M., Smith, C.B., White, P., Davison, A.N., 1976, Neurotransmitter-related enzymes and indices of hypoxia in senile dementia and other abiotrophies, Brain., 99:459.

Bowen, D.M., Allen, S.J., Benton, J.S., Goodhardt, M.J., Haan, E.A., Palmer, A.M., Sims, N.R., Smith, C.C.T., Spillane, J.A., Esiri, M.M., Neary, D., Snowdon, J.S., Wilcock, G.K., Davison, A.N., 1983, Biochemical assessment of serotonergic and cholinergic dysfunction and cerebral atrophy in Alzheimer's disease, J. Neurochem., 41:266.

Bowen, D.M., Davison, A.N., 1986, Biochemical studies of nerve cells and energy metabolism in Alzheimer's Disease, Brit. Med. Bull., 42:75.

Bowen, D.M., 1987, Neurochemistry of Alzheimer's Disease, Reviews in the Neurosciences, in press.

Bowen, D.M., Lowe, S.L., Francis, P.T., Cooper, D.N., 1987, Methionine catabolism and chromosome 21 in Alzheimer's Disease, (Abst. Second World Congress of Neuroscience, Budapest) Neuroscience, Supplement, in press.

Brattstrom, L., Englund, E., Brun, A., 1987, Does Down's syndrome support homocysteine theory of arteriosclerosis? Lancet., i:391.

Carlsson, A., Winblad, B., 1976 Influence of age and time interval between death and autopsy on dopamine and 3-methoxy-tyramine levels in human basal ganglia, J. Neurol. Transm., 38:271.

Clarke, P.B.S., Schwartz, R.D., Paul, S.M., Pert, C.B., Pert, A., 1985, Nicotinic binding in rat brain: autoradiographic comparison of $^3$H-acetylcholine, $^3$H-nicotine, and $^{125}$I-$\alpha$ bungarotoxin, J. Neurosci., 5:1307.

Davies, P., Maloney, A.J.F., 1976, Selective loss of cholinergic neurons in Alzheimer's disease, Lancet., ii:1403.

De Souza, E.B., 1986, Reciprocal changes in corticotropin-releasing factor (CRF)-like immunoreactivity and CRF receptors in cerebral cortex of Alzheimer's disease, Nature., 319:593.

Deutsch, J., 1971, The cholinergic synapse and the site of memory, Science, 174:788.

Drachman, D.A., Leavitt, J., 1974, Human memory and the colinergic system, Arch. Neurol., 30:113.

Emson, P.C., Lindvall, O., 1986, Neuroanatomical aspects of neurotransmitters affected in Alzheimer's disease, Brit. Med. Bull., 42:57.

Fine, A., Dunnett, S.B., Bjorklund, A., Iversen, S.D., 1985, Cholinergic ventral forebrain grafts into the neocortex improve passive avoidance memory in a rat model of Alzheimer's disease, Proc. Natl. Acad. Sci., 82:5227.

Flicker, C., Ferris, S.H., Crook, T., Bartus, R.T., Reisberg, B., 1985, Cognitive function in normal aging and early dementia, in: "Senile Dementia of the Alzheimer Type," J. Traber, W.H. Gispen, ed., Springer-Verlag, Berlin.

Flynn, D.D., Mash, D.C., 1986, Characterization of L-[$^3$H]nicotine binding in human cerebral cortex: comparison between Alzheimer's disease and the normal, J. Neurochem., 47:1948.

Foster, N.L., Chase, T.N., Mansi, L., Brooks, R., Fedio, P., Patronas, N.J., De Chiro, G., 1984, Cortical Abnormalities in Alzheimer's Disease, Annals Neurol., 16:649.

Francis, P.T., Palmer, A.M., Sims, N.R., Bowen, D.M., Davison, A.N., Esiri, M.M., Neary, D., Snowden, J.S., Wilcock, G.K., 1985, Neurochemical studies of early-onset Alzheimer's disease. Possible Influence on Treatment. New Eng. J. Med., 313:7.

Francis, P.T., Bowen, D.M., Lowe, S.L., Neary, D., Mann, D.M.A., Snowden, J.S., 1987, Somatostatin content and release measured in cerebral biopsies from demented patients, J. Neurol. Sci., 78:1.

Goelet, P., Castellucci, V.F., Schacher, S., Kandel, E.R., 1986, The long and the short of long-term memory - a molecular framework, Nature., 322:419.

Hebb, D.O., 1949, "The Organisation of Behavior," Wiley, New York.

Ishii, T., 1966, Distribution of Alzheimer's neurofibrillary changes in the brain stem and hypothalamus of senile dementia, Acta Neuropathol., 6:181.

Jones, E.G., Hendry, S.H.C., 1986, Co-localization of GABA and neuropeptides in neocortical neurons, Trends Neurosci., 9:71.

Kitt, C.A., Price, D.L., Struble, R.G., Cork, L.C., Wainer, B.H., Becher, M.W., Mobley, W.C., 1984, Evidence for Cholinergic Neurites in Senile Plaques, Science, 226:1443.

Kraus, J.P., Williamson, C.L., Firgaira, F.A., Yang-Feng, T.L., Nunke,

M., Francke, U., 1986, Cloning and screening with nanogram amounts of immunopurified mRNAs: cDNA cloning and chromosomal mapping of cystathionine-B-synthase and the B-subunit of propionyl-CoA carboxylase, Proc. Natl. Acad. Sci. USA., 83:2047.

Kuhar, M.J., Murrin, L.C., 1978, Sodium-dependent high affinity choline uptake, J. Neurochem., 30:15.

Lloyd, K.G., 1978, Neurotransmitter interactions related to central dopamine neurons, in, "Essays in Neurochemistry and Neuropharmacology," M.B.H. Youdim, W. Lovenberg, D.F. Sharman, J.R. Lagnado, ed., Wiley, Chichester.

Lynch, G., Baudry, M., 1984, The Biochemistry of Memory: A new and specific hypothesis, Science., 224:1057.

Mann, D.M.A., Yates, P.O., 1982, Is the loss of cerebral cortical choline acetyltransferase activity in Alzheimer's disease due to degeneration of ascending cholinergic nerve cells? J. Neurol. Neurosurg. Psych., 45:936.

May, P.C., Grey, P.M., 1985, L-homocysteic acid as an alternative cytotoxin for studying glutamate-induced cellular degeneration of Huntington's disease and normal skin fibroblasts, Life Sci., 37:1483.

McGeer, P.L., McGeer, E.G., Fibiger, H.C., Wickson, V., 1971, Neostriatal choline acetylase and cholinesterase following selective brain lesions, Brain Res., 35:308.

McKhann, G., Drachman, D., Folstein, M., Katzman, R., Price, D., Stadlan, E.M., 1984, Clinical diagnosis of Alzheimer's disease: Report of the NINCDS-ADRDA work group under the auspices of department of health and human services task force on Alzheimer's disease, Neurology., 34:939.

Neary, D., Snowden, J.S., Bowen, D.M., Sims, N.R., Mann, D.M.A., Yates, P.O., Davison, A.N., 1986 Cerebral biopsy in the investigation of presenile dementia due to cerebral atrophy, J Neurol. Neurosurg. Psychiat., 49:157.

Palmer, A.M., Procter, A.W., Stratmann, G.C., Bowen, D.M., 1986, Excitatory amino acid-releasing and cholinergic neurones in Alzheimer's Disease, Neurosci. Letts., 66:199.

Palmer, A.M., Francis, P.T., Bowen, D.M., Benton, J.S., Neary, D., Mann, D.M.A., Snowden, J.S., 1987, Catecholaminergic neurones assessed ante-mortem in Alzheimer's disease, Brain Res., in press.

Pearson, R.C.A., Esiri, M.M., Hiorns, R.W., Wilcock, G.K., Powell, T.P.S., 1985, Anatomical correlates of the distribution of the pathological changes in the neocortex in Alzheimer disease, Proc. Nat. Acad. Sci. USA., 82:4531.

Perry, E.K., 1986, The cholinergic hypothesis - ten years on, Brit. Med. Bull., 42:63.

Perry, E.K., Gibson, P.H., Blessed, G., Perry, R.H., Tomlinson, B.E., 1977, Neurotransmitter enzyme abnormalities in senile dementia, J. Neurol. Sci., 34:247.

Pope, A., Hess, H.H., Lewin, E., 1965, Microchemical pathology of the cerebral cortex in pre-senile dementia, Trans. Am. Neurol. Assoc., 89:15.

Price, D.L., Whitehouse, P.J., Struble, R.G., Clarke, A.W., Coyle, J.T., De Long, M.R., Hedreen, J.C., 1982, Basal forebrain cholinergic systems in Alzheimer's disease and related dementias, Neurosci. Commentaries, 1:84.

Procter, A.W., Bowen, D.M., 1987, Ageing, the central neocortex and psychiatric disorder, in: "Neurochemistry of Ageing," P. Davies, C.E. Finch, ed., Banbury Report, Cold Spring Harbor Laboratory, NY.

Rossor, M., Garrett, N.J., Johnson, A.L., Mountjoy, C.Q., Roth, M., Iversen, L.L., 1982, A post-mortem study of the cholinergic and

GABA systems in senile dementia, <u>Brain</u>, 105:313.

Rossor, M., Iversen, L.L., 1986, Non-cholinergic neurotransmitter abnormalities in Alzheimer's disease, <u>Brit. Med. Bull.</u>, 42:70.

St George-Hyslop, P.H., Tanzi, R.E., Polinsky, R.J., Haines, J.L., Nee, L., Watkins, P.C., Meyers, R.H., Feldman, R.G., Pollen, D., Drachman, D., Growdon, J., Bruni, A., Foncin, J-F., Salmon, D., Frommelt, P., Amaducci, L., Sorbi, S., Placentini, S., Stewart, G.D., Hobbs, W.J., Conneally, P.M., Gusella, J.F., 1987, The genetic defect causing familial Alzheimer's disease maps on chromosome 21, <u>Science</u>, 235:885.

Sims, N.R., Bowen, D.M., Allen, S.J., Smith, C.C.T., Neary, D., Thomas, D.J., Davison, A.N., 1983, Presynaptic cholinergic dysfunction in patients with dementia, J. Neurochem., 40:503.

Sims, N.R., Bowen, D.M., 1987, Recent studies of cholinergic and other neurochemical changes in early-onset Alzheimer's disease, <u>in</u>: "Cellular and Molecular Basis of Cholinergic Function," M.J. Dowdall, ed., Ellis Horwood, Chichester.

Smith, C.J., Perry, E.K., Perry, R.H., Candy, J.M., Johnson, M., Bonham, J.R., Dick, D.J., Fairbairn, A., Blessed, G., Birdsall, N.J.M., 1987, Muscarinic cholinergic receptor subtypes in hippocampus in human cognitive disorders, J. Neurochem., in press.

Tarbit, I, Perry, E.K., Perry, R.H., Blessed, G., Tomlinson, B.E., 1980, Hippocampal free amino acids in Alzheimer's Disease, <u>J. Neurochem.</u>, 35:1246.

Tomlinson, B.E., Irving, D., Blessed, G., 1981, Cell loss in the locus coeruleus in senile dementia of Alzheimer type, <u>J. Neurol. Sci.</u>, 49:419.

Tucek, S., 1985, Regulation of acetylcholine synthesis in the brain, <u>J. Neurochem.</u>, 44:11.

Walker, L.C., Kitt, C.A., DeLong, M.R., Price, D.L., 1985, Noncollateral projections of basal forebrain neurons to frontal and parietal neocortex in Primates Brain, <u>Brain.</u>, 15:307.

White, P., Goodhardt, M.J., Keet, J.P., Hiley, C.R., Carrasco, L.H., Williams, I.E.I., Bowen, D.M., 1977, Neocortical cholinergic neurons in elderly people, <u>Lancet</u>, i:668.

Wilcock, G.K., Esiri, M.M., Bowen, D.M., Smith, C.C.T., 1982, Alzheimer's disease. Correlation of cortical choline acetyltransferase activity with the severity of dementia and histological abnormalities, <u>J. Neurol. Sci.</u>, 57:407.

Winblad, B., Adolfsson, R., Gottfries, C.G., Oreland, L., Roos, B.E., 1978, Brain monoamines, monoamine metabolites and enzymes in physiological ageing and senile dementia <u>in</u>: "Recent Developments in Mass Spectrometry in Biochemistry and Medicine," A. Frigerio ed., Plenum, New York.

Whitehouse, P.J., Price, D.L., Struble, R.G., Clark, A.W., De Long, M.R., 1982, Alzheimer's disease and senile dementia: loss of neurons in the basal forebrain, <u>Science</u>, 215:1237.

Whitehouse, P.J., Martino, A.M., Price, D.L., Kellar, K.J., 1985, Reductions in nicotinic but not muscarinic cholinergic receptors in Alzheimer's disease measured using [3]H-acetylcholine, <u>Ann. Neurol.</u>, 18:145.

# SLEEP, EEG AND SLEEP DISORDERS IN ALZHEIMER'S DISEASE

P. Prinz and M. Vitiello

American Lake VAMC & Dept. of Psychiatry, Univ. of Wash.
Seattle, Washington 98195

Impairment of sleep-wake function is a common clinical
observation of demented individuals; nighttime insomnia and
wandering in cognitively impaired geriatric patients is
often a factor in a family's decision to institutionalize an
impaired relative. These clinical observations of impaired
sleep have been confirmed by objective sleep laboratory
studies. This chapter will describe these changes and
explore possible explanations including several factors
known to cause sleep disorders and examine the usefulness of sleep and EEG measures as aids in the diagnosis of
Alzheimer's Disease (AD).

## Sleep in Alzheimer's Disease

Disturbed sleep-wake function can result from a variety of
known pathologies, listed in the current nosology of sleep
disorders, or may result from dementia. Profound sleep
changes have been observed in diagnosed dementia patients
(Feinberg, et al., 1967; Prinz, et al., 1982a; Prinz, et
al., 1982b; Reynolds, et al., 1985; Eisdorfer and Cohen,
1978).
In our study of individuals with advanced stage, institutionalized AD (Prinz, et al., 1982a), frequent, lengthy
awakenings, decreased rapid eye movement (REM) sleep and
reduced EEG slow wave (SW) sleep (Stages 3 and 4) were
observed compared to aged matched normal controls. Similar
significant changes of a lesser magnitude were observed in
individuals with earlier, mild and moderate stages of AD
(Prinz, et al., 1982). Both of these studies utilized
subjects selected for minimal health problems and minimal
depression (Prinz, et al., 1982a; Prinz, et al., 1982b).
Depression was carefully controlled for since dementia often
co-exists with depression (Reifler, et al., 1982; Albert,
1981; Eisdorfer and Cohen, 1978; Haase, 1977; Libow, 1977)
and depression can cause decreased SW sleep, increased
wakefulness and altered REM sleep measures (Kupfer, et al.
1978; Reynolds, et al., 1983; Gillin, et al., 1981).

Diagnostic, demographic, cognitive and sleep measures are summarized in Tables 1, 2 and 3 for four groups: control, mild, moderate and severe probable AD patients. Our laboratory employs DSMIII and research diagnostic criteria (Prinz, et al., 1982a; Prinz, et al., 1982b) for probable AD. These diagnostic criteria have been confirmed histologically at autopsy in 15 of 17 patients (88%). Level of functional impairment was used to assign AD patients to groups, with the mild group showing some impairment of daily function, the moderate group more extensive impairment, and the severe group almost complete impairment. Results are based on nights 2 and 3 of a 72 hour stay by each subject on the Clinical Research Center, University Hospital.

Significant changes in sleep occurring in the early, mild stage of the disease include increased nighttime wakefulness, increased sleep fragmentation and reductions in SW wave sleep measures. Overall, these changes become more pronounced with increasing severity of the disease (Table 3). No changes in amounts of stage 1 or 2 sleep were observed. REM sleep measures decreased nonsignificatly in the mild stage, with further, significant reductions in more advanced stages of the disease (Table 3).

While discouraged, napping was allowed and recorded in all cases. Inclusion of nap data to create 24 hour measures of minutes of SW and minutes of REM did not alter the results shown in Table 3. Naps consisted primarily of stages 1-2 sleep and wakefulness.

Certain REM sleep measures are known to be altered in depression (Kupfer, et al., 1978; Reynolds, et al., 1983). REM latency (min sleep prior to the onset of the first REM period) and number and density of rapid eye movements in the first REM period are among the more useful biological markers for this disorder. To determine if any changes in REM measures occur in AD, we carefully examined REM sleep in a subset of nine control and nine mild, nine moderate, and nine severe AD subjects (Vitiello, et al., 1984). REM latency, REM time, and computer assessed REM activity and REM density were determined. REM sleep measures were minimally affected by mild dementia. No REM sleep variable differed significantly in comparing mild AD subjects with controls (Table 4). However, REM time and REM latency (calculated to include intervening wakefulness) were significantly affected in moderate and severe AD. This latter measure is confounded by the general increase in nighttime wakefulness due to AD (Tables 3 and 4). REM latency calculated to exclude intervening wakefulness was unaffected by dementia (Table 4), a finding in agreement with Reynolds, et al. (1985). Next, we quantitated REM activity and density measures using computer methods for possible AD effects. We failed to observe significant differences from controls, with the exception of the severest, institutionalized, AD subjects. In this group, both REM activity and density were significantly lower than controls (Table 4). The observations that mild to moderate AD has minimal effects on REM activity, density and timing of the first REM period are of particular importance given that these measures are all significantly altered by major depression. Consequently, they may prove useful in diagnostic discrimination of mild dementia from depression (Reynolds, et al., 1983; Vitiello, et al., 1984).

## EEG Variables in Dementia

The clinical EEG is sometimes altered in dementia (Obrist and Busse, 1965; Wells, 1978). Reviewing the clinical EEG measures that change across the continuum from adulthood through nondemented old age to the organic brain syndrome, Obrist and others (Mundy-Castle, 1954; Miyasaka, et al., 1978; Gordon and Sim, 1967; Johannesson, et al., 1979) noted two specific measures that appear to correlate best with the degree of mental deterioration: (1) the alpha rhythm over the occipital region or dominant occipital frequency (DOF) and (2) diffuse slow waves in the waking EEG.

DOF undergoes slowing with age from averages of 10.5 cps to of 8 - 9.5 cps in normal elderly individuals (Otomo, 1966; Brazier, et al., 1944). It should be noted that DOF differs from alpha frequency in a standard clinical EEG reading in that it is based on systematic frequency counts averaged across many epochs spanning 9-11 hours (Prinz, et al., 1982b). Our results indicate that DOF is significantly slower (below the alpha range) in mild AD than controls with progressive slowing as the disease advances (Table 5).

Diffuse slowing as evaluated qualitatively in the clinical EEG is sometimes useful in diagnosis of early AD (Gordon and Sim, 1967). Quantitative measures of diffuse slowing have been sought by ourselves and others (Miyasaka, et al., 1978; Otomo, 1966; Brazier, et al., 1944) using computer assisted waveform analyses, such as power spectra or linear modeling. We employed power spectral analyses to quantitate the activity in the delta, theta and alpha bands during waking and various stages of sleep in our subject populations. Table 5 summarizes some of the results. Of all the measures studied, delta activity in the waking EEG (D W) was most affected by AD, being significantly increased in mild AD with further increases as the disease progressed. This is consistent with observations from clinical electroencephalography. Conversely, delta abundance during SW sleep (D SW) was non-significantly reduced in mild dementia with further reductions observed in later stage AD (Table 5).

Sleep can be disrupted by many factors. One possible cause is the primary neuronal degeneration underlying AD. Because of our particular interest in the effects of primary neuronal degeneration, we undertook to control for other factors known to impair sleep.

## Sleep Disorders in Dementia

Sleep disorders have been categorized according to etiology or main features. Major categories include disorders associated with psychophysiological (tension-anxiety) states, psychiatric states (e.g., depression), drug use, sleep related respiratory dysfunction (apnea), sleep related myoclonus, medical, toxic and environmental conditions, and circadian rhythm abnormalities (shiftwork, bedrest).

Any of these disorders may affect sleep-wake function in a given dementia patient with adverse effects that may worsen the dementia. It is useful to consider whether the dementia impairs sleep directly, as opposed to increasing pathologies known to impair sleep (e.g., apnea, myoclonus).

We attempted to examine these questions, using the same study populations described earlier. The physical and history used in screening subjects minimized the likelihood of observing many sleep disorders known to exist in aged populations. In these subjects depression was minimal, history for psychophysiological insomnia was negative, subjects were drug free for one month prior to and during the study, and medical and toxic conditions were excluded (e.g., obesity, hypertension, diabetes). However, sleep related respiratory dysfunction, nocturnal myoclonus and circadian rhythm abnormalities could not be controlled for in this fashion. Consequently, these factors were assessed separately.

We examined apnea-hypopnea activity during sleep in 30 aged controls and in 15 dementia patients with mild to moderate AD (Smallwood, et al., 1983). A sex effect was observed with males demonstrating significantly more apnea-hypopnea activity. No dementia effect was observed in male groups. Because the number of female AD subjects was small (N=4), dementia effects could not be adequately assessed (Figure 1). A subsequent study of females (Frommlet, et al., 1986) observed a significant AD effect. In a similar study (Reynolds, et al., 1985), a comparable negative dementia effect was observed among male subjects; however, female dementia patients had considerably more apnea than female controls (but did not differ from male AD patients). We conclude that AD effects on apnea, while present among females, are not of great magnitude in early AD. Reynolds and coworkers observed a positive correlation between dementia severity and apnea activity, suggesting that an interaction between Alzheimer's disease and sleep apnea phenomena develop as AD progresses in severity. As Reynolds, et al. (1985), point out, widespread use of sleeping pills and other CNS depressants among cognitively impaired geriatric patients might have a deleterious effect on sleep apnea, which in turn can adversely affect cognition.

Nocturnal Myoclonus was examined by quantitating period leg movements (PLMS) resulting in arousal or lightening of sleep stage in a group of 19 controls and 18 mild stage AD patients (Prinz, et al., 1986). As shown in Table 6, no dementia or sex effects were observed. The total number of PLMS resulting in either arousal or lightening of sleep stage across the night's sleep was comparable for the controls and for the mild AD subjects. Few subjects exceeded the clinical criterion of five or more PLMS per hour of sleep.

We also assessed circadian rhythm function by monitoring 24 hour rectal temperatures in 16 controls and 28 dementia patients in the mild to moderate stages of AD (Prinz, et al., 1984). A sex effect was observed, confirming a previous study in young adults (Winget, et al., 1977) showing higher temperatures in females than males at all clock times. No dementia effect were observed; mean 24 hour temperature, amplitude of the day vs. night difference in temperature, and timing of the peak and trough of the temperature rhythm were all unaltered by AD (Table 7). It is unlikely that circadian rhythm abnormalities are induced by dementia per se, in the absence of other factors (e.g., drugs, lack of exercise).

These negative findings regarding pathologies impairing

sleep were obtained using healthier subjects in the earlier stages of dementia.  It can be expected that some AD patients will suffer from the pathologies just as in the general population of older adults.  Early diagnosis and treatment can forestall the additional decline in mental function caused by these conditions (Vitiello and Prinz, 1986).

## Early Identification of Dementia

The negative findings regarding known sleep pathologies in mild AD led us to conclude that AD sleep changes can be largely attributed to the primary neuronal degeneration that characterizes AD.  At present there are no therapeutic interventions capable of halting or slowing this process.  Earlier identification of this disease, though diagnostically difficult, is important if we are to address preventative therapeutic strategies and/or attempt intervention prior to widespread neuronal damage.  Some anatomical evidence supports the hypothesis that sleep variables may serve as markers for the early stages of AD.  Signs of neuronal degeneration occur  in AD in cortical, presynaptic cholinergic nerve terminals which originate mainly from the nucleus basalis of Meynert in the basal forebrain (McKinney, et al., 1982), a structure which may have sleep promoting properties (Sterman and Clemente, 1974).  Other brain areas considered important in sleep/wake functioning also undergo degenerative changes in AD (reviewed in Prinz, et al., 1982b).

As we have observed, sleep and EEG changes in AD do in fact appear early in the disease process.  Indeed, they may serve as markers for onset of AD as suggested by our observation that sleep and EEG variables predict well for mild dementia and for cognitive scores in the mild dementia range (Prinz, et al., 1982b).  We conducted discriminant analyses (DA) to assess the ability of the sleep and EEG variables to correctly classify subjects into control or mild dementia groups (Prinz, et al., 1982b; Vitiello, et al., 1984).  Of the sleep and waking measures utilized, percent waking of time in bed (% W TIB), and percent stage 3 and 4 of time in bed (%3-4 TIB) emerged as the best classifiers, correctly identifying 90% of the mild AD and control subjects.  When EEG and REM measures were also included in the analysis, variables such as % W TIB, DOF, and various computer-derived measures (abundance of delta EEG activity during REM sleep and during slow wave sleep) correctly classified significant percentages (65-90%) of mild dementia and control subjects (Tables 8 and 9).  These observations are of course preliminary, and definitive conclusions must await cross-validation using new subject samples.  Such validation studies are currently in progress in our laboratory.

Our current research efforts continue to evaluate how well sleep-wake and EEG measures might aid in the early diagnosis of AD, even when the clinical picture is confounded by coexisting depression.  In addition, we are examining these and similar measures in older subjects who may be at risk for dementia, to determine their potential usefulness as prognostic indicators for subsequent development of Alzheimer's Disease.

TABLE 1. CRITERIA FOR INCLUSION IN DEMENTIA RESEARCH PROJECT

Selected for inclusion will be patients who have a mild to moderate or severe senile or presenile dementia, defined as a global impairment of intellect and memory associated with organic brain disease.[1] Patients will be further selected as having probable dementia of the Alzheimer's type[2] according to the following criteria[3] (based on current and prior physical exam and history data):

1. Dementia, non-vascular type
   a. Gradual onset in later life
   b. No history of cerebrovascular accident or chronic hypertension
   c. No focal neurological signs
2. No history of
   a. Myocardial infarction or chronic hypertensive cardiovascular disease
   b. Alcoholism
   c. Major chronic or recurring psychiatric illness
   d. Parkinson's disease, Huntington's chorea, Pick's disease and related neurological disorders selectively affecting certain brain regions
   e. Chronic renal, hepatic, pulmonary or endocrine disease
   f. Syphillis or other disease affecting the central nervous system
   g. Brain damage sustained earlier from any known cause, such as hypoxia, neurotoxins or head trauma
3. Not requiring therapy for
   a. Diabetes mellitus or other major endocrine disease
   b. hypertension (less than 150/95)
4. EEG and/or CT scan confirming absence or cerebrovascular accidents or other focal intracranial pathology

Patients are included if free of temporary illness or psychoactive medication for one or more months prior to the study.

---

[1] Organic brain syndrome: acquired chronic deterioration of intellectual function secondary to damaged or lost brain tissue.

[2] Dementia resulting from primary neuronal degeneration with resultant specific neuropathologic changes similar to the classic Alzheimer's disease. Cardinal manifestations include impaired memory (greatest for recent events), impaired attention span and impaired cognition, especially abstraction, calculation, judgement and spatial relations. While disturbances of affect may also occur, these are not invariably present.

[3] These criteria are consistent with those stated in the diagnostic manual (DSM III) of the APA.

TABLE 2.  GROUP RESULTS FOR DEMOGRAPHIC, AFFECTIVE AND
COGNITIVE OF THE CONTROL (N=22) AND MILD (N=18),
MODERATE (N=16) AND SEVERE (N=10) DEMENTIA GROUPS
IN PERCENT OR MEAN SEM

|  | Control[2] | Mild[2] | Moderate[2] | Severe[2] |  |
|---|---|---|---|---|---|
|  | N=22 | N=18 | N=16 | N=10 |  |
| SEX | M=50% | M=50% | M=63% | M=100% |  |
| AGE | 69.0+1.4 | 67.8+2.2 | 70.2+1.5 | 72.8+3.5 |  |
| EDUC. (YRS.) | 14.2+1.2 | 15.2+0.8 | 15.1+0.8 | 12.6+1.5 |  |
| HAMILTON | 4.9+0.4 | 7.2+0.5 | 8.4+1.1 | * | * |
| RDC MAJOR[1] | 0% | 6.7% | 8.3% | * | * |
| RDC MINOR[1] | 18.2% | 13.3% | 8.3% | * | * |
| TOTAL DRS[3] | 137.5+1.1 | 104.9+5.0 | 35.3+8.2 |  |  |
| Attention | 35.8+0.3 | 34.4+0.7 | 15.6+3.2 |  |  |
| Initiation | 36.2+0.3 | 24.5+2.4 | 6.6+2.3 |  |  |
| Construct | 4.9+0.4 | 2.2+0.5 | 0.4+0.1 |  |  |
| Concept | 36.7+0.7 | 30.5+2.1 | 9.0+3.1 |  |  |
| Memory | 23.8+0.3 | 13.4+1.1 | 2.4+0.9 |  |  |
| BOSTON NAMING | 9.7+0.1 | 6.3+0.6 | 3.4+0.6 | * |  |
| MINI MENTAL STATUS | 29.6+0.2 | 16.7+1.3 | 5.4+0.9 | 1.3+0.6 |  |

1   Measures of depressive affect were not reliable in some
    dementia subjects; measures are reported for 15 milds
    and 12 moderates.

2   The severity grouping was based on Activity of Daily
    Living (ADL) scores (6).

3   Dementia Rating Scale (6)

*   Severe patients could not be assessed adequately.

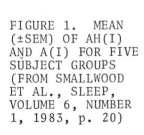

FIGURE 1.  MEAN
(±SEM) OF AH(I)
AND A(I) FOR FIVE
SUBJECT GROUPS
(FROM SMALLWOOD
ET AL., SLEEP,
VOLUME 6, NUMBER
1, 1983, p. 20)

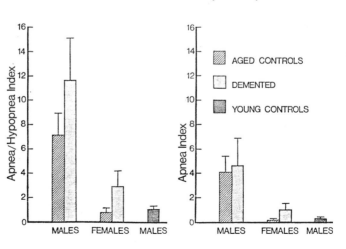

TABLE 3: SLEEP MEASURES IN CONTROL AND DEMENTIA GROUPS.
MEAN $\pm$ SEM (See group description in Table 1)

| | Control N=22 | Mild N=18 | Moderate N=16 | Severe N=10 |
|---|---|---|---|---|
| **A.  SLEEP CONTINUITY** | | | | |
| %W TIB | 21.0+1.5 | 35.7+2.0* | 40.2+4.6 | 36.5+5.0 |
| WASO | 83.4+6.2 | 151.0+11.2* | 163.6+25.3 | 170.1+28.6 |
| No. W | 13.6+1.0 | 17.7+ 1.1* | 19.6+ 2.1 | 20.6+ 3.8 |
| **B.  SLEEP ARCHITECTURE** | | | | |
| % 3-4** TIB | 8.9+1.1 | 5.0+ 0.9* | 2.4+ 0.9 | 1.8+ 1.1 |
| Min 3-4** | 40.4+4.9 | 23.7+ 4.4* | 11.5+ 4.2 | 7.2+ 4.7 |
| % REM TIB | 16.8+0.9 | 13.8+ 1.7 | 9.1+ 1.3 | 7.3+ 1.5 |
| Min REM | 77.2+4.4 | 66.9+ 8.6 | 44.0 +7.3 | 33.4+ 6.1 |

VARIABLE DEFINITIONS

SLEEP CONTINUITY

% W TIB:   Percent time awake expressed as a ratio to time in bed (TIB).
WASO:      Waking after sleep onset; min awake between sleep onset and final morning awakening.
No. W:     Number of wakes $\geq$ 1 min during sleep.

SLEEP ARCHITECTURE

% 3-4 TIB:   Percent time stages 3 and 4 sleep expressed as a ratio to TIB.
Min 3-4:     Minutes of stages 3 and 4 sleep.
% REM TIB:   Percent time REM sleep expressed as a ratio to TIB.
Min REM:     Minutes of REM sleep for entire night.

1.   Time in bed was similar across all groups (456+8.1, 486.6+14.6, 455.5+26.3, and 475.3+23.8 min., respectively).

*    Mild groups differs from control, $p < 05$.

**   Strict criteria were used in rating: delta waves of 75 V peak to peak were required for rating of stages 3 or 4.

TABLE 4.   REM LATENCY AND REM SLEEP MEASURES (X + SEM) OF
          THE FOUR STUDY GROUPS FOR REM PERIODS 1, 2 AND 3,
          AND FOR THE TOTAL NIGHT

| Variable | Control(n) | Mild (n) | Moderate (n) | Severe(n) |
|---|---|---|---|---|
| REM Latency | | | | |
|   REM LAT* | 67.2+ 8 | 86.5+13 | 125.2+18 | 111.5+25 |
|   REM LATS | 53.8+ 8 | 53.2+ 8 | 70.3+14 | 57.5+16 |
| REM period | | | | |
|   REMP  1 | 13.6+ 3 | 21.2+ 3 | 14.8+ 4 | 5.9+ 2 |
|   2* | 23.0+ 4 | 19.3+ 3 | 12.5+ 4 | 8.6+ 2 |
|   3 | 24.5+ 5 | 18.4+ 3 | 17.0+ 4 | 13.2+ 5 |
|   T* | 85.9+ 9 | 66.4+11 | 51.2+10 | 30.4+ 6 |
| REM activity | | | | |
|   REMA  1 | 20.3+ 7 | 53.3+20 | 33.4+20 | 5.4+ 2 |
|   2 | 30.4+ 7 | 39.6+16 | 53.0+35 | 12.3+ 7 |
|   3 | 57.5+25 | 19.0+ 7 | 27.4+17 | 5.6+ 4 |
|   T | 36.9+35 | 124.1+32 | 108.2+51 | 26.0+13 |
| REM density | | | | |
|   REMD  1 | 1.2+0.3 | 2.2+.4 | 1.8+0.6 | 0.7+.3 |
|   2 | 1.7+0.4 | 1.8+.6 | 2.5+1.2 | 1.3+.7 |
|   3 | 2.0+0.7 | 0.9+.3 | 1.3+0.5 | 0.7+.3 |
|   T | 1.8+0.4 | 1.9+.5 | 1.5+0.5 | 0.7+.3 |

*  Moderate and Severe groups differ from controls, p<0.05.
   T tests comparing mild and control groups were non-
   significant for all measures shown.

REM MEASURES DEFINED

| | |
|---|---|
| REM LAT: | REM latency; min from sleep onset to first REM period including waking. |
| REM LATS: | REM latency; min from sleep onset to first REM period, not including waking. |
| REMA T: | REM activity total night.  Number of REM's(12) during all REM periods. |
| REMA 1: | REM activity in 1st REM period only. |
| REMD T: | REM density, total night.  REMA/min REM for all REM periods. |
| REMD 1: | REM density, 1st REM period only. |
| REM PER 1: | Min REM in the first REM period. |

TABLE 5.  GROUP RESULTS FOR EEG MEASURES (Mean $\pm$ SEM)

| EEG Measures | Control N=22 | Mild N=18 | Moderate N=16 | Severe N=10 |
|---|---|---|---|---|
| DOF | $9.10\pm.15$ | $7.8\pm.3$* | $6.62\pm.42$ | $6.40\pm.45$ |
| D W | $223\pm50$ | $635\pm115$* | $831\pm132$ | $1,078\pm151$ |
| D SW | $5,020\pm632$ | $3,892\pm318$ | $2,204\pm253$ | $2,530\pm382$ |

* Mild differs from control group, $p<05$.

VARIABLE DEFINITIONS:

DOF:  Dominant occipital frequency in the quiet, waking EEG when rhythmicity is most pronounced.

DW:   EEG abundance (power) in the delta band (0.5 to 4 Hz) during waking (C3 vs. A2).

DSW:  As above, during a slow wave sleep sample that best approximates stage 4 for each subject.


TABLE 6.  PERIODIC LEG MOVEMENTS (PLMS) AND MYOCLONUS INDEX (MI, OR NUMBER OF PLMS PER HOUR OF SLEEP) IN MALE (M) AND FEMALE (F) GROUPS OF CONTROLS (CONT) AND ALZHEIMER'S DISEASE (AD) PATIENTS.  MI>5 IS THE PROPORTION OF THE TOTAL GROUP HAVING MORE THAN 5 PLMS PER HOUR OF SLEEP

| | | MI | PLMS | MI > 5 |
|---|---|---|---|---|
| M | AD | $2.7\pm2$ | $15.0\pm9$ | 2/9 |
| | CONT | $1.7\pm0.8$ | $11.0\pm6$ | 1/9 |
| F | AD | $1.5\pm0.7$ | $8.0\pm3$ | 0/8 |
| | CONT | $1.6\pm1$ | $9.7\pm7$ | 0/10 |

TABLE 7.  TWENTY-FOUR-HOUR RECTAL AND RECTAL EQUIVALENT
TEMPERATURE IN AGED NORMALS AND IN ALZHEIMER'S
DEMENTIA.  RESULTS FROM COSINOR ANALYSES, WITH
COMPARATIVE YOUNG NORMAL SUBJECT DATA (34)

| Group | Mean 24-hr deg. C | | Amplitude Max-Min deg. C | |
|---|---|---|---|---|
| | M | SEM | M | SEM |
| Aged, healthy men (n=8)[a] | 37.25 | .07 | .96 | .07 |
| Alzheimer's men (n=16)[a] | 37.14 | .07 | 1.06 | .14 |
| Aged, healthy women (n=8)[a] | 37.17 | .07 | .80 | .14 |
| Alzheimer's women (n=12)[a] | 37.35 | .07 | .86 | .06 |
| Winget's young women (n=12) | 37.45 | .12 | .72 | .04 |
| Winget's young men (n=37) | 37.02 | .05 | .93 | .03 |

Time (hrs. min.)

| Group | Peak Temperature | | Lights Out | |
|---|---|---|---|---|
| | M | SEM | M | SEM |
| Aged, healthy men (n=8)[a] | 1704 | 0138 | 2326 | 049 |
| Alzheimer's men (n=16)[a] | 1629 | 0122 | 2259 | 116 |
| Aged, healthy women (n=8)[a] | 1600 | 0135 | 2318 | 022 |
| Alzheimer's women (n=12)[a] | 1600 | 0137 | 2229 | 031 |
| Winget's young women (n=12) | 1626 | | 2400 | |
| Winget's young men (n=37) | 1644 | | 2200 | |

[a]Mesor, amplitude, and acrophase data based on cosinor
analysis.  Amplitude and phase results based on significant cosinor fits only; n=8,8,8, and 9 for male control,
male Alzheimer's, female control, and female Alzheimer's
groups, respectively.

### TABLE 8. VARIABLE GROUPINGS AND DEFINITIONS USED IN DISCRIMINANT ANALYSES

A. Sleep Continuity

1. % W TIB:   Percent time awake expressed as a ratio to time in bed (TIB).
2. WASO:      Waking after sleep onset; min awake between sleep onset and final awakening
3. No. W:     Number of wakes ≥ 1 min during sleep.

B. Sleep Architecture

1. % 3-4 TIB:   Percent time stages 3 and 4 sleep expressed as a ratio to TIB.
2. Min 3-4:     Minutes of stages 3 and 4 sleep.
3. % REM TIB:   Percent time REM sleep expressed as a ratio to TIB.
4. Min REM:     Minutes of REM sleep for entire night.

C. REM Measures

1. REM LAT:    REM latency; min from sleep onset to first REM period.
2. REM LATS:   REM latency; min from sleep onset to first REM excluding waking.

D. EEG Frequency

1. DOF:   Dominant occipital frequency in the quite, waking EEG when rhythmicity is most pronounced.

E. EEG Abundance (Power) in the Less Synchronized EEG

1. D W:    in delta band during waking
2. T W:    in theta band during waking
3. A W:    in alpha band during waking
4. D REM:  in delta band during REM
5. T REM:  in theta band during REM
6. A REM:  in alpha band during REM

F. EEG Abundance (Power) in the More Synchronized EEG

1. D NR:   in delta band during non-REM
2. T NR:   in theta band during non-REM
3. A NR:   in alpha band during non-REM
4. D SW:   in delta band during 3-4 sleep
5. T SW:   in theta band during 3-4 sleep
6. A SW:   in alpha band during sleep

TABLE 9.  RESULTS OF STEPWISE DISCRIMINANT ANALYSES
(DA's). THE BEST SIGNIFICANT DISCRIMINATOR
FOR EACH VARIABLE GROUP (SHOWN) WAS
ENTERED IN THE OVERALL DISCRIMINANT MODEL
FOR CLASSIFYING CONTROLS VS. MILD DEMENTIA
SUBJECTS (A-F). "WAKE EEG" GROUP INCLUDED DOF,
DW, TW AND AW

| Group | Significant Variables | $Rc^2$ | %Corr. Classified |
|-------|----------------------|--------|-------------------|
| A: | % W TIB | .696 | 82.5 |
| B: | % 3-4 TIB | .401 | 65.0 |
| C: | REM LAT | .332 | 62.5 |
| D: | DOF | .527 | 75.0 |
| E: | D REM | .527 | 77.5 |
| F: | D SW | .318 | 76.5 |
| A+B | % W TIB | | |
| | %3-4 TIB | .733 | 90.0 |
| E+F: | D REM | | |
| | D SW | | |
| | A SW | .691 | 85.0 |
| WAKE EEG: | DOF | | |
| | DW | .614 | 80.0 |
| A-F: | % W TIB | | |
| | DOF | .764 | 85.0 |

RESULTS OF SIMULTANEOUS DA USING FIRST 6 VARIABLES ABOVE

| Group | Significant Variables | $Rc^2$ | %Corr. Classified |
|-------|----------------------|--------|-------------------|
| A-F: | % W TIB | | |
| | % 3-4 TIB | | |
| | DOF | | |
| | D SW | | |
| | D REM | | |
| | REM LAT | .811 | 92.5 |

1.  Depression (RDC diagnosis) and sex failed to enter
    into each analysis.

2.  Correlation between the discriminant variable(s) and
    the group variable.

# REFERENCES

1.  Association of Sleep Disorders Centers, Diagnostic Classification of Sleep and Arousal Disorders, First Edition, prepared by the Sleep Disorders Classification Committee, Roffwarg H, Chairman, Sleep 2:1-137, 1979.

2.  Brazier M, Finesinger F and Jacob E: Characteristics of the electroencephalogram. A study of the occipital cortical potentials in 500 norma adults. J Clin Invest 23:303-311, 1944.

3.  Feinberg U, Koresko R, and Heller N: EEG Sleep patterns as function of normal and pathological aging in man. J Psych Res, 5:107, 1967.

4.  Frommlet M, Prinz P, Vitiello M, Ries R and Williams D: Sleep Hypoxemia and Apnea are Elevated in Females With Alzheimer's Disease. Sleep Research, 1986.

5.  Gillin J, Duncan W, Murphy D, Post R, Wehr T, Goodwin F, Wyatt R, and Bunney W: Age-related changes in sleep and depressed and normal subjects. Psychiat Res 4:73, 1981.

6.  Gordon E and Sim M: The EEG in presenile dementia. J Neurol Neurosurg Psychiat 30:285, 1967.

7.  Johannesson G, Brun A, Gustafson I, and Ingvar D: EEG in presenile dementia related to cerebral blood flow and autopsy findings. Acta Neurol Scand 56:89, 1977.

8.  Johannesson G, et al.: EEG and cognitive impairment in presenile dementia. Acta Neurological Scandinavia 59:225-240, 1979.

9.  John E: Neurometric evaluation of brain dysfunction related to brain disorders. In Melin K (ed.): Second Workshop on Memory Functions, Acta Neurologica Scandinavia, Supplement 89, 64:87-100, 1981.

10. Katzman R and Karasu T: Differential diagnoses of dementia. In Fields W (ed.), Neurologic and Sensory Disorders in the Elderly, Stratton Inter-Continental Medical Book Corp., New York, 1975.

11. Kaszniak W, Fox J, and Bandell, D: Predictors of mortality in presenile and senile dementia. Ann Neurol 3:246, 1978.

12. Kupfer D, Spiker O, Coble P, and Shaw D: Electroencephalographic sleep recordings and depression in the elderly. J Am Geriat Soc 26:2:53-57, 1978.

13.  McKinney M, Kedreen J, and Coyle J:  Cortical cholinergic innervation: Implications for pathophysiology and treatment of Alzheimer's disease.  In Corkin S, et al. (eds.): Alzheimer's Disease: A Report of Progress (Aging, Vol. 19), Raven Press, New York, 1982.

14.  Miyasaka M, et al.:  The mental deterioration in the aged and the computerized EEG analysis.  Folia Psychiatrica et Nurological Japonica 32, 1:95-108, 1978.

15.  Mortimer J, Schuman L and French L:  Epidemiology of dementing illness.  In J Mortimer and L Schuman (eds.): The Epidiomology of Dementia, Oxford University Press, New York, 3024, 1981.

16.  Mundy-Castle, A, et al.:  The EEG in the senile psychoses.  EEG and Clinical Neurophysiology 6:245-252, 1954.

17.  Obrist W and Busse E:  The electroencephalogram in old age.  In Wilson W (ed.): Applications of Electroencephalography in Psychiatry: A Symposium. Durham, NC, Duke University Press, 1965.

18.  Obrist W:  EEG changes in normal aging and dementia. Brain Function in Old Age, 102-111, Bayer-Symposium VII, Springer-Verlag, 1979.

19.  Otomo E:  Electroencephalography in old age: Dominant alpha pattern.  Electroenceph Clin Neurophysiol 21:489, 1966.

20.  Prinz P, Peskind E, Vitaliano P, Raskind M, Eisdorfer C, Zemcuznikov N, and Gerber C:  Changes in the sleep and waking EEG in nondemented and demented elderly.  J Amer Geriatr Soc. 30:86-93, 1982a.

21.  Prinz P, Vitaliano P, Vitiello M, Peskind R, Bokan J, and Gerber C:  Sleep, EEG and mental function changes in dementia.  Neurobiology of Aging, 3:4, 361-370, 1982b.

22.  Prinz P, Christie C, Smallwood R, Vitaliano P, Bokan J, Vitiello M, and Martin D:  Circadian Temperature Variation in Healthy Aged and in Alzheimer's dementia.  Journal of Gerontology 39:30-35, 1984.

23.  Prinz P, Frommlet M, Vitiello M, Ries R and Williams D:  Periodic Leg Movements are Unaffected by Mild Alzheimer's Disease.  Sleep Research, 1986 (in press).

24.  Reifler B, Larson E, and Hanley R:  Coexistence of Cognitive impairment and depression in geriatric outpatients.  American Journal of Psychiatry 139:5, 623-26, 1982.

25. Reynolds C, Spiker D, Hanin I, and Kupfer D: Electroencephalographic sleep, aging, and psychopathology: New data and state of the art. Biol Psychiatr 18:139-155, 1983.

26. Reynolds C, Kupfer D, Taska L, Hoch C, Spiker D, Sewitch D, Zimmer B, Marin R, Nelson J, Martin D, and Morycz R: EEG Sleep in Elderly Depressed, Demented and Healthy Subjects. Biol Psychiatry 20:431-442, 1985.

27. Reynolds, C, Kupfer D, Taska L, Hoch C, Sewitch D, Restifo K, Spiker D, Zimmer B, Marin R, Nelson J, Martin D, and Morycz R: Sleep apnea in Alzheimer's dementia: Correlation with mental deterioration. J Clin Psychiatry 46:257-261, 1985.

28. Smallwood R, Vitiello M, Giblin E, and Prinz P: Sleep apnea: Relationship to age, sex and Alzheimer's dementia. Sleep 6:16-22, 1983.

29. Vitiello M, Kukull W, and Prinz P: Sleep/Waking and EEG pattern classification of Alzheimer's dementia. Sleep Research 13:213, 1984.

30. Vitiello M, Bokan J, Kukull W, Muniz R, Smallwood R, and Prinz P: Rapid eye movement sleep measures of Alzheimer's-type dementia patients and optimally healthy aged individuals. Biological Psychiatry 19:721-734, 1984.

31. Vitiello M and Prinz P: Aging and Sleep Disorders, in Williams and Karacan (eds.), Sleep Disorders: Diagnosis and Treatment, Second Edition, John Wiley and Sons, Inc., New York, 1986.

32. Wells C: Chronic brain disease: An overview. American Journal of Psychiatry 135:1-47, 1978.

33. Winget C, Deroshia C, Vernikos-Danellis J, Rosenblatt W, and Hetherington N: Comparison of circadian rhythm in male and female humans. Waking and Sleeping 1:356-363, 1977.

# ON POSSIBLE RELATIONSHIPS BETWEEN ALZHEIMER'S DISEASE, AGE-RELATED MEMORY LOSS AND THE DEVELOPMENT OF ANIMAL MODELS

Raymond T. Bartus[1,2] and R. L. Dean[1]

[1]Department of CNS Research, American Cyanamid Company
Medical Research Division, Lederle Laboratories
Pearl River, NY  10965

[2]New York University Medical Center
New York, NY  10016

## INTRODUCTION

Aged humans, and other mammals, exhibit a variety of bio-behavioral changes ranging from decreases in muscle tone and motor coordination to impairments of sensory and cognitive abilities. Among the earliest, most consistent, and potentially most devasting of these changes are deficits in memory and related cognitive functions.

Senile dementia (especially Alzheimer's disease) is recognized as the most serious malady associated with age related cognitive decline. It is considered to be the number one health problem by the National Institute on Aging (NIA) (Goldsmith, 1984) and is considered by organizations within both the executive (USDHHS, 1984) and legislative branches of the federal government to be reaching epidemic proportions in the United States (OTA, 1985). The incidence at age 65 is one out of ten, and increases to approximately one out of three by age 85 (USDHHS, 1984). Because this latter segment of our population is experiencing the most dramatic increases in absolute and relative numbers, problems associated with dementia are complicated even further and will undoubtedly worsen during the next decade. The disease progresses insidiously, eventually destroying the functional capacity of the brain. This is first manifested in loss of memory and in other cognitive disturbances, but eventually progresses to the point where its victims are unable to perform the simplest tasks and can no longer care for themselves (Reisberg, Ferris, & Crook, 1982). Most often this leads to institutionalization or a similar radical solution, at tremendous emotional and financial burdens to families and society (Anderson, 1981; Cowell, 1983; Gwyther & Blazer, 1984).

Despite the tremendous attention directed toward the memory loss and related cognitive disturbances of Alzheimer's disease, age-related cognitive disturbances are hardly restricted to Alzheimer's patients. For example, it is now becoming recognized that even normal aging is associated with a selective loss of certain mental abilities, especially those requiring or involving memory. In fact, impairments in memory for recent events appear to be the price paid by members of all mammalian species that are successful in surviving into the post-reproductive, senescent years (Bartus & Dean, 1985).  In humans, normal age-related loss of memory is considered to be one of the most consistent and de-humanizing consequences of aging (Kral, 1978; Weinberg, 1980; Crook, Bartus, Ferris, Whitehouse, Cohen & Gershon, 1986).  The number of patient to physician complaints is also high, with approximately 90% of people over age 65 expressing concern (Zelinsky, in press).

Although the decline in memory ability in normal aging in no way approaches the more severe and broader loss of mental capacity seen in Alzheimer's disease, the effects on the individual and family can be dramatic, nevertheless (e.g., see Bartus, 1986; Crook, et al. 1986).

Despite the obvious financial and emotional consequences of age-related cognitive impairments and the clear projections for increased incidence as population longevity increases, there is no currently available treatment with established therapeutic efficacy.  The search for such therapies has been hampered by the complexity of the nervous system and our limited knowledge of the biological basis of normal cognition, as well as by difficulties in identifying and establishing the functional importance of age-related neurobiological changes.

In other words, progress continues to be retarded by the lack of a solid foundation of basic information and a clearly defined direction for systematic inquiries.  Historically, the biomedical community has been helped in similar situations by the application of data from animal models.  The underlying question addressed in this paper is whether our understanding of the neurobiology of aging is sufficiently advanced and sophisticated to permit data from animals to be utilized by medicinal chemists, pharmacologists and clinicians, in the search for effective treatments for age-related cognitive disturbances.

Efforts to develop valid and reliable animal models of geriatric congitive deficiencies have only recently begun to attract widespread attention.  Past isolated attempts to use animal models of geriatric memory generally were hampered by poorly founded rationales and inade-quate empirical support for their underlying assumptions (Bartus, Flicker & Dean, 1983).  Consequently, there is little genuine consensus regarding the best approach to adopt, although almost everyone would agree that the ultimate animal model for geriatric memory disturbances has yet to be developed.  Nevertheless, research spanning the last few years has produced significant progress which may have important impli-cations for geriatric assessment of memory.

ON THE LIMITATIONS AND EXPECTANTCIES OF CURRENT ANIMAL MODELS

Although there may be some general agreement regarding what factors or variables are likely to be important in developing effective animal models, in the final analysis the value of any model will depend not on the inherent logic of the principles which guided its development, but on its ability to make meaningful predictions about the clinical condi-tion it was designed to study.  In this regard, it is important to consider exactly what specific questions the model is being asked to answer and exactly what types of predictions are being made in the study of the diseases.

One issue which is clearly relevant, but which has received insuf-ficient recognition, is the fact that the study of any disease involves numerous, interdependent levels of analysis.  With regard to neurode-generative diseases like Alzheimer's, these levels of study would in-clude such categories as etiologic factors, molecular biology and pharmacology, neural functional disturbances, neurobehavioral deficits, and specific behavioral or clinical measurements (Bartus & Dean, 1985).  Certainly, investigations which focus attention on areas at opposite ends of this spectrum will differ radically in terms of the nature of the questions asked, the types of studies performed, and the answers obtained.

For example, studies of the role of neurotoxic, genetic, immunological and viral influences upon the progression of Alzheimer's disease would seem to be necessary in order to understand the etiology of Alzheimer's disease. Similarly, examination of the development and consequences of neurofibrillary tangles, senile plaques, and possible changes in DNA, RNA, and protein synthesis, may help identify the molecular mechanisms responsible for the progressive neuronal damage. Alternatively, although the identification of disturbances in neural function and biochemical processes may reveal little about the root cause of the disease, they may help establish important final common pathways responsible for the primary symptomatic cognitive disturbances. This insight should, in turn, suggest effective strategies for more immediate, shorter-term treatment of the disease's major symptomatology. Additionally, this research might ultimately reveal areas of selective vulnerability to the disease which may help expand our understanding of how the etiologic variables produce their progressive damage.

It should be apparent, therefore, that just as the level of inquiry will greatly affect the types of questions asked and studies performed, it will also affect the nature and intended purpose of any model employed, as well as the particular considerations used in developing or selecting the model. For example, when the etiology and pathogenesis of neurodegenerative diseases are considered, specialized cell lines, tissue cultures and other molecular approaches provide valuable tools for addressing the issues of concern. At the same time, the usefulness or relevance of these tools to understanding the nature of the clinical symptoms or neurological variables involved is often less clear.

Alternatively, neurobehavioral models of the type described in previous papers (e.g., Bartus, Flicker, Dean, Fisher, Pontecorvo, & Figueiredo, 1986; Kordower & Gash, 1986; Olton, 1985), involving artificial brain lesions in animals, may not be appropriate for many questions, but could prove to be quite useful for studying possible relationships between relevant neural dysfunctions and behavioral deficits, as well as for evaluating potential pharmacological treatment approaches for the primary symptomatology. In other words, although such models will neither mimic the etiology nor much of the neuropathology associated with Alzheimer's disease, properly placed lesions (e.g. of nucleus basalis; septal-hippocampal-entorhinal complex; locus coeruleus) can provide animal models which share certain, important neurodegenerative, neurochemical and even behavioral deficits characteristic of Alzheimer's diseased patients.

From this perspective, it is apparent that even aged animals may serve as useful models for certain specific types of questions concerning Alzheimer's disease. While it is well-recognized that animals do not contract Alzheimer's disease, and most aged animals develop few of the neuropathological features of the disease, these differences may only be important for certain types of questions. For example, it seems unlikely that aged animals would offer much information about the root cause of the disease or the primary variables involved in the pathogenesis of Alzheimer's disease. However, because aged animals share certain neurochemical deficiencies with Alzheimer's disease patients (Bartus, et al. 1982; Zornetzer, 1985), and because aged animals suffer memory deficits which are conceptually similar to loss of memory observed in the earliest stages of Alzheimer's disease (Bartus & Dean, 1985; Bartus et al. 1982), aged animals might be useful in investigations of the neural basis of the memory loss and in evaluations of potential treatment approaches. In fact, this viewpoint has been raised and briefly discussed in prior publications (Bartus & Dean, 1985; Bartus, Flicker & Dean, 1983).

Presumably, as more is learned about degenerating human diseases, and more sophisticated approaches are adopted in the development and application of animal models, differences between the clinical condition and the animal model will decrease significantly, as will differences in the issues addressed at various levels of inquiry. In the meantime, however, it would seem that serious confusion might be reduced and certain pseudo issues avoided by properly recognizing that clear differences exist among current levels of inquiry. These differences have important implications with regard to the specific questions addressed, the assumptions made, the short-term goals set, the optimal species or specimens used, and the type of model employed. Since the present paper is concerned primarily with age-related memory loss, the remainder of the text will restrict itself to means of using animals to develop in vivo models of this behavioral loss, as one essential component to studying the problem.

ON THE SIMILARITY OF CROSS-SPECIES MEMORY LOSSES AND THE USE OF AGED ANIMALS

Of the many approaches to developing animals models of age-related memory disturbances, one that is gaining increasing popularity involves the use of aged animals. During the last several years, a number of laboratories have tested relatively healthy, aged animals on numerous, behavioral tasks and have demonstrated that a progressive, age-related loss of memory represents one of the most consistent and robust behavioral changes (Bartus & Dean, 1985). Perhaps this phenomenon is most clearly revealed in the series of studies published with nonhuman primates by a number of laboratories over the last two decades (Bartus, 1979; Bowden & Williams, 1984; Davis, 1978; Dean & Bartus, 1986). These studies convincingly demonstrate that while aged primates suffer deficits on a number of behavioral paradigms, other behaviors appear to be relatively spared by the effects of age. Moreover, the most impressive deficit occurs on tasks involving recent, or trial-specific memory, typically measured by requiring monkeys to remember the spatial location of a visual stimulus over brief intervals of time (Dean & Bartus, 1986). Control tests suggest the deficit is at least partly dependent on memory for recent (but not immediate) information and relatively independent of other potentially confounding variables. For example, the magnitude of this deficit is generally small at short retention intervals, but increases dramatically as the duration of the retention interval is increased. Additionally, age-related dysfunctions in motivation, sensory processing, and motor performance do not adequately account for the behavioral deficit. Rather, the inability of the aged monkeys to perform accurately on the longer retention intervals appears to reflect a genuine dysfunction in mnemonic mechanisms mediating the storage, maintenance, or retrieval of information. This deficit in recent, trial-specific memory contrasts markedly with the lack of age effects observed on the longer-term retention of well-learned stimulus-reinforcement associations formed through multiple trial experiences.

In view of comparisons in various studies that equated past and current living conditions between age groups, these nonhuman primate data suggest that the age-related loss of recent memory is dependent, at least in part, upon a biological dysfunction. Further, replications in both New World and Old World monkeys underscore the generality of this phenomenon (Dean & Bartus, 1986). Additionally, a number of clinical laboratories have recently begun to develop human test paradigms which are conceptually similar to those used in nonhuman primate laboratories, and these human studies have confirmed the existence of similar age-related deficits in non-demented elderly volunteers (Oscar-Berman & Bonner, 1985; Flicker et al. 1985; Flicker et al. 1984; Moss & Albert, 1984).

In sum, the series of studies performed with aged monkeys and humans demonstrates that: (a) certain common behavioral losses exist in both demented and non-demented elderly humans and nonhuman primates, (b) a loss of recent memory is generally recognized as one of the earliest and most severe behavioral consequences in each group, and (c) it is likely that common biological factors contribute to the problem.

Although more difficult to ascertain, studies with aged rodents generally support the idea that specific behavioral deficits develop with advanced age, with a loss of recent, trial-specific memory being among the more prevalent (Bartus, Flicker & Dean, 1983; Kubanis, Gobbel & Zornetzer, 1981). To be certain, comparisons of rodents to humans are often more difficult, and extrapolating behavioral data from one to the other seems, at least superficially, more hazardous and complicated. At a minimum, the more primitive behavioral repetoire of the rodent makes the paradigms that can be used to test it necessarily more distant from human behavior (as it is conventionally viewed today) and limits the number and elegance of additional tests that can be performed. Further, it is more difficult to establish experimental control of the rodents' behavior in learning/memory paradigms, requiring the use of strongly adversive stimuli (such as electrical shock) when punishment and negative reinforcement are used, or severe physiological states of deprivation (reduction to 65-80% of ad lib body weight is common) when positive reinforcement is used (Bartus & Dean, 1985). Notwithstanding these serious obstacles, data from a number of laboratories suggest some degree of analogy exists in the type of memory loss which occurs in aged humans and nonhuman primates versus that which apparently exists in aged rats and mice.

A number of laboratories have tested various aged groups of rats and mice on a variety of behavioral paradigms. Of all the behaviors measured, the most striking deficits in both aged mice and rats occur on retention of a simple, single-trial passive avoidance task (Bartus, Flicker & Dean, 1983). Control tests showed that the deficits could not be explained on the basis of differences in shock threshold, activity levels, or other confounding factors, but rather reflected an impairment in ability to remember the learned aversive event for sufficiently long periods of time. For example, it has been shown that differences in motor activity and shock response threshold cannot explain the age-related differences in retention. Further, the performance of the aged rodent was comparable to that of the young rodent when retention was tested within one hour after training but gradually worsened as the interval of time between training and retention testing was increased. Thus, despite the relative crudeness of the passive avoidance procedure, these findings strongly suggest that a memory-related phenomenon is involved in this age deficit (Bartus, 1982).

The robustness of the age-related deficit is particularly striking when one considers that the passive avoidance procedure is basically a simple task for the subjects to perform. It is well established that with all things equal, the less complex a task is for aged subjects to perform, the smaller the age-related deficit generally observed. Thus, the robustness of this deficit suggests that this particular procedure may measure some fundamental aspect of neurological aging in the rodent. At the same time, it is interesting and noteworthy that a simple and effective means of eliminating the passive avoidance deficit in aged rats is simply to arrange the procedure so that it requires rats more than a single trial to learn the task (Bartus, 1982). In this multi-pretrial version of the procedure, aged rats are able to learn the task at about the same rate as young rats and retention is comparable, even when measured 2 weeks after training.  Of course, one of the more salient operational differences between recent, trial-specific memory and long-term, repetitive trial memory, involves the consistent repetition of the event to be remembered.  Thus, the data from this variation of the passive avoidance paradigm support the idea that a selective vulnerability of recent memory also occurs with advanced age in rodents.

Further, these rodent data are reminiscent of prior data in non-human primates in which controlled comparisons demonstrated significant effects of age when the behavioral paradigm required temporary, non-practiced recall of stimulus events over short intervals of time, but no deficits when the paradigm required trial by trial learning of reinforcement contingencies and subsequent tests of recall days later.  In fact, on a more general level, the passive avoidance deficit shares certain operational similarities with the primary age-related deficits in both human and nonhuman primates (Bartus & Dean, 1985).  That is, some of the more robust and consistent deficits observed in aged members of several mammalian species, including humans, occur (1) in situations where the event to be remembered is brief and discrete; (2) when little or no opportunity for practice or rehearsal exists; and (3) over a relatively rapid temporal span, with retention often declining markedly within minutes, and usually within hours (Bartus & Dean, 1985).  Taken together, the data suggest that a conceptually similar type of age-related memory decline may exist across various members of the mammalian class.

The similarity in certain primary memory deficits in aged animals and aged humans presents a number of potentially important implications.  First, the variety of mammalian species exhibiting the deficits, and the varied paradigms employed, argue strongly that a common biological component most likely contributes to the behavioral symptoms.  This, in turn, implies that studying aged animals which are inflicted with these neurobehavioral disturbances might provide meaningful information for helping to understand the complex problem of cognitive disturbances in elderly humans.  Finally, animal models derived from these efforts might be used to help develop pharmacological approaches to the problem and evaluate specific drug candidates to determine which might deserve more exhaustive and difficult testing in human patients.  A number of previous reviews (Bartus, Dean, Beer, 1983; Bartus & Dean, 1985; Bartus, Flicker & Dean, 1983) have described some of the early efforts to accomplish these goals.

## ON THE USE OF ANIMALS WITH DISCRETE BRAIN LESIONS

Although the research described above argues that it may be possible to gain some insight into certain types of treatment approaches for Alzheimer's disease from the study of normally aged animals, there is little question that greater predictability might be achieved with an animal model that shares more of the neuropathological and abberant neurochemical characteristics found in Alzheimer patients.  Earlier attempts to induce neurofibrillary tangles in animals artificially via aluminum (Crapper and Dalton, 1972; 1973) have been disappointing, neither providing greater insight into the nature of the disease nor leading to more effective means of testing drugs to treat its symptoms.  Other attempts to produce an animal model through injection of presumed transmissible agents may continue to hold promise, but have so far been equally disappointing (Klatzo, et al. 1965; Wisniewski, et al. 1975).

More recently, however, evidence of severe deterioration in the nucleus basalis of Meynert in Alzheimer and other demented patients

(Whitehouse, et al. 1981; 1982; Rogers, et al. 1985) has given new momentum to the development of potential animal models of the disease. This formerly obscure brain region is recognized as providing the major extrinsic cholinergic input to the cortex (Johnston, et al. 1979) and its degeneration in Alzheimer's disease most likely accounts for the severe loss of cortical CAT activity and other cholinergic markers which now characterize the brain from Alzheimer patients. Artificial destruction of this brain region in animals would certainly not be expected to produce an exact model of Alzheimer's disease, including such classic neuropathological features as senile plaques and neurofibrillary tangles. Nevertheless it would provide an animal model that shares many of the other CNS deficiencies associated with the disease, including loss of cortical CAT activity, reduced cortical high affinity choline uptake, and degeneration of basal forebrian cholinergic neurons. Furthermore, destruction of the homologous brain region in animals provides a means of determining the functional consequences of such nucleus basalis degeneration, thus providing one empirical test of its possible role in the cognitive loss of Alzheimer's disease and other degenerative disorders. If loss of CAT-containing cholinergic neurons in the basal forebrain can be causally linked to a specific decline in memory, then it might be possible to use animals with the perturbation as a valid model of the primary neurobehavioral characteristics of Alzheimer's disease. Such an animal model might greatly facilitate the search for alternative pharmacological approaches and help reduce the number of candidates for human testing.

Within the last few years a number of laboratories have studied the behavioral consequences of destroying cholinergic neurons originating in the NBM. Of course, one goal of this research is to develop an animal model of some of the primary neurobehavioral symptoms of Alzheimer's disease. Although it is still too early to determine how successfully this goal will be met, the studies being conducted are producing some intriguing results and raising a number of interesting empirical issues. The first issue involves the question the role the NBM (and its cortical cholinergic projections) may play in mediating memory. It has been shown that destruction of this brain region can produce a profound loss of memory for recent events, while leaving other types of memory relatively unimpaired (see Bartus, et al. 1985). Thus, these data clearly support the idea that this group of neurons (and their cortical cholinergic efferents) play an important and potentially quantifiable role in mediating recent memory. Certainly, the observation of a gradual behavioral recovery observed by several laboratories (Bartus, et al. 1986; Bartus et al. 1985; Dunnett, 1985; Hepler, et al. 1985; Ridley, et al. 1985) by no means invalidates the functional implications of the lesion effects initially observed. Indeed, there exist numerous examples of comparable recovery of behavioral function following brain lesions (Finger & Stein, 1982; Lashley, 1929; LeVere, 1980). Rather, the specificity and severity of the memory loss initially inflicted by the lesion strongly implicates some role for the nucleus and its pathway in mediating recent memory. This conclusion remains valid in spite of the eventual recovery that occurred with extensive training, and independent of whether or not any neural compensatory changes might ever be found.

The second issue concerns the role that cell loss in the nucleus basalis (and its presumed relationship to decreased cortical CAT activity) may play in the early symptoms of Alzheimer's and other neurodegenerative diseases. Certainly, the profound and specific loss of memory following damage to the basal forebrain-cortical cholinergic system provides a strong argument for a possible role. Moreover, the operational similarities between the artificially-induced deficit and the memory loss found to occur spontaneously in aged rodents, primates, humans and early-stage Alzheimer patients, make the argument for an important role even more compelling. At the same time, however, complete recovery of the memory deficit has been observed, which is certainly contrary to the prognosis given for patients with Alzheimer's disease, or any of the degenerative diseases in question. A major question which presents itself is whether recovery would occur if the lesion had been given to older animals which suffer a number of additional, age-related neurofunctional disturbances (Bartus, 1979; Bartus, et al. 1982; 1985; Kubanis, Gobbel & Zornetzer, 1981), possibly including a reduced capacity to recover lost neurobehavioral function (Mufson & Stein, 1980; Stein & Firl, 1976). Also of interest would be the effects of combining lesions of the basal forebrain with other areas also implicated in Alzheimer's disease (such as the hippocampus or locus coeruleus). Clearly pertinent to this point are recent preliminary findings in monkeys which suggest that although more robust and reliable effects are obtained with combined septum/NBM lesions, recovery of the deficit still occurs after several months of training (Mishkin, et al. 1985).

From a similar perspective, the question of the functional significance of the classic neuropathology of Alzheimer's disease (i.e. neurofibrillary tangles and amyloid plaques) must be considered; perhaps this neuropathology must coexist with the neurodegeneration to cause the severe and permanent loss of cognitive function characteristic of diseases such as Alzheimer's. In other words, given the apparent complexity of these diseases and their clinical manifestations, it seems reasonable to consider that simultaneous degeneration of a number of brain regions, or the existence of a number of different pathologies, may be required to produce not only the profound and permanent loss of memory and related cognitive skills, but also the insidious progression of the symptoms seen in these diseases.

Finally, from a different perspective, might it be possible to significantly reduce the functional loss associated with Alzheimer's disease by providing intense, routine practice and remedial training of daily living skills? Clearly, attention to these many issues must be a concern for future research.

In summary, additional experimental work in both primates and rodents, as well as with postmortem tissue from various demented and non-demented patient populations, is clearly needed. Future studies should help clarify the role that various brain regions play in mediating behavior, and their relationship to the cognitive loss associated with aging and dementia. Although it is unreasonable to expect studies with animals to unravel single-handedly the complex mysteries of human Alzheimer's and other dementing diseases, information gained from such studies, and new thinking generated by the questions raised, should ultimately contribute to a more complete understanding. Whether the preliminary drug studies (Davis, et al. 1982; Ridley et al, 1986; Murray & Fibiger, 1985) which have thus far employed NBM-lesioned animals will develop into a legitimate means of directing pharmaceutical development and clinical decisions remains to be clarified by additional, extensive studies.

ACKNOWLEDGEMENT

The authors gratefully acknowledge the clerical assistance of Rhonda J. Sheppard in the preparation of this manuscript.

REFERENCES

Anderson, O. W., 1981, The social strategy of disease control: the case of senile dementia, in: "Clinical Aspects of Alzheimer's Disease and Senile Dementia," N. E. Miller and G. D. Cohen, eds., Raven Press, NY.

Bartus, R. T., Flicker, C., Dean, R. L., Fisher, S., Pontecorvo, M. and Figueiredo, J., 1986, Behavioral and biochemical effects of nucleus basalis magnocellularis lesions: implications and possible relevance to understanding or treating Alzheimer's disease, in: "Progress in Brain Research," Vol 70, E. Fliers, ed., Elsevier, NY.

Bartus, R. T., Pontecorvo, M. J., Flicker, C., Dean, R. L. and Figueiredo, J. C., 1986, Behavioral recovery following bilateral lesions of the nucleus basalis does not occur spontaneously, Pharmacol Biochem & Behav., 24:1287-1292.

Bartus, R. T., 1986, Drugs to treat age-related cognitive disorders: on the threshold of a new era in the pharmaceutical industry? in: "Treatment Development Strategies for Alzheimer's Disease," T. Crook, R. T. Bartus, S. Ferris, and S. Gershon, eds., Powley Assoc. Inc., Madison, CT.

Bartus, R. T. and Dean, R. L., 1985, Developing and utilizing animal models in the search for an effective treatment for age-related memory disturbances, in: "Physiological Aging and Dementia," C. Gottfries, ed., Karger Press, Basle.

Bartus, R. T., Flicker, C., Dean, R. L., Pontecorvo, M. J., Figueiredo, J. and Fisher, S. K., 1985, Selective memory loss following nucleus basalis lesions: long term behavioral recovery despite persistent cholinergic deficiencies, Pharmacol Biochem Behav., 23:125-135.

Bartus, R. T., Dean, R. L. and Beer, B., 1983, An evaluation of drugs for improving memory in aged monkeys: implications for clinical trials in humans, Psychopharmacol Bull., 19:168-184.

Bartus, R. T., Flicker, C. and Dean, R. L., 1983, Logical principles for the development of animal models of age-related memory impairments, in: "Assessment for Geriatric Psychopharmacology," T. Crook, S. Ferris, and R. T. Bartus, eds., Mark Powley Assoc. Inc., Canaan, CT.

Bartus, R.T., Dean, R. L., Beer, B. and Lippa, A. S., 1982, The cholinergic hypothesis of geriatric memory dysfunction, Science 217:408-417.

Bartus, R. T., 1982, The one-trial passive avoidance procedure as a possible marker of aging, in: "Biological Markers of Aging," M.E. Reff and E.L. Schneider, eds., Publication No. 82-2221, (April).

Bartus, R. T., 1979, Effects of aging on visual memory, sensory processing and discrimination learning in the non-human primate, in: "Aging, Vol 10: Sensory Systems and Communication in the Elderly," J. M. Ordy, and K. Brizzee, eds., Raven Press, NY.

Cowell, D. D., 1983, Senile dementia of the Alzheimer's type: a costly problem, J Geriatrics Soc., 31:61.

Crapper, D. R. and Dalton, A. J., 1973, Aluminum induced neurofibrillary degeneration, brain electrical activity and alteration in acquisition and retention, Physiol Behav., 10:935-945.

Crapper, D. R. and Dalton, A. J., 1972, Alterations in short-term retention, conditioned avoidance response acquisition and motivation following aluminum induced neurofibrillary degeneration, Physiol Behav., 10:925-932.

Crook, T., Bartus, R. T., Ferris, S., Whitehouse, P., Cohen, G. D., and Gershon, S., 1986, Age-associated memory impairment: proposed diagnostic criteria and measures of clinical change, Develop Neuropsychol. (in press)

Davis, K. L., Mohs, R. C., Davis, B. M., Levy, M. I., Horvath, T. B., Ronsberg, G. S., Ross, A., Rothpearl, A. and Rosen, W., 1982, Cholinergic treatment in Alzheimer's disease: implications for future research, in: "Aging, Vol 19: Alzheimer's Disease, A Report of Progress in Research," S. Corkin, K. L. Davis, J. H. Growdon, E. Usdin, and R. J. Wurtman, eds., Plenum Press, NY.

Davis, R. T., 1978, Old monkey behavior, Exp Gerontol., 13:237-250.

Dean, R. L. and Bartus, R. T., 1986, Behavioral models of aging in nonhuman primates, in: "Handbook of Psychopharmacology, Vol 20: Psychopharmacology of the Aging Nervous System," L. L. Iverson, S. D. Iversen, and S. H. Synder, eds., Plenum Press, NY. (in press)

Dunnett, S. B., 1985, Comparative effects of cholinergic drugs and lesions of nucleus basalis or fimbria-fornix on delayed matching in rats, Psychopharmacology (Berlin) 87:357-363.

Finger, S. and Stein, D. G., 1982, "Brain Damage and Recovery: Research and Clinical Perspectives, Academic Press, NY.

Flicker, C., Dean, R., Bartus, R. T. and Fisher, S. H., 1985, Animal and human memory dysfunctions associated with aging, cholinergic lesions, and senile dementia, in: "Memory Dysfunctions: An Integration of Animal and Human Research from Preclinical and Clinical Perspectives," D. S. Olton, E. Gamzu, and S. Corkin, eds., Ann NY Acad Sci., Vol 444.

Flicker, C., Bartus, R. T., Crook, T. H. and Ferris, S. H., 1984, Effects of aging and dementia upon recent visuospatial memory, Neurobiol Aging. 5:275-283.

Goldsmith, M. F., 1984, Youngest institute addresses aging problems, J Amer Med Assoc., 252:2315-2317.

Gwyther, L. P. and Blazer, D. G., 1984, Family therapy and the dementia patient, Amer Family Physician. 29:149-156.

Hepler, D. J., Wenk, G. L., Cribbs, B. L., Olton, D. S. and Coyle, J. T., 1985, Memory impairments following basal forebrain lesions. Brain Res., 346:8-14.

Johnston, M. V., McKinney, M. and Coyle, J. T., 1979, Evidence for a cholinergic projection from neurons in basal forebrain. Proc Nat'l Acad Sci., USA 76:5392-5396.

Klatzo, I., Wisniewski H. and Streicher, E., 1965, Experimental production of neurofibrillary degeneration. J Neuropath Exp Neurol., 24:187-199.

Kordower, J. H. and Gash, D. M., 1986, Animals and experimentation: an evaluation of animal models of Alzheimer's and Parkinson's disease, Integr Psychiatry. 4:64-80.

Kral, V. A,. 1978, Benign senescent forgetfulness, in: "Alzheimer's disease: Senile Dementia and Related Disorders," R. Kataman, R. D. Terry, and K. L. Bick, eds., Raven Press, NY.

Kubanis, P., Gobbel, G. and Zornetzer, S. F., 1981, Age-related memory deficits in Swiss mice, Behav Neural Biol., 32:241-247.

Lashley, K. S., 1929, "Brain Mechanisms and Intelligence: A Quantitative Study of Injuries to the Brain," University of Chicago Press, Chicago, IL.

LeVere, T. E., 1980, Recovery of function after brain damage: a theory of the behavioral deficit, Physiol Psychol., 8:297-308.

Mishkin, M., Aigner, T. G. and Aggleton, J., 1985, Neurobiology of memory in primate brain, Thirteenth International Congress of Gerontology Abstracts.

Mufson, E. J. and Stein, D. G., 1980, Behavioral and morphological aspects of aging: an analysis of rat frontal cortex, in: "The Psychobiology of Aging: Problems and Perspectives," D. G. Stein, ed., Elsevier, NY.

Murray, C. L. and Fibiger, H. D., 1985, Learning and memory deficits after lesions of the nucleus basalis magnocellularis: reversal by physostigmine, Neurosci., 14:1025-1032.

Office of Technology Assessment, United States Congress, 1985, Technology and Aging in America, Washington, DC.

Olton, D. S., 1985, Strategies for the development of animal models of human memory impairments, in: "Memory Dysfunctions: An Integration of Animal and Human Research from Preclinical and Clinical Perspectives," D. S. Olton, E. Gamzu, and S. Corkin, eds., Ann NY Acad Sci., Vol 444.

Oscar-Berman, M., Bonner, R. T., 1985, Matching- and delayed matching-to- sample performance as measures of visual processing, selective attention, and memory in aging and alcoholic individuals, Neuropsychologia. 23(5):639-651.

Reisberg, B., Ferris, S. H. and Crook, T., 1982, Signs, symptoms and course of age-associated cognitive decline, in: "Alzheimer's Disease: A Report of Progress in Research," S. Corkin, K. L. Davis, J. H. Growdon, E. Usdin, and R. J. Wurtman, eds., Raven Press, NY.

Ridley, R. M., Murray, T. K., Johnson, J. A. and Baker, H. F., 1986, Learning impairment following lesion of the basal nucleus of Meynert in the marmoset: modification by cholinergic drugs, Brain Res., 376:108-116.

Ridley, R. M., Baker, H. F., Drewett, B. and Johnson, J. A., 1985, Effects of ibotenic acid lesions of the basal forebrain on serial reversal learning in marmosets, Psychopharmacology (Berlin). 86:438-443.

Rogers, J. D., Brogan, D. and Mirra, S. S., 1985, The nucleus basalis of Meynert in neurological disease: a quantitative morphological study, Ann Neurol., 17:163-170.

Stein, D. G. and Firl, A. C., 1976, Brain damage and reorganization of function in old age, Exp Neurol., 52:157-167.

U.S. Department of Health and Human Services, 1984, Alzheimer's Disease: Report of the Secretary's Task Force on Alzheimer's Disease. (DHHS Publication No. [ADM]84-1323. US Government Printing Office, Washington, DC.

Weinberg, J., 1980, Geriatric psychiatry, in: "Comprehensive Textbook of Psychiatry/III," (3rd ed., Vol. III), H. I. Kaplan, A. M. Freedman, and B. J. Sadock, eds., Williams & Williams, Baltimore, MD.

Whitehouse, P. L., Price, D. L., Struble, R. G., Clark, A. W., Coyle, J. T. and DeLong, M. R., 1982, Alzheimer's disease and senile dementia: Loss of neurons in basal forebrain, Science. 215:1237-1239.

Whitehouse, P. J., Price, D. L., Clark, A. W., Coyle, J. T. and DeLong, M. R., 1981, Alzheimer's disease: evidence for selective loss of cholinergic neurons in the nucleus basalis, Ann Neurol., 10:122-126.

Wisniewski, H. M., Bruce, M. E. and Fraser, H., 1975, Infection etiology of neuritic (senile) plaques in mice, Science. 190:1108-111.

Zelinsky, D., 1986, Complaints of memory loss in community dwelling elderly, in: "The Handbook of Clinical Memory Assessment in Older Adults," L. Poon, ed., American Psychological Assoc., Washington, DC. (in press)

Zornetzer, S. F., 1985, Catecholamine system involvement in age-related memory dysfunction, in: "Memory Dysfunctions: An Integration of Animal and Human Research from Preclinical and Clinical Perspectives," Vol 444, D. S. Olton, E. Gamzu, and S. Corkin, eds., Ann NY Acad Sci.

SEROTONIN, ALZHEIMER'S DISEASE AND LEARNING AND MEMORY IN ANIMALS

Howard J. Normile and Harvey J. Altman

Department of Psychiatry
Wayne State University School of Medicine
Detroit, MI  48207

Alzheimer's disease (AD) is the most tragic and devastating neurologic disorder of the elderly, characterized by personality deterioration and a variety of cognitive disabilities highlighted by memory loss.  The earliest symptom of the disease - an inability to remember recent events - eventually advances to a vegetative state in which the victim may be totally unresponsive, incontinent, incapable of self-care and bedfast.  The memory deficit progresses to where even friends and family members become unrecognizable.  The progression of the disease is highly idiosyncratic, it may take years or only months before it reaches its final stages.  Death then follows.

It is estimated that 5% of the individuals over the age of 65 have AD, affecting perhaps 20% of the persons who reach age 80.  During the next decade, the disease will reach epidemic proportions, simply due to the increasing age of the population.  The disorder is more prevalent in women than in men and there appears to be an increased risk among first-order relatives of AD patients.

During the last few years, research efforts relating to the diagnosis, cause, and treatment of AD have accelerated rapidly.  This is partly due to the increased awareness of the impact of AD, in terms of its prevalence, the emotional pain and personal burden experienced by the victim's family, and the financial cost of institutional care for the patient.  Unfortunately, despite intensive research activity by numerous investigators from a variety of disciplines, the cause of AD is unknown and there is no accepted treatment that can cure or stop the progression of AD.

RESEARCH STRATEGIES

A number of different experimental approaches have been used in the search for an effective treatment of Alzheimer type dementia.  Although each approach involves independent areas of clinical and basic research, it is hoped that the information generated will converge and help identify efficacious treatment strategies for the memory dysfunctions associated with AD.

The first and most frequent approach is the postmortem examination of the brain's of AD patients in an attempt to identify those chemical features that differ quantitatively or qualitatively from healthy age-matched subjects. While this approach may appear straightforward and uncomplicated, considerable care must be taken to account for those changes associated with aging, rather than AD, as well as the possibility that postmortem changes (time interval between death and chemical assessment) may influence the results. In addition, inconsistencies in the neurochemical determinations, observed either within or between laboratories, may indicate the existence of subgroups of AD patients and/or improper patient screening procedures.

A second approach, associated with the first, attempts to determine if the chemical abnormalities observed in AD contribute to the symptomatology. That is, demonstrating that a reduction in chemical X occurs in AD does not establish a functional relation between chemical X and the memory impairments. This approach involves basic research aimed at developing an understanding of the role of chemical X in normal learning/memory processes. In addition, the development of relevant animal models by employing experimental manipulations designed to mimic the disease state in normal animals could help establish the relation between the chemical deficit and the memory disturbance, while simultaneously providing an efficient means to develop, test and refine potential pharmacological treatments.

Another approach to the development of effective treatment strategies for memory dysfunctions in general is the attempt to discover "memory-enhancing" agents. The approach differs from the latter in that it is independent of any theoretical assumptions concerning the cause of the disease or its symptoms. Similarly, the mechanism of action by which the pharmacological agents exert their positive effects may be unknown. This approach is simply a search for memory-enhancing agents whose use may prove efficacious for the treatment of one or more types of dementia. The focus of this approach is on animal behavioral tests in order to develop pharmacological agents that (1) enhance learning and memory of normal animals and/or (2) enhance or protect learning and memory in animals with either a naturally occurring deficit (old animals, poor learners) or a deficit induced by some experimental manipulation (CNS lesions, CNS hypoxia). The potential therapeutic agent may not necessarily have any direct action on the processes underlying learning/memory, but rather produce its positive response indirectly by influencing related processes such as arousal, attention or motivation.

THE CHOLINERGIC HYPOTHESIS

An example of how information derived from these separate experimental approaches can evolve into a working hypothesis is provided by what has come to be known as the "cholinergic hypothesis" of geriatric memory disorders. The foundation for this hypothesis stems from the efforts of numerous investigators in different research disciplines and includes both human and animal experimentation. Early work in the 1960's began to generate evidence supporting an important role for the cholinergic nervous system in learning and memory. A number of investigators showed that experimental manipulations designed to disrupt cholinergic neurotransmission impaired memory in both animals and humans (Longo, 1966; Deutsch and Rocklin, 1967; Dundee and Pandit, 1972). Conversely, increased cholinergic activity was found to enhance memory in young subjects (Davis et al., 1978; Sitaram et al., 1978; Flood et al., 1983).

In the mid 1970's Drachman and Leavitt (1974) reported that the anticholinergic-induced memory deficit observed in young, healthy subjects was quite similar to that found in aged, demented individuals. During this period, three independent laboratories (Bowen et al., 1976; Davies and Maloney 1976; Perry et al., 1977) reported reduced levels of the acetylcholine synthesizing enzyme, choline acetyltransferase (ChAT) in postmortem brains of AD patients, (ChAT is confined to cholinergic cells and

is a viable postmortem marker of the integrity of cholinergic neurons).
Moreover, the reduced levels of ChAT were shown to be correlated with the
density of senile plaques (the major neuropathologic symptom of AD) and with
the severity of dementia exhibited before death (Perry et al., 1978). In
addition, a deficiency in the acetylcholine degradatory enzyme,
acetylcholinesterase, has been observed in brain tissue from AD patients
(Pope et al., 1965; Davies and Maloney, 1976; Atack et al., 1983).

Recently, a cholinergic animal model has been developed that shares
some of the neurochemical and behavioral disturbances associated with AD.
The major source of cholinergic input to the cortex appears to arise from
perikarya located in the nucleus basalis of Meynert (Johnston et al., 1979;
Fibiger, 1982). A loss of a specific population of cells within this region
of the brain has been reported to occur in AD (Whitehouse et al., 1981;
Candy et al., 1983). Destruction of the homologous area in the rat has been
shown to significantly lower cortical ChAT and produce performance deficits
in certain types of memory tasks (Laconte et al., 1982: Flicker et al.,
1983; Friedman et al., 1983; Altman et al., 1985).

This substantial body of information suggests that disturbances in the
cholinergic nervous system occur in AD and that the associative memory
dysfunction may be specifically related to impaired cholinergic function.
In addition, these data suggest the possibility that therapeutic
interventions designed to augment cholinergic neurotransmission might
improve memory in AD patients. Unfortunately, clinical trials aimed at
increasing cholinergic activity have not produced any effective therapy for
AD (Bartus et al., 1982; Brinkman et al., 1982), although trials with
acetylcholinesterase inhibitors are somewhat encouraging and warrant further
investigation (Summers et al., 1981; Beller et al., 1985).

In addition to the continued search for an effective cholinomimetic
agent for use in the treatment of AD, the contributions of other
neurotransmitter systems to the memory disturbances associated with the
disease are also being pursued. That is, there is emerging neurochemical
evidence that AD is a multidimensional disease, possibly affecting a number
of neurotransmitter systems. Furthermore, the cholinergic nervous system is
not the only neurotransmitter system suspected of playing an important role
in the processing of information. Accordingly, a considerable amount of
research effort is currently being directed toward understanding the
relation, if any, between Alzheimer's type dementia and the various chemical
changes reported to occur in AD.

The remainder of this chapter will focus on one such system, the
serotonergic nervous system. Changes in this system have been reported to
occur in AD and will be summarized. How these changes may or may not be
related to some of the clinical symptomatology of the disease will be
addressed by reviewing the results of animal studies which have examined the
effects of altered serotonergic activity on the performance of animals in
various learning and memory tasks. The purpose of the ensuing discussion is
not to suggest a "serotonergic hypothesis" for geriatric memory disorders.
Rather, it serves to provide a summary of data derived from several areas of
research and identify any functional relations that may exist between the
changes in the serotonergic nervous system and the memory disturbances
associated with AD.

SEROTONIN AND ALZHEIMER'S DISEASE

Changes in the functional and structural integrity of the serotonergic
nervous system in AD is indicated by several lines of evidence. Ishii
(1966) was first to report that serotonergic cells in the raphe nuclei of AD
patients frequently showed dense neurofibrillary tangle formation. The

dorsal raphe (DR) nucleus and the median raphe (MR) nucleus were severely affected. Recent studies have reported metabolic abnormalities and cell loss in the raphe (Mann and Yates, 1983; Yamamoto and Hirano, 1985). Although there is some disagreement regarding the relative contribution of these two midbrain nuclei to the serotonin innervation of distinct brain regions, there is general agreement that cells originating in the DR and MR form the major ascending serotonergic pathways of the brain. Based on histochemical fluorescence and autoradiographic tracing techniques, the DR-MR complex appears to project to the striatum, substantia nigra, thalamus, hippocampus, amygdala-olfactory area as well as the temporal, parietal, piriform, cingulate, and frontal cortices (Azmithia, 1978; O'Hearn and Molliver, 1984; Steinbusch, 1984). In addition, there appears to be a wide range of afferents to both the DR and MR, including projections from the hypothalamus, septal-hippocampus complex, locus coeruleus, cingulate cortex and sensorimotor cortex (Azmitia, 1978).

Several investigators have found that serotonin and/or its metabolite, 5-hydroxy-3-indoleacetic acid (5-HIAA) are significantly lower in many areas of postmortem AD brains. Bowen et al. (1979, 1983) reported significant reductions of serotonin in the temporal lobe of AD patients. Winblad et al. (1982) reported marked reductions of serotonin in the hippocampus and hypothalamus, as well as the cingulate, temporal and frontal cortices (Adolfsson et al., 1979; Winblad et al., 1982; Cross et al., 1983). A recent study which investigated the levels of a number of neurotransmitters and their metabolites in 22 regions of histologically verified AD brains found a reduction in the levels of serotonin and 5-HIAA in nine and eight regions, respectively (Arai et al., 1984).

Examination of CSF from patients with a clinical diagnosis of AD have also shown a significant reduction in 5-HIAA levels (Gottfries et al., 1969; Argentiero and Tavolato, 1980, Palmer et al., 1984). In a recent study, Volicer et al. (1985) reported detection of "abnormal forms" of serotonin and its precursor, 5-hydroxytryptamine, in the CSF of AD patients using a novel multisensor coulometric detection system. In addition, turnover of serotonin, as measured in CSF by loading test with probenecid, has been reported to be reduced in AD patients (Gottfries and Ross, 1973). Probenecid blocks passage of acid metabolites across membranes resulting in an accumulation of the metabolites in the CSF and thereby provides an index of serotonin turnover. The blunted rise in CSF 5-HIAA following probenecid thus indicates a reduced or disturbed metabolism of serotonin in the brain. It should be noted, however, that the clinical relevance of alterations in CSF 5-HIAA in AD is uncertain since a large portion of the metabolite is derived from serotonin released within the spinal cord (Bulat and Zivcovic, 1971; Garelis et al., 1974).

Biochemical markers of the serotonergic synapse also appear to be significantly reduced in cortical brain tissue from AD patients. The uptake of serotonin in biopsy samples of temporal cortex was found to be reduced by 72% in AD (Benton et al., 1982; Bowen et al., 1983). Another measurement considered to reflect the integrity of serotonergic terminals is the binding of imipramine. Imipramine binding sites are thought to be associated (although not exclusively) with the serotonin uptake complex. A significant reduction in imipramine binding has been observed in autopsy samples of temporal cortex from AD patients (Bowen et al., 1983).

A significant reduction in the number of serotonin receptors has also been reported to occur in AD (Bowen et al., 1979; Bowen et al., 1983; Cross et al., 1984; Reynolds et al., 1984). Using 3H-LSD (which binds to both serotonin S1 and S2 receptors), Bowen et al. (1979) observed a significant reduction in serotonin receptors in the temporal cortex of postmortem AD brains. More recent studies suggest that the reduction in serotonin receptors is somewhat selective to the S2 receptor subtype. That is, Cross et al. (1986) found that the number of S2 receptors in the temporal cortex was significantly reduced to 57% of controls with no change in the number of S1 receptors. Although reductions in the S1 receptor have been reported (Bowen et al., 1983; Briley et al., 1986), it has been suggested that these changes appear to be associated with only the more severe (early onset) AD cases. For example, Cross et al. (1984) observed a significant reduction in S1 receptors in the temporal cortex, hippocampus and amygdala of AD patients that died at an early age (less than 75 years). These reductions were not significant to AD patients who died over the age of 75. Both of these age groups, however, showed significant reductions in the number of S2 receptors.

While the studies above provide evidence for a loss of pre- and post-synaptic markers of serotonin in AD, the markers are not affected to the same degree in all areas of the brain. For example, in the study by Arai et al. (1984), only 8 of the 22 brain regions examined demonstrated significant reductions in both serotonin and 5-HIAA. Similarly, Cross et al. (1984) reported that serotonin binding to its S1 receptor was significantly reduced in only 3 of the 10 regions assayed. These findings may indicate that the neurofibrillary tangle formation in the raphe nuclei and any concomitant dysfunction in serotonergic neurons originating in the raphe may be secondary to the changes occurring in their projection sites. That is, if abnormalities in the raphe nuclei were the primary changes in AD, then one would expect to observe a somewhat uniform reduction in serotonergic presynaptic markers in many, if not all, of the brain regions innervated by neurons originating in the raphe nuclei.

The data summarized above suggest that serotonergic neurotransmission may be impaired in AD. The consequences of impaired serotonergic activity in terms of the functional deficits in AD may be derived partly from the results of animal studies designed to assess the effects of altered serotonergic activity on learning and/or memory. It should be emphasized that the experimental manipulations employed in the studies summarized below were not used in an attempt to mimic those changes reported to occur in AD. Rather, the studies were generally designed to examine and/or characterize the role, if any, of serotonin in the physiological processes underlying information processing.

SEROTONIN, LEARNING AND MEMORY

A number of observations support a role for brain serotonin in learning and the processing and retrieval of acquired information. This evidence is mainly derived from studies in which depletion of serotonin was found to affect the performance of animals in a variety of learning/memory paradigms. For example, combined electrolytic lesions of the DR and MR nuclei impaired the acquisition of an unsignalled one-way conditioned avoidance response (Lorens et al., 1976; Srebro and Lorens, 1975; Hole and Lorens, 1975), the acquisition and extinction of a straight-alley food-reinforced task (Asin et al., 1979) and the reversal of a Y-maze discrimination habit (Srebro et al., 1975). Electrolytic lesions of both the DR and MR nuclei have been shown to significantly reduce whole forebrain serotonin concentrations (Hole and Lorens, 1975; Srebro and Lorens, 1975) and produce regional reductions in the hippocampus and striatum (Lorens et al., 1976). Electrolytic lesions of the MR nucleus alone have been shown to produce effects similar to those seen after lesions of both midbrain nuclei. Thus, electrolytic MR lesions impaired the acquisition of an unsignalled one-way conditioned avoidance response (Srebro and Lorens, 1975), the acquisition of both a straight-alley food-reinforced single alternation task (Asin et al., 1979) and a T-maze successive brightness discrimination task (Asin et al., 1979) as well as the acquisition of an 8-arm radial maze task (Asin et al., 1979; Asin et al., 1985). Destruction of the MR nucleus also appears to produce retrograde amnesia since MR lesions have been shown to impair retention of a preoperatively learned spatial discrimination task (Wirtshafter and Asin, 1983). The MR nucleus appears to be the primary origin of septal-hippocampal serotonin, also sending fibers to the thalamus, hypothalamus and neocortex (Bobillier et al., 1975; Azmitia and Segal, 1978). Accordingly, electrolytic MR lesions have been reported to significantly reduce serotonin levels in the hippocampus, thalamus, hypothalamus and frontal cortex (Jacobs et al., 1974; Lorens and Guldberg, 1974). It may be relevant that in AD, neurons within the MR nuclei frequently contain dense tangle formation (Ishii, 1966) and that levels of serotonin/5-HIAA have been shown to be significantly reduced in number of brain regions including the hippocampus, thalamus, hypothalamus as well as the temporal and frontal cortices (Adolfsson et al., 1979; Bowen et al., 1979; Winblad et al., 1982; Cross et al., 1983).

In addition to electrolytic lesions of the midbrain raphe nuclei, pharmacological interventions that deplete brain serotonin have been reported to impair the performance of animals in certain types of learning and memory paradigms. For instance, depletion of brain serotonin with the serotonin synthesis inhibitor p-chlorophenylalanine (PCPA) has been reported to impair both active (Valzelli and Pawlowski, 1979) and passive (Stevens et al., 1969) avoidance learning. Likewise, serotonin depletion by the neurotoxin p-chloroamphetamine (PCA) impaired active avoidance acquisition (Ogren et al., 1976). Moreover, interference with serotonergic neurotransmission by either acute or chronic administration of serotonergic receptor antagonists prior to training has been reported to impair active (Hano et al., 1981) and passive (Bammer, 1982; Normile and Altman, 1985) avoidance responding.

While the above results tend to support the view impaired serotonergic function could contribute to the memory dysfunctions in AD, there are a number of reasons why such an interpretation may be premature or at least, simplistic:

1. The effect of serotonin depletions dependent on the type of task used for testing. For example, combined electrolytic lesions of the DR and MR nuclei have been shown to impair the acquisition and retention of an unsignalled one-way active avoidance response (Srebro and Lorens, 1975) and facilitate the acquisition of a signalled two-way active avoidance response (Lorens and Yunger, 1974, Srebro and Lorens, 1975). Moreover, PCA-induced serotonin depletion has been reported to impair signalled two-way active avoidance responding (Ogren et al., 1976), have no effect on unsignalled one-way active avoidance acquisition (Ogren and Johnsson, 1985) and even enhance spatial discrimination learning (Altman et al., 1985).

2. The effect of serotonin depletion is dependent on the procedure by which the depletion is accomplished. That is, electrolytic raphe nuclei lesions have been shown to impair one-way unsignalled active avoidance acquisition (Srebro and Lorens, 1975; Lorens et al., 1976). On the other hand, acquisition was facilitated following depletion of serotonin induced by PCPA (Ogren et al., 1981) while reductions in brain serotonin following PCA administration were without effect (Ogren and Johansson, 1985).

3. Intracranial injections of 5,7-dihydroxytryptamine (5,7-DHT) have failed to affect the performance of animals in a number of tasks. The hydroxylated indoleamines produce a rather selective degeneration of central serotonergic neurons and their terminal systems. Unlike electrolytic raphe nuclei lesions, 5,7-DHT injected into the vicinity of the DR and MR nuclei was found not to affect the acquisition of an unsignalled one-way active avoidance response (Lorens et al., 1976). Similarly, electrolytic midbrain

raphe lesions have been shown to retard the acquisition of a spatial discrimination task (Wirtshafter and Asin, 1983). Intramidbrain 5,7-DHT did not produce the same effect (Asin et al., 1985). Intracranial administration of 5,7-DHT has also been reported to have no significant effect on signalled two-way active avoidance acquisition (Ogren et al., 1981) and the performance of animals in both a delayed spatial alternation task (Asin and Fibiger, 1984) and a one-trial passive avoidance task (Montanaro et al., 1981). These data suggest, in part, that the effects of electrolytic midbrain raphe lesions on information processing may not be due to raphe nuclear damage per se and exemplifies the fact that different experimental manipulations designed to impair serotonergic function can differentially affect performance.

In summary, the available data suggest that the effects of reduced brain serotonin or interference with serotonergic neurotransmission depend on both the experimental methods employed to alter serotonergic activity and the nature of the behavioral task used for testing the animal. It is possible that the different results produced by the various manipulations are caused by different degrees of serotonin depletion and/or regional variations in serotonin levels. Furthermore, since many of the serotonin depletion methods necessitate their use days to weeks prior to behavioral assessment, it is also possible that depletion-induced changes in non-serotonergic systems may contribute to the different effects observed. Finally, the discrepancies observed following reduced serotonergic activity may reflect alterations in sensory processing, locomotor activity and/or task-dependent motivation. That is, a large number of data implicate serotonin in functions such as sleep (Jouvet, 1969), nociception (Roberts, 1984), locomotion (Brodie and Shore, 1957) and appetite (Bundell, 1984). Altered serotonergic activity may produce changes in any one or more of these non-associative processes. This would likely differentially effect the performance of animals in various types of tasks that employ different sensory cues and/or reinforcement contingencies.

FUTURE DIRECTIONS

Although a strong case can be made for the importance of cholinergic dysfunction in the development of the cognitive impairment in AD, and that any effective treatment should involve restoration of cholinergic function, it is becoming increasingly evident that other neurotransmitter systems are affected in AD. Therefore, any neurotransmitter suspected of having a role in the processing of information should be examined for its possible contribution to the cognitive decline in patients with AD. The present chapter has focused on the serotonergic nervous system. However, when compared to the amount of basic and clinic research efforts directly or indirectly relating to other systems (cholinergic, noradrenergic), there is a paucity of research directed toward serotonin - its role in information processing and the symptomatology of AD. Clearly, additional systematic research is required to define and clarify the specific role of the serotonergic nervous system in the processes underlying learning and memory and any contribution that this system may have in the cognitive deficits associated with AD.

Serotonin, learning and memory. There are presently several critical methodological problems with regard to the tools employed to investigate the role of serotonin in learning and memory. For example, 5,7-HDT can cause significant reductions in spinal serotonin levels (Lorens et al., 1976) and can have a substantial neurotoxic action on norepinephrine neurons which can partially, but not totally, be counteracted by pretreatment with norepinephrine uptake blockers (Bjorklund et al., 1975; Hole et al., 1976) Likewise, PCPA is not specific for serotonin and can cause significant reductions in the concentrations of norepinephrine and dopamine (Koe and

Weissman, 1966; Ogren et al., 1981). Electrolytic lesions are not selective for serotonin containing neurons since damage can occur to fibers of passage and non-serotonergic perikarya within the raphe nuclei (Lorens, 1978; Ochi and Shimizu, 1978). Even the serotonergic receptor antagonists demonstrate an affinity for non-serotonergic receptors (Janssen, 1981; Leysen et al., 1981). These observations may not only account for the discrepancies in the results, but also exemplify the need for the development of newer and more selective pharmacological agents that alter serotonergic function.

Further research should be directed toward identifying the specific brain regions or pathways that may be important in the serotonergic-induced response. This could be accomplished by lesioning specific pathways and/or their terminal areas and by the regional application of pharmacological agents that altar serotonergic neurotransmission. In addition, it is clear that multiple types of serotonin receptors exist and that their distribution in the brain is not uniform (Aghajanian and Wang, 1978; Peroutka and Snyder, 1979; Blackshear et al., 1981; Peroutka et al., 1981; Biegon et al., 1986). While elucidation of the role of serotonin in information processing may be complicated by the use of agents that simultaneously activate/antagonize multiple serotonin recognition sites, the use of receptor-specific pharmacological probes may help identify the type of receptor involved in the serotonin-mediated response.

The possible interaction between the serotonergic nervous system and other neurotransmitter systems suspected of having a significant role in information processing needs to be investigated. That is, there exists a substantial body of evidence supporting an anatomical/functional interaction between serotonin and other neurotransmitter systems (Brodie and Shore, 1957; Euvard et al., 1977; Samanin et al., 1978; Baraban and Aghajanian, 1981), including the processes underlying learning and memory (Kruglikov, 1982; Vanderwolf and Baker, 1986; Normile and Altman, 1986; Ogren et al., 1986). It is possible that serotonin modulates the activity of other systems that are critically involved in information processing. Consequently, alterations in serotonergic function may indirectly affect the processing of information by directly influencing the activity of other neurotransmitter systems.

The contribution of several non-learning or non-associative factors (nociception, motivation, locomotion, perception) to the serotonergic-induced effect needs to be examined. That is, studies involving the effects of serotonergic manipulations on the performance of animals in various tasks should be designed (when possible) to simultaneously evaluate whether changes in non-associative factors may be partly responsible for the observed change in performance.

Serotonin and AD. Obviously, continued research effort must be directed toward identifying and characterizing the changes that occur in the serotonergic nervous system in AD. This research should not only focus on the regional changes that occur, but also the quantitative and temporal relation of these changes to those of other transmitter systems. Such an analysis may identify subgroups of AD patients and ultimately provide a rationale for a combination treatment strategy. It should be mentioned that the lack of significant reduction in serotonin levels in a particular brain region may not exclude its involvement in the symptomatology of AD. That is, serotonin has been shown to have both excitatory and inhibitory actions on central neurons (Haigler and Aghajanian, 1974; Wang and Aghajanian, 1977). In addition, procedures designed to enhance serotonergic activity have been reported to impair avoidance responding (Eassman, 1973; Fibiger et al., 1978; Ogren and Johansson, 1985) and discrimination learning (Wooley and Vander Hoeven, 1963; Wetzel et al., 1980). Accordingly, if serotonin possesses an inhibitory action on other neuronal systems more vulnerable to the disease process (e.g., the cholinergic nervous system), then its normal degree of inhibition may be enhanced by the concomitant reduction in cholinergic efficiency. Therefore, the regional balance (or imbalance) between neurotransmitter systems may be more relevant to the clinical symptoms of the disease than a change in the level of any single neurotransmitter.

## REFERENCES

Adolfsson, R., Gottfries, C.G., Roos, B.E. and Winblad, B., 1979, Changes in the brain catecholamines in patients with dementia of Alzheimer type, British Journal of Psychiatry, 135: 216-223.

Aghajanian, G.K. and Wang, R.Y., 1978, Physiology and pharmacology of central serotonergic neurons, in: "Psychopharmacology: A Generation of Progress," M.A. Lipton, A. DiMascio and K.F. Killam, eds., Raven Press, New York.

Altman, H.J., Crosland, R.D., Jenden, D.J. and Berman, R.F., 1985, Further characterization of the nature of the behavioral and neurochemical effects of lesions to the nucleus basalis of Meynert in the rat, Neurobiology of Aging, 6: 125-130.

Altman, H.J., Normile, H.J. and Ogren, S.O., 1985, Facilitation of discrimination learning in the rat following cytotoxic lesions of the serotonergic nervous system, Society for Neuroscience, Abstract, 11: 874.

Arai, H., Kosaka, K. and Iizuka, R., 1984, Changes of biogenic amines and their metabolites in postmortem brains from patients with Alzheimer-type dementia, Journal of Neurochemistry, 43: 388-393.

Argentiero, V. and Tavolato, B., 1980, Dopamine and serotonin metabolite levels in the cerebrospinal fluid in Alzheimer's presenile dementia under phospholipids, Journal of Neurology, 224: 53-58.

Asin, K.E., Wirtshafter, D. and Kent, E.W., 1975, Straight alley acquisition and extinction and open field activity following discrete electrolytic lesions of the mesencephalic raphe nuclei, Behavioral and Neural Biology, 25: 242-256.

Asin, K.E., Wirtshafter, D. and Kent, E.W., 1979, Discrimination learning and reversal following electrolytic median raphe lesions, Society for Neuroscience, Abstract 5: 269.

Asin, K.E. and Fibiger, H.C., 1984, Spontaneous and delayed spatial alternation following damage to specific neuronal elements within the nucleus medianus raphe, Behavioral Brain Research, 13: 241-250.

Asin, K.E., Wirtshafter, D. and Fibiger, H.C., 1985, Electrolytic, but not 5,7-dihyidroxytryptamine, lesions of the nucleus medianus raphe impair acquisition of a radial maze task, Behavioral and Neural Biology, 44: 415-424.

Atack, J.R., Perry, E.K., Bonham, J.R., Perry, R.H., Tomlinson, B.E., Blessed, G. and Fairbairn, A., 1983, Molecular forms of acetylcholin-esterase in senile dementia of Alzheimer type: Selective loss of the intermediate (10S) form, Neuroscience Letters, 40: 199-205.

Azmitia, E.C. and Segal, M., 1978, An autoradiographic analysis of the differential ascending projections of the dorsal and median raphe nuclei in the rat, Journal of Comparative Neurology, 179: 641-668.

Bammer, G., 1982, Pharmacological investigations of neurotransmitter involvement in passive avoidance responding: A review and some new results, Neuroscience and Biobehavioral Reviews, 6:247-296.

Baraban, J.M. and Aghajanian, G.K., 1981, Noradrenergic innervation of serotonergic neurons in the dorsal raphe: Demonstration by electron microscopic autoradiography, Brain Research, 204: 1-11.

Bartus, R.T., Dean, R.L., Beer, B. and Lippa, A.S., 1982, The cholinergic hypothesis of geriatric memory dysfunction, Science, 217: 408-417.

Beller, S.A., Overall, J.E., and Swann, A.C., 1985, Efficacy of oral physostigmine in primary degenerative dementia, Psychopharmacology, 87: 147-151.

Benton, J.S., Bowen, D.M., Allen, S.J., Haan, E.A., Davison, A.N., Neary, D. Murphy, R.P. and Snowden, J.S., 1982, Alzheimer's disease as a disorder of the isodendritic core, Lancet, i: 456.

Biegon, A., Kargman, S., Snyder, L. and McEwen, B.S., 1986, Characterization and localization of serotonin receptors in human postmortem brain, Brain Research, 363: 91-98.

Bjorklund, A., Baumgarten, H.G. and Rensch, H.G., 1975, 5,7-dihydroxytrypt-amine: Improvement of its selectivity for serotonin neurons in the CNS by pretreatment with desipramine, Journal of Neurochemistry. 24: 833-835.

Blackshear, M.A., Steranka, L.R. and Sanders-Bush, E., 1981, Multiple serotonin receptors: Regional distribution and effect of raphe lesions, European Journal of Pharmacology, 76: 325-334.

Blundell, J.E., 1984, Serotonin and appetite, Neuropharmacology, 23: 1537-1551.

Bobillier, P., Petitjean, F., Salvert, D., Ligier, M. and Sequin, S., 1975. Differential projections of the nucleus raphe dorsalis and nucleus raphe centralis as revealed by autoradiography, Brain Research, 85: 205-210.

Bowen, D.M., Smith, C.B., White, P. and Davison, A.N., 1976, Neurotrans-mitter-related enzymes and indices of hypoxia in senile dementia and other abiotrophies, Brain, 99: 459-496.

Bowen, D.M., White, PO., Spillane, J.A., Goodhardt, M.J., Curzon, G., Iwangoff, P., Meier-Ruge, W. and Davison, A.N., 1979, Accelerated aging or selective neuronal loss as an important cause of dementia?, Lancet, i: 11-14.

Bowen, D.M., Allen, S.J., Benton, J.S., Goodhardt, M.J., Haan, E.A., Palmer, A.M., Sims, N.R., Smith, C.C.T., Spillane, J.A., Esira, G.K., Neary, D., Snowdon, J.S., Wilcock, G.K. and Davison, A.N., 1983, Biochemical assessment of serotonergic and cholinergic dysfunction and cerebral atrophy in Alzheimer's disease, Journal of Neurochemistry, 41: 266-272.

Briley, M., Chopin, P. and Moret, C., 1986, New concepts in Alzheimer's disease, Neurobiology of Aging, 7:57-62.

Brinkman, S., Pomara, N., Goodnick, P., Domino, E. and Gerhson, S., 1982, Dose-ranging study of lecithin in the treatment of primary degenerative dementia (Alzheimer's disease), Journal of Clinical Psychopharmacology, 2: 281-285.

Brodie, B. and Shore, P., 1957, A concept for a role of serotonin and norepinephrine as chemical mediators in the brain, Annuals of the New York Academy of Science, 66: 631-642.

Bulat, M. and Zivcovic, N., 1971, Origin of 5-hydroxyindoleacetic acid in the spinal fluid, Science, 173: 738-740.

Candy, J.M., Perry, R.H., Perry, E.K., Irving, D., Blessed, G., Fairbairn, A.F. and Tomlinson, R.L., 1983, Pathological changes in the nucleus of Meynert in Alzheimer's and Parkinson's diseases, Journal of Neuroscience, 54: 277-289.

Cross, A.J., Crow, T.J., Johnson, J.A., Joseph, M.H., Perry, E.K., Perry, R.H., Blessed, G. and Tomlinson, B., 1983, Monoamine metabolism in senile dementia of Alzheimer type, Journal of Neurological Science, 60: 383 392.

Cross, A.J., Crow, T.J., Johnson, J.A., Perry, E.K., Perry, R.H., Blessed, G. and Tomlinson, B.E., 1984, Studies on neurotransmitter receptor systems in cortex and hippocampus in senile dementia of the Alzheimer-type, Journal of Neurological Science, 64: 109-117.

Cross, A.J., Crow, T.J., Ferrier, I.N. and Johnson, J.A., 1986, The selectivity of the reduction of serotonin S2 receptors in Alzheimer-type dementia, Neurobiology of Aging, 7: 3-7.

Davies, P. and Maloney, A.J.F., 1976, Selective loss of central cholinergic neurons in Alzheimer's disease, Lancet, ii: 1403.

Davis, K.L., Mohs, R.C., Tinklenberg, J.R., Pfefferbaum, A., Hollister, L.E. and Kopell, B.S., 1978, Physostigmine: Improvement of long-term memory processes in normal humans, Science, 20: 272-274.

Deutsch, J.A. and Rocklin, R., 1967, Amnesia induced by scopolamine and its temporal variations, Nature, 216: 89-90.

Drachman, D.A. and Leavitt, J., 1974, Human memory and the cholinergic system: A relationship to aging, Archives of Neurology, 30: 113-121.

Dundee, J.K.W. and Pandit, S.K., 1972, Anterograde amnesic effects of pethidine, hyoscine and diazepam in adults, British Journal of Pharmacology, 44: 140-144.

Essman, W.B., 1973, Age dependent effects of 5-hydroxytryptamine upon memory consolidation and cerebral protein synthesis, Pharmacology, Biochemistry and Behavior, 1: 7-14.

Euvard, C., Javoy, F., Herbet, A. and Glowinski, J., 1977, Effect of quipazine, a serotonin-like drug, on striatal cholinergic interneurons, European Journal of Pharmacology, 41: ;281-289.

Fibiger, H.C., 1982, The organization and some projections of cholinergic neurons of the mammalian forebrain, Brain Research Reviews, 4: 327-388.

Fibiger, H.C., Lepiane, F.G. and Phillips, A.G, 1978, Disruption of memory produced by stimulation of the dorsal raphe nucleus: Mediation by serotonin, Brain Research, 155: ;380-386.

Flicker, C., Dean, R.L., Watkins, D.L., Fischer, S.K. and Bartus, R.T., 1983, Behavioral and neurochemical effects following neurotoxic lesions of a major cholinergic input to the cerebral cortex in the rat, Pharmacology, Biochemistry and Behavior, 18: 973-991.

Flood, J.F., Smith, G.G. and Cherkin, A., 1983, Memory retention: Potentiation of cholinergic drug combinations in mice, Neurobiology of Aging, 4: 37-43.

Friedman, E., Lerer, B. and Kuster, J., 1983, Loss of cholinergic neurons in rat neocortex produces deficits in passive avoidance learning, Pharmacology Biochemistry and Behavior, 19: 309-312.

Fuxe, K., Ogren, S.O. Agnati, L.F., Jonsson, G. and Gustafsson, J.A., 1978, 5,7-Dihydroxytryptamine as a tool to study the functional role of central 5-hydroxytryptamine neurons, in: "Serotonin Neurotoxins," J.H. Jacoby and L.D. Lytle, eds., The New York Academy of Sciences, New York.

Garelis, E., Young, S.H. and Lal, S., 1974, Monoamine metabolites in lumbar CSF: The question of their origin in relation to clinical studies, Brain Research, 79: 1-8.

Gottfries, C.G., Cottfries, I. and Roos, B.E., 1969, Homovanillic acid and 5-hydroxyindoleacetic acid in the cerebral spinal fluid of patients with senile dementia, presenile dementia and Parkinsonism, Journal of Neurochemistry, 16: 1341-1345.

Haigler, H.J. and Aghajanian, G.K., 1974, Lysergic acid diethylamide and serotonin: A comparison of effects on serotonergic neurons and neurons receiving serotonergic input, Journal of Pharmacological and Experimental Therapeutics, 188: 688-699.

Hano, J., Vetulani, J. Sansone, M. and Olivero, A., 1981, Changes in action of tricyclic and tetracyclic antidepressants: Desipramine and mianserin, on avoidance behavior in the course of chronic treatment, Psychopharmacology, 73: 265-268.

Hole, K. and Lorens, S.A., 1975, Response to electric shock in rats: Effects of selective midbrain raphe lesions, Pharmacology, Biochemistry, and Behavior, 3: 95-102.

Hole, K., Fuxe, K. and Jonsson, G., 1976, Behavioral effects of 5,7-dihydroxytryptamine lesions of ascending 5-hydroxytryptamine pathways, Brain Research, 107: 385-399.

Ishii, I., 1966, Distribution of Alzheimer's neurofibrillary changes in the brain stem and hypothalamus of senile dementia, Archives of Neuropathology, 6: 181-187.

Jacobs, B.L., Wise, W.D. and Taylor, K.M., 1974, Differential behavioral and neurochemical effects following lesions of the dorsal or median raphe nuclei in rats, Brain Research, 79-353-361.

Janssen, P.A.J., 1981, The pharmacology of specific, pure and potent serotonin 5-HT2 or S2-antagonists, Eight International Congress of Pharmacology, Tokyo (Japan), July 19-24.

Johnston, M.V., McKinney, M. and Coyle, J.T., 1979, Evidence for a cholinergic projection to the neocortex from neurons in basal forebrain, Proceedings of the National Academy of Science, 76: 5392-5396.

Jouvet, M., 1969, Biogenic amines and the states of sleep, *Science*, 163: 32-34.

Koe, B.K. and Weissman, A., 1966, p-Chlorophenylalanine: A specific depletor of brain serotonin, *Journal of Pharmacological and Experimental Therapeutics*, 154: 499-516.

Kruglikov, R.I., 1982, On the interaction of neurotransmitters in processes of learning and memory. in: "Neuronal Plasticity and Memory Formation," C.A. Marsan and H. Matthies, eds., Raven Press, New York.

Leysen, J.E., Awouters, F., Kennis,L., Laduron, P.M., Vandenberk, J. and Janssen, P.A.J., 1981, Receptor binding profile of R-41,468, a novel antagonist at 5-HT2 receptors, *Life Sciences*, 28: 1015-1022.

LoConte, G., Bartolini, L., Casamenti, F., Marconcini-Pepeu, I. and Pepeu, G., 1982, Lesions of cholinergic forebrain nuclei: Changes in avoidance behavior and scopolamine actions, *Pharmacology, Biochemistry and Behavior*, 17: 933-937.

Longo, V.G., 1966, Behavioral and electroencephalographic effects of atropine and related compounds, *Pharmacological Reviews*, 18: 965-966,

Lorens, S.A., 1978, Some behavioral effects of serotonin depletion depend on method: A comparison of 5,7-dihydroxytryptamine, p-chlorophenylalanine, p-chloroamphetamine, and electrolytic raphe lesions, in: "Serotonin Neurotoxins, J.H. Jacoby and L.D. Lytle, eds., New York Academy of Sciences, New York.

Lorens, S.A. and Guldberg, H.C., 1974, Regional 5-hydroxytryptamine following selective midbrain raphe lesions in the rat, *Brain research*, 78: 45-56.

Lorens, S.A. and Yunger, L.M., 1974, Morphine analgesia, two-way avoidance, and consummatory behavior following lesions in the midbrain raphe nuclei in the rat, *Pharmacology, Biochemistry and Behavior*, 2: 215-221.

Lorens, S.A., Guldberg, H.C., Hole, K., Kohler, C. and Srebro, B., 1976, Activity, avoidance learning and regional 5-hydroxytryptamine following intrabrain stem 5,7-dihydroxytryptamine and electrolytic midbrain raphe lesions in the rat, *Brain Research*, 108: 97-113.4

Mann, D.M.A. and Yates, P.O., 1983, Serotonin nerve cells in Alzheimer's disease, *Journal of Neurological and Neurosurgical Psychiatry*, 46: 96.

Montanaro, N., Dall'Olio, R. and Gandolfi, O., 1981, Reduction of ECS-induced retrograde amnesia of passive avoidance conditioning after 5,7-dihydroxytryptamine median raphe nucleus lesion in the rat, *Neuropsychobiology*, 7: 56-67.

Normile, H.J. and Altman, H.J., 1985, The effects of serotonergic receptor blockade on learning and memory in mice, Society for Neuroscience, Abstract, 11: 875.

Normile, H.J. and Altman, H.J., 1986, Evidence for a possible interaction between noradrenergic and serotonergic neurotransmission in the retrieval of a previously learned aversive habit in mice, *Psychopharmacology*, 92: 388-392.

Ochi, J. and Shimizu, K., 1978, Occurrence of dopamine-containing neurons in the midbrain raphe nuclei of the rat, *Neuroscience*, 8: 317-320.

Ogren, S.O., Kohler, C., Ross, S.B. and Srebro, B., 1976, 5-hydroxytryptamine depletion and avoidance acquisition in the rat. Antagonism of the long-term effects of p-chloroamphetamine with a selective inhibitor or 5-hydroxytryptamine uptake, Neuroscience Letters, 3: 341-347.

Ogren, S.O., Fuxe, K., Archer, T., Hall, H., Holm, A.C. and Kohler, C., 1981, Studies on the role of central 5-HT neurons in avoidance learning: A behavioral and biochemical analysis. in: "Serotonin: Current Aspects of Neurochemistry and Function," B. Gabay, S. Issidorides, M.R., Alivisatos, S.G.A., eds., Plenum Press, New York.

Ogren, S.O. and Johansson, C., 1985, Separation of the associative and non-associative effects of brain serotonin released by p-chloroamphetamine: Dissociable serotonergic involvement in avoidance learning, pain and motor function, Psychopharmacology, 86: 12-26.

Ogren, S.O., Altman, H.J. and Bartfai, T., 1987, Alaproclate potentiation of muscarinic agonist evoked tremor, salivation and enhanced recall, in: Synaptic Transmitters and Receptors," S. Tucek, ed., John Wiley & Sons, Chichester, U.K. (In press).

O'Hearn, E. and Molliver, M.E., 1984, Organization of raphe-cortical projections in the rat: A quantitative retrograde study, Brain Research Bulletin, 13: 7i09-726.

Palmer, A.M., Sims, N.S., Bowen, D.M., Neary, D., Palo, J., Wikstrom, J. and Davison, A.N., 1984, Monoamine metabolite concentrations in lumbar cerebrospinal fluid of patients with histology verified Alzheimer's dementia, Journal of Neurological and Neurosurgical Psychiatry, 47: 481-484.

Peroutka, S.J. and Snyder, S.H., 1979, Multiple serotonin receptors: Differential binding of 3H-serotonin, 3H-lysergic acid diethylamide and 3H-spiroperidol, Molecular Pharmacology, 16: 687-699.

Peroutka, S.J., Lebovitz, R.M. and Snyder, S.H., 1981, Two distinct central serotonin receptors with different physiologic functions, Science, 212: 827-829.

Perry, E.K., Perry, R.H., Blessed, G. and Tomlinson, B.E., 1977, Necropsy evidence of central cholinergic deficits in senile dementia, Lancet, i: 189.

Perry, E.K., Tomlinson, B.E., Blessed, G. Bergmann, K., Gibson, P.H. and Perry R.H., 1978, Correlation of cholinergic abnormalities with senile plaques and mental test scores in senile dementia, British Medical Journal, 2: 1457-1459.

Pope, A., Hess, H.H. and Levin, E, 1965, Neurochemical pathology of the cerebral cortex in presenile dementias, Transactions of the American Neurological Association, 89: 15-16.

Quirion, R., Richard, J. and Dam, T.V., 1985, Evidence for the existence of serotonin type-2 receptors on cholinergic terminals in rat cortex, Brain Research, 333: 345-349.

Reynolds, G.P., Arnold, L., Rossor, M.N., Iversen, L.L., Mountjoy, C.Q. and Roth, M., 1984, Reduced binding of (3H)ketanserin to cortical 5-HT2 receptors in senile dementia of the Alzheimer type, Neuroscience Letters, 44: 47-51.

Roberts, M.H.T., 1984, 5-Hydroxytryptamine and antinociception, Neuro-pharmacology, 23: 1529-1536.

Samanin, R., Quattrone, A., Prei, G., Ladinski, H. and Consolo, S., 1978, Evidence for an interaction between serotonergic and cholinergic neurons in the corpus striatum and hippocampus of the rat brain, Brain Research, 151: 73-82

Sitaram, N., Weingartner, H. and Gillin, K.C., 1978, Human serial learning enhancement with arecoline and impairment with scopolamine, Science, 201: 274-276.

Srebro, B. and Lorens, S.A., 1975, Behavioral effects of selective midbrain raphe lesions in the rat, Brain Research, 89: 303-325.

Srebro, B. Jellestad, F. and Lorens, S.A., 1975, Activity, avoidance behavior, and spatial reversal learning after midbrain raphe lesions, Experimental Brain Research, 23: 193.

Steinbusch, H.W.M., 1984, Serotonin-immunoreactive neurons and their projection in the CNS, in: "Handbook of Chemical Neuroanatomy," A. Bjorklund, T. Hokfelt and M.J. Kuhar, eds., Elsevier, New York.

Stevens, D.A., Flechter, L.D. and Resnick, O., 1969, The effects of p-chlorophenylalanine, a depletor of brain serotonin, on behavior: Retardation of passive avoidance learning, Life Science, 8: 379-385.

Summers, W.K., Viesselman, J.O., Marsh, G.M. and Candelora, K., 1981, Use of THA in treatment of Alzheimer-like dementia: Pilot study in twelve patients, Biological Psychiatry, 16: 145-153.

Valzelli, L. and Pawlowski, L., 1979, Effect of p-chlorophenylalanine on avoidance learning of two differentially housed mouse strains, Neuro-psychobiology, 5: 121-128.

Vanderwolf, C.H. and Baker, G.B., 1986, Evidence that serotonin mediates non-cholinergic neocortical low voltage fast activity, non-cholinergic hippocampal rhythmical slow activity and contributes to intelligent behavior, Brain Research, 374: 342-356.

Volicer, L., Langlais, P.J., Matson, W.R., Mark, K.A. and Gamache, P.H., 1985, Serotonergic system in dementia of the Alzheimer type, Archives of Neurology, 42: 1158-1161.

Wetzel, W., Getsova, V.M., Jork, R. and Matthies, H., 1980, Effect of serotonin on Y-maze retention and hippocampal protein synthesis in rats. Pharmacology, Biochemistry and Behavior, 12: 319-322.

Whitehouse, P.J., Price, D.L., Clark, A.W., Coyle, J.T. and DeLong, M.R., 1981, Alzheimer's disease: Evidence for a selective loss of cholinergic neurons in the nucleus basalis, Annals of Neurology, 10: 122-126.

Winblad, B., Adolfsson, R., Carlsson, A. and Gottfries, C.G., 1982, Biogenic amines in brains of patients with Alzheimer's disease. in: "Alzheimer's Disease: A Report of Progress. Vol. 19, Aging," S. Corkin, K.L. Davis, J.H. Growdon, E. Usdin and R.J. Wurtman, eds., Raven Press, New York.

Wirtshafter, D. and Asin, K.E., 1983, Impaired radial maze performance in rats with electrolytic median raphe lesions, Experimental Neurology, 79: 412-412.

Wooley, D.W. and Van der Hoeven, T., 1963, Alteration in learning ability caused by changes in cerebral serotonin and catecholamines, <u>Science,</u> 139: 610-611.

Yamamoto, T., Hirano, A., 1985, Nucleus raphe dorsalis in Alzheimer's disease: Neurofibrillary tangles and loss of large neurons, <u>Annals of Neurology,</u> 17: 573-577.

# INTRACRANIAL CHOLINERGIC DRUG INFUSION IN PATIENTS WITH ALZHEIMER'S DISEASE

Robert E. Harbough

Section of Neurosurgery, Department of Surgery
Dartmouth-Hitchcock Medical Center
Hanover, N.H. 03756

Improved understanding of the chemical aspects of brain function during the last two decades has changed our concepts of a number of neurologic diseases (Snyder, 1984; Harbough, 1985a). Unfortunately, clinical application of this information has been plagued by longstanding problems with drug delivery to the brain. Neurosurgery may have a role to play in previously non-surgical neurologic disease by the ability of neurosurgeons to overcome problems with drug delivery to the brain. Neurotransmitter augmentation by regional infusion of drugs into the central nervous system may open a whole new field of neurosurgical endeavor.

Presented here is a brief review of problems encountered when attempting to deliver drugs to the brain. Experience with intracranial cholinomimetic drug infusion in patients with Alzheimer's disease will be used as a model for delineating the rationale, benefits, and risks of central drug infusion as a means of overcoming these problems.

## DRUG DELIVERY TO THE BRAIN IN PATIENTS WITH ALZHEIMER'S DISEASE

The clinical presentation of patients with Alzheimer's disease has been clearly delineated (Reisberg, 1983). In addition to the well documented memory dysfunction, these patients also exhibit alterations in attention, language, mood, psychomotor abilities, food intake, and sleep patterns. How much of this behavioral dysfunction is due to neurochemical abnormalities is a subject of controversy (Bartus et al., 1986). Before considering the rationality of any drug therapy, one should consider the evidence for neurochemical brain dysfunction in patients with Alzheimer's disease.

The short-term memory dysfunction in patients with Alzheimer's disease may be due to anatomical disruption of afferent and efferent hippocampal fibers resulting in isolation of the hippocampi from the rest of the brain. If this proves to be the case, then drug therapy is unlikely to have clinically meaningful effects on short-term memory.

However, there is also substantial evidence to suggest that some symptoms of patients with Alzheimer's disease may be secondary to neurochemical abnormalities. An extensive literature on this subject has been reviewed elsewhere (Carlson, 1983). The well-documented decrease of brain cholinergic activity in such patients has been of particular interest. Evidence for a cholinergic hypothesis of Alzheimer's disease and treatment approaches based on this hypothesis have also been extensively reviewed (Bartus et al., 1986). There does seem to be adequate evidence for neurochemical abnormalities to justify treatment approaches that attempt to manipulate cholinergic neurotransmitter levels in Alzheimer's disease patients.

Even if the symptoms of Alzheimer's disease can be ameliorated by increasing brain cholinergic activity, there are still substantial difficulties to be overcome in delivering a cholinomimetic substance to the brain (Harbough, 1985b). These include adverse systemic side effects, peripheral inactivation or metabolism of drugs, inadequate blood-brain barrier penetration, erratic drug absorption, serum protein binding, and poor patient compliance. Because of these difficulties we began investigating the possibility of delivering a muscarinic agonist to the brain by means of continuous intracranial infusion (Harbough et al., 1984). All clinical trails were approved by the committee for the protection of human subjects at our institution.

Earlier experience with implantable drug delivery devices (Coombs et al., 1983; Harbough et al., 1982) has shown that such an approach was technically possible. The potential advantages, rationale, and potential risks of central drug infusion will be briefly discussed. The mechanism of the implantable pump (Intermdeics-Infusaid, Inc., Norwood, MA) has been previously presented (Harbough et al., 1982; Harbough et al., 1984) and will be reviewed.

The potential advantages of intracranial drug infusion are numerous. Direct infusion of drugs into the cerebral ventricles bypasses the problems of systemic side effects, peripheral drug inactivation, poor drug absorption, serum protein binding, inadequate blood-brain barrier penetration, and poor patient compliance. However, intrathecal drug administration has by and large been ineffective (Aird, 1984). Therefore, the first question to be addressed regarding central drug infusion is whether drugs achieve adequate brain penetration from the cerebrospinal fluid.

In many ways the cerebrospinal fluid is an ideal drug delivery medium, with little protein binding and decreased enzymatic activity compared to plasma (Wood, 1980). The subarachnoid space penetrates the brain by means of the Virchow-Robins spaces, and substances in the cerebrospinal fluid enter the brain extracellular fluid by diffusion (Blasberg et al., 1975). However, the extent of drug penetration into the brain depends not only on the drug being used, but also on the method of administration.

Most clinical trials of central drug administration have employed single or intermittent bolus injections into the subarachnoid space or ventricular system. Of all the ways to deliver drugs to the central nervous system, this is probably the worst. Bolus injections initially result in very high cerebrospinal fluid drug concentrations and relatively limited parenchymal penetration (Blasberg et al., 1977). In addition, a single bolus of drug is likely to be more toxic and less effective than more frequent smaller doses (Bleyer et al., 1978). However, even with bolus administration, drugs will penetrate the parenchyma and, as cerebrospinal fluid is cleared by bulk flow, diffuse back into the subarachnoid space (Blasberg et al., 1977). In situations where high drug concentrations in the cerebrospinal fluid or immediately adjacent parenchyma are desired (carcinomatous meningitis, spinal anesthesia/analgesia, chemical rhizotomy), bolus injections are effective. However, if deeper diffusion into parenchyma is desired, longer term infusion is necessary (Blasberg et al., 1975).

Intravascular administration of drugs that cross the blood-brain barrier shows a rapid onset of action due to the short circulation time and extensive vascular-central nervous system interface (Aird, 1984). However, drugs administered into the cerebrospinal fluid require much longer for adequate diffusion into the parenchyma (Lee and Olszewski, 1960). As the duration of central drug administration increases, the depth of parenchymal penetration, even of large protein molecules, also increases (Brightman and Reese, 1968). Therefore, to adequately evaluate the effectiveness of central drug administration, infusions must be carried out over a period of days to weeks (Blasberg, 1975).

The site of infusion within the central compartment may also be of significance. Drug penetration into the parenchyma may occur more readily through the ependymal than the pial surface (Rall, 1968), and drugs administered into the subarachnoid space may not enter the ventricular system (Bleyer and Poplack, 1978). Therefore, intraventricular drug infusion is a more reasonable approach for achieving diffuse brain penetration than is lumbar intrathecal administration. Conversely, if one wishes to confine drug effect to the spinal cord with minimal effects at higher levels of the neuraxis, then intraspinal infusion may be beneficial (Harbough, 1982; Coombs et al., 1983). Thus, some relatively restricted neuropharmacologic effects can be achieved. Theoretically, with stereotaxic cannula placement and very low flow rate infusion devices, delivery of minute quantities of drugs to very circumscribed regions of brain parenchyma is possible.

When evaluating the effectiveness of central drug administration, the choice of drug is as important as the method of delivery. The ability of a drug to cross the blood-brain barrier is more likely to be detrimental than beneficial if the drug is given as a continuous central infusion. Drugs which readily cross brain capillaries can be readily cleared from the central nervous system when infused into the cerebrospinal fluid (Blasberg, 1975). The use of such drugs may be valuable if high local concentrations in tissue adjacent to the subarachnoid space or ependyma is desired. However, if deeper parenchymal penetration is the goal, then lipid insoluble, polar molecules are better candidates for infusion (Blasberg, 1975).

When considering drugs for long-term central infusion, chemical and biological stability become important criteria. For continuous infusion via an implantable pump, the infused drug must be stable at body temperature for at least as long as the time between pump refills. In addition, if widespread diffusion of active drug into parenchyma is desired, then the infused drug cannot be rapidly metabolized within the central nervous system or cerebrospinal fluid. This last consideration may not apply to local intraparenchymal infusion where a steep concentration gradient of active drug could be beneficial. Our clinical experience at Dartmouth with implantable infusion devices for central drug administration may serve to illustrate some of the points raised above (Harbough et al., 1982; Coombs et al., 1983; Harbough et al., 1984; Harbough, 1985b; Harbough et al., submitted for publication).

Previous attempts at increasing brain cholinergic activity in patients with Alzheimer's disease by administration of acetylcholine precursors, cholinesterase inhibitors, or systemic cholinergic agonists had been attended by the difficulties with drug delivery to the brain discussed earlier in this paper (Bartus et al., 1986). Intracranial cholinergic drug infusion was started as a means of testing the validity of the cholinergic hypothesis and as an attempt at therapy for a devastating neurologic disease with no known treatment.

The drug delivery system used consists of a Intermedics-Infusaid implantable pump connected to a Silastic intracranial catheter. The pump consists of a discoid titanium shell containing a metal bellows drug chamber and an underlying charging fluid chamber. Vapor pressure generated by a two-phase fluorocarbon in the charging fluid chamber compresses the bellows, forcing the drug through an outlet flow restrictor and into the outflow catheter. After implantation, the drug chamber can be refilled percutaneously via an inlet septum. Each pump has a preset flow rate and drug dosage is varied by changing the concentration of the infusate.

A stable, water soluble, pure muscarinic agonist which is not degraded by cholinesterases was sought for infusion. Bethanechol chloride (Urecholine; Merck, Sharp and Dohme), an ester of a choline-like compound, has significant muscarinic activity without nicotinic agonist properties, is not hydrolyzed by cholinesterases, and is freely soluble and stable in water. The drug is commercially available as a sterile solution with no preservatives and has a neutral pH.

Following toxicity studies in dogs, a preliminary clinical trial was approved by the committee for the protection of human subjects at our institution (Harbough et al., 1984). All patients in our study had a history of progressive memory, cognitive, and social dysfunction for at least three years and demonstrated moderately severe to severe cognitive decline. A thorough clinical, laboratory, and radiologic evaluation was carried out to exclude other causes of progressive dementia. If a patient was then felt to be an acceptable candidate for the study, informed consent was obtained from the patient and the family before proceeding.

Under general anesthesia, patients were positioned and draped as of ventriculoperitoneal shunt placement. A small frontal craniotomy was done, a cortical biopsy taken for light and electron microscopic documentation of Alzheimer's disease (Harbough, in press), and the intrathecal catheter placed (Harbough et al., 1984). The pumps were sutured in a subcutaneous abdominal pocket and the outflow catheters tunneled subcutaneously and connected to the intracranial catheters with straight metal connectors. Connections were secured with nonabsorbable ligatures and the incisions were closed. Pumps were refilled percutaneously at three-week intervals on an outpatient basis.

As mentioned earlier, the problems of systemic drug inactivation, serum protein binding, drug absorption and poor blood-brain barrier penetration are avoided by delivering a muscarinic agonist into the ventricular system. The use of an implantable continuous infusion pump permits long-term intracranial infusion of drug or placebo on an outpatient basis and avoids any problems of patient compliance. Pump flow rates ranged from 1 to 2 ml/day. Systemic side effects were not encountered.

For patients with Alzheimer's disease, drug distribution to the hippocampi, locus coeruleus, reticular nucleus of the thalamus, and cerebral cortex was desired. Therefore, for the reasons outlined above a drug that does not cross the blood-brain barrier, infused into the ventricular system, was chosen.

The potential advantages of central drug infusion have been discussed. There are, however, some potential disadvantages which require equal consideration. These include the operative risks of catheter placement and pump implantation and the risk of increased neurotoxicity.

As for any neurosurgical procedure, the risks of catheter placement and pump implantation include anesthetic complications, hemorrhage, and infection. Although all these risks are low, there is probably an irreducible minimum and some complications must be anticipated.

The risk of neurotoxicity with intracranial drug infusions must also be considered. Before considering intracranial to intraspinal infusion of drugs in patients, toxicity studies in animals are mandatory. Although such toxicity studies decrease the risk of human neurotoxicity, some unexpected reactions to drug infusions in patients are likely to occur. We have now been infusing bethanechol chloride intracranially in patients with Alzheimer's disease for more than 30 months (Harbough et al., submitted for publication). One patient developed a reversible Parkinsonian syndrome or rigidity and bradykinesia and another developed a reversible cerebrospinal fluid inflammatory response which may or may not have been related to drug infusion (Harbough et al., 1984; Harbough, submitted for publication). Experience with more patients infused for longer periods of time will be necessary before any accurate figures on the risk of neurotoxicity are available. However, to date, drug infusions appear to be well tolerated (Harbough, submitted for publication).

The feasibility of intracranial and intraspinal administration of neurotransmitter analogues has been demonstrated (Harbough et al., 1982; Coombs et al., 1983; Harbough et al., 1984; Harbough, 1984; Harbough, submitted for publication). However, the value of these therapeutic endeavors over presently available therapy remains to be proven (Harbough et al., 1982; Coombs et al., 1983; Harbough et al., 1984; Harbough, submitted for publication). We are conducting studies of the effects of intracranial bethanechol infusion on activities of daily living and neuropsychologic test scores in a double-blind, placebo-controlled crossover design. Preliminary studies show family reports of decreased confusion, increased initiative, and improvements in activities of daily living during the drug infusion, but no subjective improvement in short-term memory has been reported (Harbough et al., 2984). A double-blind study at another institution has shown similar results (Personal communication, R.D. Penn, 1986). Long-term follow-up on our initial four patients suggests that improvement in function is maintained for at least two years (Harbough, submitted for publication).

Clearly, a great deal more work needs to be done to determine if central cholinergic drug infusion has a therapeutic effect in patients with Alzheimer's disease, and if so, how this effect is achieved. However, I think this technique of drug delivery to the brain will be of greater importance than the outcome of any single clinical trail.

SUMMARY

Increasing evidence documents the importance of neurochemistry in normal and pathologic brain function. This information suggests innovative therapeutic approaches for previously untreatable neurologic disease by manipulation of brain chemistry. Neurosurgery may have a role to play in allowing drug delivery to the brain, either diffusely or within anatomically restricted areas. Neurotransmitter augmentation by drug infusion may open entirely new fields of neuropharmacology and functional neurosurgery.

In relation to Alzheimer's disease, experience with intracranial
cholinergic drug infusion suggests that this treatment approach does improve
behavior in some patients. Double-blind studies, long-term follow-up
studies and animal trials searching for an ideal cholinergic drug for
infusion are underway.

## REFERENCES

Aird, R.B., 1984, A study in intrathecal, cerebrospinal fluid-to-brain
exchange, Exp. Neurol., 86: 342-358.

Bartus, R.T., Dean, R.L. and Fisher, S.K., 1986, Cholinergic treatment for
age-related memory disturbances: Dead or merely coming of age? in:
"Treatment Development Strategies for Alzheimer's Disease," T. Crook,
R.T. Bartus, S. Ferris and S. Gershon, eds., Mark Powley Assoc., New
Canaan, Connecticut. pp 421-450.

Blasberg, R.G., Patlak, C.S. and Fentermacher, J.D., 1975, Intrathecal
chemotherapy: Brain tissue profiles after ventriculocisternal perfusion,
J. Pharmacol. Exp. Ther., 195: 73-83.

Blasberg, R.G., Patlak, C.S. and Shapiro, W.R., 1977, Concentration x time
methotrexate in cerebrospinal fluid and brain after intraventricular
administration, Cancer Treat. Rep., 61: 633-641.

Bleyer, W.A. and Poplack, D.G., 1978, Clinical studies on the central
nervous system pharmacology of methotrexate, in: "Clinical Pharmacology
of Antineoplastic Drugs," H.M. Pinedo, ed., Elsevier, Amsterdam.

Bleyer, W.A., Poplack, D.G. and Simon, R.M., 1978, Concentration x time
methotrexate via a subcutaneous reservoir: A less toxic regimen for
intraventricular chemotherapy of central nervous system neoplasms, Blood,
51: 835-842.

Brightman, M.W. and Reese, R.S., 1969, Junctions between intimately apposed
cell membranes in the vertebrate brain, J. Cell Biol., 40: 814-822.

Carlson, A., 1983, Changes in neurotransmitter systems in the aging brain
and in Alzheimer's disease, in: "Alzheimer's Disease: The Standard Desk
Reference," B. Reisberg ed., The Free Press, New York. pp 100-106

Coombs, D.W., Saunders, R.L., Gaylor, M.S. et al., 1984, Preliminary report:
Intracranial cholinergic drug infusion in patients with Alzheimer's
disease, Neurosurgery, 15: 514-518.

Harbough, R.E., 1985a, Neural transplantation vs central neurotransmitter
augmentation in diseases of the nervous system, Neurobiol. Aging, 6:
164-166.

Harbough, R.E., 1985b, Continuous central drug infusion to the central
nervous system: Treatment for Alzheimer's and chronic pain syndrome,
Neuro. Views: Trends in Clinical Neurology, 1: 5-7.

Harbough, R.E., Brain biopsy in Alzheimer's disease: Surgical techniques
and indications, Bull Clin. Neurosci. (in press).

Harbough, R.E., Coombs, D.W., Saunders, R.L. et al., 1982, Implanted
continuous epidural morphine infusion system: Preliminary report, J
Neurosurg., 56: 803-806.

Harbough, R.E., Culver, C.M., Roberts, D.W.,et al., Long term follow-up of intracranial cholinergic drug infusion in Alzheimer's disease patients. (submitted for publication)

Harbough, R.E., Roberts, D.W., Coombs, D.W. et al., 1984, Preliminary report: Intracranial cholinergic drug infusion in patients with Alzheimer's disease, Neurosurgery, 15: 514-518.

Lee, J.C. and Olszewski, J., 1960, Penetration of radioactive bovine albumin from cerebrospinal fluid into brain tissue, Neurology, 10: 814-822.

Rall, D.P., 1968, Transport through the ependymal linings, Progress in Brain Research, 29: 159-167.

Reisberg, B., 1983, Clinical presentation, diagnosis, and symptomatology of age associated cognitive decline and Alzheimer's disease, in: "Alzheimer's Disease: The Standard Desk Reference," B. Reisberg, ed., The Free Press, New York. pp 173-187.

Snyder, S.H., 1984, Drug and neurotransmitter receptors in the brain, Science, 224: 22-31.

Wood, J.H., 1980, Physiology, pharmacology and dynamics of cerebrospinal fluid, in: "Neurobiology of Cerebrospinal Fluid," J.H. Wood, ed., Plenum Press, New York.

# NEURAL IMPLANTS: A STRATEGY FOR THE TREATMENT OF ALZHEIMER'S DISEASE

Don Marshall Gash

Department of Neurobiology and Anatomy
University of Rochester Medical Center
Rochester, New York 14642

## INTRODUCTION

Following the seminal studies of Stenevi et al. (1976) and Lund and Hauschka (1976), the techniques of neural transplantation have been increasingly employed to study regeneration and recovery of function in the mammalian brain. Experiments, primarily using fetal rodent donor tissue, have demonstrated that neural grafts can survive and develop relatively normal cytoarchitectural features, neurochemical properties and synaptic relationships when implanted into a host nervous system (for a review see Gash et al., 1985). Neural transplants have been found to be effective in ameliorating neurological deficits in rodent model systems of Parkinson's disease (Perlow et al., 1979), Huntington's disease (Isacson et al., 1984), neuroendocrine disorders (Gash et al., 1980; Krieger et al., 1982) and cognitive deficits (Low et al., 1982; Dunnett et al., 1982). These successes with transplants in rodents have led to suggestions that neural transplants might be of therapeutic value in treating human neurological disorders, including neurodegenerative disorders associated with aging such as Alzheimer's disease and Parkinson's disease (Backlund et al., 1985; Gash et al., 1985). The present paper will review recent studies on transplants in rodents with cognitive deficits, and discuss the potential of using transplants in treating Alzheimer's disease.

## NEURAL TRANSPLANTATION

Stenevi et al. (1976), in investigating the optimal conditions for neural graft survival, found that the best results were obtained when fetal central nervous system neurons were placed next to a rich vascular supply. In fact, a review of the literature reveals that almost every area of the fetal brain can be successfully transplanted if care is taken with procedural details (see for example Olson et al., 1984). In contrast, mature CNS neurons have never been found to survive in transplants (Saltykow, 1905; Wenzel and Barlehner, 1969; Stenevi et al., 1976). The reason fetal CNS neurons survive grafting procedures while adult neurons do not, is probably related to several factors. First, fetal neurons are less affected by low oxygen levels than mature neurons (Jilek, 1970) and grafting procedures necessarily involve periods of anoxia until an adequate blood supply is established by the transplant. Secondly, fetal neurons seem to survive best when they are taken during a rapid growth phase and before connections are established with target tissues (Boer et al., 1985). By choosing the optimal period in development, neurons can be dissected from the donor embryonic brain without damaging axonal and dendritic processes and thus prejudicing their survival. Also, the millieu of the damaged host brain apparently contains growth and survival factors which promote the viability of the grafted cells (Nieto-Sampedro et al., 1984) and fetal tissue may be especially responsive to these factors. Finally, the brain is classified as an "immunologically priviledged site" because allogeneic grafts are either not rejected or are rejected at a slower rate in the brain then in other sites in the body (Freed, 1985; also see Mason et al. 1985).

Other donor tissues have also been employed in neural grafts. In sharp contrast to CNS donor tissues, mature neurons from the peripheral nervous system (e.g. superior cervical ganglion) readily survive implantation into the brain (Ranson, 1914; Stenevi et al., 1976; Rosenstein and Brightman, 1984). In fact, a number of recent studies have concentrated on using the adrenal medulla (which can be considered in many ways to be a modified sympathetic ganglion), for transplants into rodents and nonhuman primates with movement disorders related to Parkinson's disease (Freed et al., 1981; Morihisa et al., 1984). Adrenal transplants have been moderately successful in the rodent model of Parkinson's disease (Freed et al., 1981). However, the viability of adrenal medulla grafts in nonhuman primates has been disappointing; only a few to several hundred adrenal medullary cells could be identified in implantation sites in adult Rhesus monkey hosts (Morihisa et al., 1984). Swedish clinicians have attempted adrenal medulla autografts in four Parkinsonian patients with very limited success (Backlund et al., 1985).

In addition to fetal CNS tissue and grafts of peripheral origin, our group (Gash et al., 1985; Kordower et al., 1986) and others (Jaeger, 1985) have begun to examine the properties of cultured cell lines to determine their suitability as donor tissues in neural implants. In a recent study involving five adult African green monkeys. We tested the ability of cells from a human neuroblastoma cell line, IMR-32 to survive for prolonged periods when implanted into the nonhuman primate hippocampus (Gash et al., 1986a). The IMR-32 cells were selected for this study because (i) they synthesize several neurotransmitters including acetylcholine, norepinephrine, dopamine, and serotonin (Gupta et al., 1985), (ii) the cells can be induced to differentiate in vitro with the appropriate chemical treatment (Bottenstein, 1981; Gupta et al., 1985) and (iii) IMR-32 cells only weakly express the major human transplantation antigens (Lampson et al., 1983). We found that the grafted IMR-32 cells remained differentiated in the host brain for the longest time periods examined, 270 days (Gash et al., 1986a). Processes from the grafted cells could be identified coursing into the host brain. Our results imply that neuroblastoma cells possess many of the properties desired for donor tissue in neural implants.

## Cognitive Dysfunctions and Neural Implants

Several research groups, including ours, have tested the ability of neural implants to alleviate cognitive dysfunctions in rodents. Improved performance following transplantation has been found on passive avoidance behavior tests and in memory as measured by performance on various maze tasks (see Table 1). For example, maze performance in rats has repeatedly been shown to be affected by lesions which disrupt septal cholinergic fibers innervating the hippocampus (Crutcher et al., 1983). In an elegant series of experiments, Björklund and his colleagues have shown that fetal septal grafts are capable of providing cholinergic reinnervation of the hippocampus and dentate gyrus of adult rats which closely mimics the original pattern of innervation anatomically (Björklund and Stenevi, 1977), biochemically (Kelly et al., 1985) and electrophysiologically (Segal et al., 1985). Such septal transplants effectively ameliorate maze performance deficits in septohippocampal lesioned adult rats (Dunnett et al., 1982).

## Table 1:

### Cognitive Improvements in Rodents Following Neural Transplantation

| Animal | Deficits Measured | Graft | Reference |
|---|---|---|---|
| septohippocampal-lesioned adult female rats | maze performance | fetal septal-diagonal band | Low et al., 1982; Dunnett et al., 1982 |
| aged female rats | maze performance | fetal septal-diagonal band | Gage et al., 1984 |
| hippocampal lesioned adult male rats | maze performance | fetal hippocampus | Kimble et al., 1986 |
| frontal cortex lesioned adult male rats | maze performance | fetal frontal cortex | Labbe et al., 1983 |
| nucleus basalis lesion | passive avoidance, maze performance | fetal ventral forebrain | Fine et al., 1985; Dunnett et al., 1985 |
| aged male rats | passive avoidance | fetal locus coeruleus | Collier et al., 1985, 1986 |

Recently, Fine et al. (1985) have used cholinergic neural transplants to reverse passive avoidance deficits in rats created by unilateral nucleus basalis lesions. The importance of this study is its potential relevance to Alzheimer's disease. It has been consistently observed that neurodegenerative changes occur in the nucleus basalis of Alzheimer's patients and these changes are assumed to be responsible for the dramatic reductions of cortical cholinergic enzymes which characterize this disease.

As in humans, significant variations are found in the performance of aged rats on various motor and cognitive tasks (Gash et al., 1984, Collier et al., 1985; Collier et al., 1986). We have found that aged rats with reduced noradrenaline levels in the locus coeruleus also show an impaired passive avoidance response. Fetal locus coeruleus grafts improve (prolong) passive avoidance behavior in these aged animals. As with the above study of Fine et al., our experiments are potentially relevant to Alzheimer's disease. Post-mortem analysis of human Alzheimer's tissues indicate that the deterioration of brain noradrenergic systems may contribute to severe learning and memory impairments which characterize the end state of the disease. Our studies, in concordance with others, suggest a potential application for neural transplants in the therapeutic treatment of Alzheimer's disease.

### Future Directions

Is there a clinic role for neural transplantation in treating Alzheimer's disease? While the results from the preliminary studies on rodents are encouraging, they only provide a general outline for developing transplantation strategies for treating humans. In our opinion (see Kordower and Gash, 1986), one essential step in assessing the potential therapeutic role of neural transplantation is to conduct grafting studies on nonhuman primates with Alzheimer's-like cognitive dysfunctions. The primate brain, especially the cerebral cortex, is more complex and shows a higher level of organization than in rodents. Both man and nonhuman primates (but not rodents) possess a large, convoluted telencephalon which is intimately involved in higher cognitive functions. Alzheimer's disease has been characterized as a cortical dementia and animals possessing a well-developed cerebral cortex resembling the human brain would seem to be essential for its study.

Several research groups, including ours, are now attempting to develop a valid nonhuman primate model of Alzheimer's disease. We (Kordower, Bartus, Okawara, and Gash, in preparation) have begun by mapping three dimensional arrangements of the cholinergic and catecholaminergic systems in the Cebus apella monkey brain. Neuronal subsets of these systems, including cholinergic neurons in the nucleus basalis and noradrenergic neurons in the locus coeruleus, have been found to be severely affected in Alzheimer's disease. We have also begun to systematically lesion brain regions, such as the nucleus basalis, which consistently demonstrate degenerative changes in Alzheimer's disease and then evaluate the neurochemical and neuropathological consequences of these lesions. The purpose of these studies is to determine which lesions, or set of lesions, creates Alzheimer-like alterations in Cebus monkeys. By having the appropriate animal model, new therapeutic strategies, such as neural transplantation, can be developed. In addition, by studying the experimental conditions which produce Alzheimer-like changes in the primate brain, new insights should be gained into the events occuring in the early stages of Alzheimer's disease in man. The early events in the development of Alzheimer's disease are poorly understood at present. As discussed elsewhere (Gash et al., 1986), the key for any successful treatement of Alzheimer's disease probably lies in the early detection and early clinical intervention.

## ACKNOWLEDGEMENTS

I wish to thank Kim A. Gesell and Nancy Bales for secretarial assistance. Research from my laboratory was supported, in part, by the Brain Fund and NIH grant NS15109.

## REFERENCES

Boer, G.J., Gash, D.M., Dick, L.B., and Schluter, N., 1985, Vasopressin neuron survival in neonatal Brattleboro rats: Critical factors in graft development and innervation of the host brain. Neurosci., 15: 1087-1109.

Backlund, E.O., Granberg, P.O., Hamberger, B., Sedvall, G., Seiger, A. and Olson, L., 1985, Transplantation of adrenal medullary tissue to the striatum in Parkinsonism. in: Neural grafting in the Mammalian CNS, (A.Bjorklund and U. Stenevi, eds.), Elsevier Science Publishers, Amsterdam. pp 551-556.

Bjorklund, A., 1985, Functional reactivation of the deafferented hippocampus by embryonic septal grafts as assessed by measurements of local glucose utilization. Exp. Brain Res., 58: 570-579.

Bjorklund, A., and Stenevi, U., 1977, Reformation of the severed septohippocampal cholinergic pathway in the adult rat by transplanted septal neurons. Cell Tiss. Res., 185: 289-302.

Bottenstein, J.E., 1981, Differentiated properties of neuronal cell lines in: Functionally Differentiated Cell Lines, (G.H. Sato, ed.), A.R. Liss, New York. pp 155-184.

Collier, T.J., Gash, D.M., Bruemmer, V., and Sladek, J.R., Jr., 1985, Impaired regulation of arousal in old age and the consequences for learning and memory: Replacement of brain norepinephrine via neuron transplants improves memory performance in aged F344 RATS. in: Homeostatic Functions in the elderly (B.B. Davis and W.G. Good, Eds.), Raven Press, New York. pp 99-110.

Collier, T.J., Gash, D.M., and Sladek, J.R., Jr., 1986, Norepinephrine deficiency and behavioral senescence on aged rats: Transplanted locus coeruleus neurons as an experimental replacement therapy. Proc. N.Y. Acad. Sci. (in press).

Crutcher, K.A., Kesner, R.P. and Novak, J.M., 1983, Medial septal lesions, radial arm maze performance and sympathetic sprouting: A study of recovery of functions. Brain Res., 262: 91-98.

Dunnett, S.B., Low, W.C., Iversen, S.D., Stenevi, U., and Bjorklund, A., 1982, Septal transplants restore maze learning in rats with fornix-fimbria lesions. Brain Res., 251: 335-348.

Dunnett, S.B., Toniolo, G., Fine, A., Ryan, C.N., Bjorklund, A., and Iversen, S.D., 1985, Transplantation of embryonic ventral forebrain neurons to the neocortex of rats with lesions of nucleus basalis magnocellularis - II. Sensorimotor and learning impairments. Neurosci., 16: 787-797.

Fine, A., Dunnett, S.B., Bjorklund, A., and Iversen, S.D., 1985, Cholinergic ventral forebrain grafts into the neocortex improve passive avoidance memory in a rat model of Alzheimer disease. Proc. Natl. Acad. Sci (USA) 82: 5227-5230.

Freed, W.J., 1985, Transplantation of tissues to the cerebral ventricles: Methodological details and rate of graft survival. in: Neural grafting in the Mammalian CNS, (A. Bjorklund and U. Stenevi, Eds.), Elsevier, Amsterdam. pp 31-40.

Freed, W.J., Morihisa, J.M., Spoor, E., Hoffer, B.J., Olson, L., Seiger, A., and Wyatt, R.J., 1981, Transplanted adrenal chromaffin cells in rat brain reduce lesion-induced rotational behavior. Nature, 292: 351-352.

Gage, F.H., Bjorklund, A., Stenevi, U., Dunnett, S.B., Kelly, P.A.T., 1984, Intrahippocampal septal grafts ameliorate learning impairments in aged rats. Science, 225: 533-536.

Gash, D.M., Collier, T.J. and Sladek, J.R., Jr., 1984, Neural tranplantation: A review of recent developments and potential applications to the aged brain. Neurobiol. Aging, 6: 131-150.

Gash, D.M., Notter, M.F.D., Dick, L.B., Kraus, A.L., Okawara, S.H., Wechkin, S.W., and Joynt, R.J., 1985, Cholinergic neurons transplanted into the monkeys. in: Neural Grafting in the Mammalian CNS, (A.Bjorklund and U. Stenevi, Eds.), Elsevier, Amsterdam. pp 596-603.

Gash, D.M., Notter, M.F.D., Okawara, S.H., Kraus, A.L. and Joynt, R.J., 1986a, Amitotic Neuroblastoma Cells used for Neural Implants in Monkeys. Science (in press).

Gash, D.M., Notter, M.F.D., and Kordower, J., 1986b, Cognitive dysfunctions and neural implants in: Treatment Development Strategies for Alzheimer's Disease, (R. Bartus, S. Ferris, S. Gershon, T. Crook, Eds.) (in press).

Gash, G.M., Sladek, J.R., Jr., Sladek, C.D., 1980, Functional development of grafted vasopressin neurons. Science, 210: 1367-1369.

Gupta, M., Notter, M.F.D., Felten, S., Gash, D.M., 1985, Differentiation characteristics of human neuroblastoma cells in the presence of growth modulators and antimitotic drugs. Dev. Brain Res., 19: 21-29.

Isacson, O., Brudin, P., Kelly, P.A.T., Gage, F.H., and Bjorklund, A., 1984, Functional neuronal replacement by grafted striatal neurones in the ibotenic acid-lesioned rat striatum. Nature, 311: 458-460.

Jaeger, C.B., 1985, Immunocytochemical study of PC12 cells grafted to the brain of immature rats. Exp. Brain Res., 59: 615-624.

Jilek, L., 1970, The reaction and adaptation of the central nervous system to stagnant hypoxia and anoxia during ontogeny. in: Developmental Neurobiology (W.A. Himwich, Ed.), C.C. Thomas, Springfield, IL pp 331-369.

Kelly, P.A.T., Gage, F.H., Ingvar, M., Lindvall, O., Stenevi, U., and Kimble, D.P., Bremiller, R. and Stickrod, G., 1986, Fetal brain implants improve maze performance in hippocampal-lessioned rats. Brain Res., 363: 358-363.

Kordower, J.H. and Gash, D.M., 1986, Animals and experimentation: An evaluation of animal models of Alzheimer's and Parkinson's disease. Integr. Psychiatry, 4: 64–80.

Kordower, J., Notter, M.F.D., Yeh, H.H., and Gash, D.M., 1986, An in vivo and in vitro assessment of differentiated neuroblastoma cells as a source donor tissue for transplantation. Ann. N.Y. Acad. Sci. (in press).

Krieger, D.T., Perlow, M.J., Gibson, M.J., Davies, T.F., Zimmerman, E.A., Ferin, M., and Charlton, H.M., 1982, Brain grafts reverse hypogonadism of gonadotropin-releasing hormone deficiency. Nature, 298: 468–47.

Labbe, R., Firl, A., Jr., Mufson, E.J., and Stein, D.G., 1983, Fetal rat brain transplants: Reduction of cognitive deficits in rats with frontal cortex lesions. Science, 221: 470–472.

Lampson, L.A., Fisher, C.A., and Whelan, J.P., 1983, Striking paucity of HLA-A,B,C and 2-macroglobulin on human neuroblastoma cell lines. J. Immunol., 130: 2471–2478.

Low, W.C., Lewis, P.R., Bunch, S.T., Dunnett, S.B., Thomas, S.R., Iversen, S.D., Bjorklund, A., and Stenevi, U., 1982, Functional recovery following neural transplantation of embryonic septal nuclei in adult rats with septohippocampal lesions. Nature, 300: 260–262.

Mason, D.W., Charlton, H.M., Jones, A., Parry, D.M., and Simmonds, S.J., 1985, Immunology of allograft rejection in mammals. in Neural Grafting in the Mammalian CNS (A. Bjorklund and U. Stenevi, Eds.), Elsevier, Amsterdam. pp. 91–98.

Morihisa, J.M., Nakamura, R.K., Freed, W.J., Mishkin, M., and Wyatt, R.J., 1984, Adrenal medulla grafts survive and exhibit catecholamine-specific fluorescence in the primate brain. Exp. Neurol., 84: 643–653.

Nieto-Sampedro, M., Whittemore, S.R., Needels, D., Larson, J., and Cotman, C.W., 1984, The survival of brain transplants is enhanced by extracts from injured brain. Proc. Natl. Acad. Sci.(USA), 81: 6250–6254.

Olson, L., Bjorklund, H., and Hoffer, B.J., 1984, Camera Bulbi Anterior: New vistas on a classic locus for neural tissue transplantation. in Neural Transplants: Development and Function, (J.R. Sladek, Jr., and D.M. Gash, Eds.), Plenum Press, New York. pp 125–165.

Perlow, M.F., Freed, W.F., Hoffer, B.J., Seiger, A. Olson, L., and Wyatt, R.J., 1979, Brain grafts reduce motor abnormalities produced by destruction of nigrostriatal dopamine system. Science, 204: 643–647. Ranson, S.W., 1914, Transplantation of the spinal ganglion with observations on the significance of the complex types of spinal ganglion cells. J.Comp. Neurol., 24: 547–558.

Rosenstein, J.M., and Brightman, M.W., 1984, Some consequences of grafting autonomic ganglia to brain surfaces. in Neural transplants: Development and Function (J.R. Sladek, Jr., and D.M. Gash, Eds.), Plenum Press, New York. pp 424–443.

Saltykow, S., 1905, Versuche uber gehirnreplantation, zugleich ein beitrag zur kenntniss der vorgange an den zelligen gehirnelementen. Arch. Psychiat. Berl., 40: 329–388.

Segal, M., Bjorklund, A., and Gage, F.H., 1985, Transplanted septal neurons make viable cholinergic synapses with a host hippocampus. Brain Res., 336: 302–307.

Stenevi, U., Bjorklund, A., and Svendgaard, N.A., 1976, Transplantation of central and peripheral monoamine neurons to the adult rat brain: Techniques and conditions for survival. Brain Res., 114: 1–20.

Wenzel, J. and Barlehner, E., 1969, Zur regeneration des cortex cerebri bei mus musculus. II. Morphologische befunde regenerattiver vorgange nach replantation eines cortexabschnittes. A. Mikro-anat Forsch., 81: 32–70.

# TREATMENT OF THE DEPRESSED ELDERLY PATIENT

Carl Salzman

Associate Professor of Psychiatry
Harvard Medical School
Director of Psychopharmacology
Massachusetts Mental Health Center

## INTRODUCTION

Treatment of the depressed elderly patient requires careful appraisal of the nature and severity of the patient's affective disturbance. A program is then selected that will offer the optimum balance between the disruptive effect of the symptoms and the antidepressant treatments, most of which have a high potential for toxicity in older people. Milder depressions may be successfully treated with psychotherapy or the psychostimulants. More severe depressive states usually require treatment with cyclic antidepressants, monoamine oxidase inhibitors, or electroconvulsive therapy. Antidepressant treatment is often undertaken in patients with cardiovascular disease or preexisting cognitive dysfunction, which emphasizes the need for special care in treating this population.

## Treatment with Psychotherapy

Comprehensive reviews of the literature on the psychotherapeutic treatment of depression in the elderly have emphasized the importance of this approach, the need for therapist optimism, and the various techniques that may be helpful for the older patient (Steuer, 1982; Charatan, 1985). There have been no controlled studies, however, of the therapeutic efficacy of individual psychotherapy in the treatment of depressed elderly patients. Jarvik (1982) has demonstrated that after 26 weeks, group psychotherapy provided some benefit for most patients over the age of 55 although it was completely therapeutic in only 12% of patients as compared with 45% of patients who had a complete response to imipramine. Gallagher and Thompson (1983) have published a clinical report on the effectiveness of psychotherapy in both endogenous as well as non-endogenous elderly outpatients; both brief and cognitive therapy was highly effective in older out patients with non-endogenous depression; endogenously depressed patients responded less well.

These reports suggest that for the mildly dysphoric or depressed elderly patient without delusions or marked vegetative symptoms, psychotherapy, in one form or another, may help relieve depressive symptoms. Psychotherapy may also be of help to the older person who is recovering from a depression, as well as for improving coping strategies to help diminish stress that might trigger another depressive episode. Psychotherapy may also be helpful in improving antidepressant drug-taking compliance in an older patient who might otherwise not wish to take a side-effect producing drug.

There are no reports suggesting that psychotherapy has therapeutic benefit in the treatment of older patients with severe depressions characterized by marked vegetative signs, or depressions with delusions. These depressions, which may be life-threatening, usually must be treated with pharmacotherapy or electroconvulsive therapy,

## Psychomotor Stimulants

Some elderly persons, although not clinically depressed, appear to have lost a zest for life and have become apathetic, withdrawn and progressively disinterested in their surroundings. Elderly patients with chronic medical diseases may become so discouraged and demoralized that they appear resigned to death and cease to participate in their rehabilitative treatment. Despite the severity of their dysphoria, these patients may not fulfill the diagnostic criteria for true depression and may not respond to antidepressant therapy. CNS stimulants such as methylphenidate and amphetamines are sometimes useful (for brief periods) for apathetic, withdrawn, disheartened, or demoralized older people (Kaplitz, 1975; Kayton, 1980).

The prescription of stimulants to older patients (especially very old patients) requires a careful medical examination to rule out cardiovascular disease and hypertension; both of these conditions are relative contraindications (depending on the severity of these illnesses) to stimulant prescription (Salzman and van der Kolk, 1984). Since stimulants may adversely interact with a number of other drugs that are likely to be taken by older patients (e.g, guanethidine, vasopressors, oral anticoagulants, anticonvulsants, imipramine, desipramine, (Jenike, 1985), a careful drug history must also be taken and stimulants not prescribed in conjunction with these other drugs.

Low doses of stimulants are often beneficial. Starting doses of 2.5 to 5 mg of methylphenidate may be prescribed for older patients; the drug should be given in the morning; if given in the late afternoon, evening, or nighttime, it may cause insomnia. If well tolerated, the dosage may be increased by 2.5 to 5 mg every 2 or 3 days until a total daily dosage of 20 mg is reached.

The most common side effects of stimulants are tachycardia and mild increases in blood pressure. Methylphenidate is preferred to amphetamines because of lower cardiovascular toxicity. Stimulants given to patients who are demented, whether or not they are depressed do not appreciably improve any cognitive function, and may aggravate behavioral symptoms associated with dementia such as agitation, paranoia, restlessness, insomnia and assaultiveness (Salzman, 1981).

## Cyclic Antidepressants

For most elderly patients whose depression is not immediately life-threatening, who are not delusional, and who do not have a physical illness that would contraindicate their use, cyclic antidepressants remain the first choice of treatment. Although several comparative drug trials have been conducted there are no studies that demonstrate the therapeutic superiority or inferiority of any cyclic antidepressant in the elderly depressed patient (Gerner, 1984). Selection of a particular antidepressant, therefore, depends on four factors other than differential efficacy; 1) alteration of the pharmacokinetic disposition of antidepressant drugs by the aging process; 2) history of prior response to a given drug; 3) the patient's physical health, and 4) knowledge of the side effects profiles of the various antidepressant drugs.

1)  Altered Disposition of Antidepressants

The aging process diminishes the efficiency of the hepatic microsomal enzyme system so that metabolism of antidepressants is delayed, and drugs accumulate in the body and blood stream. Antidepressants whose metabolic pathways include demethylation (tertiary amines: amitriptyline, imipramine, doxepin, trimipramine) are particularly vulnerable to the aging process since demethylation is impaired. This leads to higher plasma levels of the non-demethylated compound as compared with its demethylated metabolite (secondary amines: nortriptyline, desipramine, desmethyldoxepin, desmethylimipramine); since the non-demethylated compounds tend to be more toxic, these tertiary amines produce more frequent and more severe side effects in older patients (Salzman, 1984). In addition to decreased demethylation leading to higher ratios of tertiary:secondary amines, both compounds increase in the blood stream as a consequence of the reduced hepatic metabolism and decreased clearance. These increased plasma levels, in older people, as compared with levels produced in younger adults taking comparable doses, also predispose the older patient to toxicity unless prescribing doses are lower to accommodate these metabolic changes. Not all studies, however, support the assumption of increased steady state concentrations with age. Cutler (1981), for example, found that concentrations of desipramine, and of the hydroxy desipramine metabolite were not increased in the elderly, suggesting that not all antidepressants may be equally affected by the aging process. Other studies of desipramine (Ziegler and Biggs, 1977; Bertilsson et al., 1979; Nelson et al., 1982; Nelson et al., 1982) also failed to find an increase in steady state plasma concentrations of nortriptyline or amitriptyline.

Decreased metabolic efficiency in the aging liver also reduces drug clearance so that antidepressants, as a group, remain at least twice as long in the body as they do in younger adults (Salzman, 1984b). Recent pharmacokinetic data regarding the new antidepressant fluoxetine, did not demonstrate any lengthening of elimination half-life. However, in both young as well as old subjects, the half-life was approximately four days; in older patients, such long acting compounds may predispose the older patient to an increased risk of toxicity (Lemberger, 1985).

Plasma protein binding of antidepressants may also be altered in the elderly, although the clinical consequences of such alteration is not clear. There is convincing evidence to demonstrate a decrease in serum albumin levels with advanced age (especially past the age of 80) and similar data to show, as would be expected, that binding to albumin is decreased (Salzman, 1984b). However, antidepressant binding to albumin is low affinity; high affinity binding occurs to alpha-1-acid glycoprotein (Javaid et al., 1983), and the effect of age on this protein is not clear. Some data suggests that this protein may increase with age (Abernathy and Kerzner, 1984) offsetting the decrease in albumin binding. Clinically, it has been suggested that one of the reasons for increased antidepressant sensitivity among older patients is decreased protein binding, which leads to a higher plasma fraction of unbound (and therefore potentially toxic as well as therapeutic) drug (Salzman, 1982; 1984b).

The relationship between prescribing dose, plasma level and therapeutic response in older patients remains unclear. For reasons outlined above, lower doses probably produce plasma levels equivalent to those that would be produced by higher doses in younger recipients, although careful studies have not been conducted, and there is wide variation among older individuals. Jarvick et al., (1982), for example, found that 75 mg/day of imipramine or doxepin was more therapeutic than higher doses of imipramine or desipramine for severely depressed delusional elderly patients, but half of the patients had to discontinue the study due to intolerable side effects or worsening clinical condition.

In general, therapeutic response in the elderly is associated with plasma levels in the therapeutic range, and there are not studies to suggest that older patients respond to subtherapeutic (by young adult standards) plasma levels. Friedel (1975), for example, has shown that elderly responders to doxepin had higher blood levels than nonresponders; Ward et al., (1982) similarly showed that higher levels of both doxepin and desmethyldoxepin were associated with therapeutic response in older patients. Smith (1980) reported that elderly responders to nortriptyline had plasma concentrations within the therapeutic range for all adult patients. Nelson et al., (1985) found that elderly patients did not respond to lower desipramine levels; therapeutic levels were required.

Taken together, these data suggest that therapeutic plasma levels of antidepressant are required for efficacy in older patients, but that smaller doses may be needed in some patients to achieve these levels. Once taken, antidepressants, as a class of drugs, tend to remain longer in the body of older people than younger adults, thereby prolonging the time for possible side effects.

## 2)   History of prior response

Although there are no controlled research observations regarding response to a previously effective antidepressant, it is a frequent clinical observation that patients often respond a second time to a drug that has been previously effective.

## 3)   Physical Health

Since the side effect profiles of cyclic antidepressants differ, some drugs may be especially toxic in patients with certain physical diseases. This is particularly true for older patients with cardiac conduction disorders. Although these drugs tend to reduce cardiac arrhythmias at therapeutic plasma levels, at higher levels, they prolong electrical conduction through the Purkinje fibers resulting in a widening of the QRS complex on the electrocardiogram. At toxic levels, the QRS may be longer than 100 msec and heart block, ventricular arrhythmias and death may result. Since it is likely that all antidepressants ultimately share cardiac toxicity given sufficient plasma drug level, it is important to ensure that levels do not enter the range of potential cardiac toxicity. Studies of the relationship between the electrocardiogram and antidepressants have demonstrated that the QRS complex begins to widen as the cardiotoxic drug level is approached. Thus, monitoring antidepressant treatment with pretreatment; and serial EKG's; may be especially useful in the older patient, particularly when cardiac conduction disease exists (Salzman, 1985c).

Older patients with narrow angle glaucoma or bowel disease, or men with prostatic hypertrophy may all react to the anticholinergic properties of antidepressants with an aggravation of symptomatology. All older patients are especially susceptible to the central effects of cholinergic blockade by antidepressants; the toxic manifestations including agitation, disorientation, decreased recent memory, and in more severe cases delirium and hallucinations. These symptoms may be misdiagnosed as evidence of rapidly progressing dementia, metastatic carcinoma, or "senility" (Salzman, 1985b).

## Differential Side Effect Profile

There are no convincing data to suggest that any one antidepressant is therapeutically superior to any other. There are differences, however, among individual antidepressants as well as between groups of pharmacologically similar antidepressants in the frequency and intensity of side effects that are produced. Tertiary amines, as a group, produce more frequent and more severe side effects. Among the secondary amines (antidepressants that have already been demethylated), desipramine and nortriptyline are usually recommended for the older patient because they produce somewhat less frequent and less severe (but not absent!) side effects (Salzman, 1985a; 1985b; Salzman and van der Kolk, 1984). The newest antidepressant, fluoxetine, has been reported in one study of elderly patients, to be as effective as doxepin; its side effect profile suggests that it is non-sedating and has no anticholinergic effects (Feighner, 1985). Additional studies in elderly patients are needed, however, before the role of fluoxetine as an antidepressant for older patients becomes clear.

Although the prescribing generalizations just outlined are generally true, they may not apply to any individual patient, and they may be ignored when careful dose and plasma level monitoring are possible. For example, studies have shown that amitriptyline, generally considered the most toxic antidepressant for older patients, may be prescribed with safety as well as efficacy when blood levels are carefully monitored (Robinson, 1981; Ahles et al., 1984; Preskorn and Mac, 1985).

Side effects can be minimized in some elderly patients by careful dosing. As already noted, older patients are more likely to develop elevated plasma drug levels per given dose because of pharmacokinetic alterations due to aging.

## Monoamine Oxidase Inhibitors

MAO inhibitors have been used with increasing frequency for the non-delusional elderly depressed patient who has not responded to cyclic antidepressants (Ashford and Ford, 1976). MAO inhibitors, like stimulants, may also be useful for the elderly patient who is not severely depressed, whose depression is not characterized by severe vegetative signs, or whose affective state is characterized by apathy, anergia and anhedonia. Brain levels of MAO are increased with age suggesting a special usefulness for these drugs in the elderly (Salzman, 1984a). However, there are no data to implicate increased MAO as a cause of depression in the elderly.

Response to MAO inhibitors in the elderly, as in younger adult patients, is correlated with degree of enzyme inhibition. Georgotas et al., (1983) found that monoamine oxidase inhibitors were very therapeutic when MAO inhibition was greater than 80%. Inhibition of platelet MAO activity may also be correlated with plasma levels of some MAO inhibitors. For example, studies of the pharmacology of phenelzine, showed that older patients tended to have higher plasma drug levels than younger patients, particularly during the first two weeks of treatment. The higher plasma level may result from an age-related decrease in the apparent volume of distribution of phenelzine in the elderly as well as a slower rate of phenelzine metabolism and clearance (Robinson, 1981).

The side effects of MAO inhibitors that may be especially troublesome for the older patient are orthostatic hypotension, sedation and aggravation of dementia. The latter effect may not occur in mildly demented patients (Jenike, 1986), but is frequently encountered in the moderately or severely demented older patient (Salzman, 1986). MAO inhibitors often also stimulate the older patient. In addition to aggravating the cognitive impairment of dementia, they can produce restlessness, agitation, paranoia, and insomnia. MAO inhibitors may also be difficult to prescribe to some older outpatients because of their questionable ability to adhere to the tyramine restricted diet. Since older patients are likely to be taking several drugs simultaneously (Salzman, 1984), the risk of serious drug interactions with MAO inhibitors and drugs containing stimulants may increase the risk of stroke or myocardial infarction in this population.

There is no evidence for therapeutic superiority of any one MAO inhibitor over another in elderly patients. Phenelzine, the most commonly prescribed MAO inhibitor, is associated with sedation and orthostatic hypotension in contrast to tranylcypromine, which is known for its stimulant properties. Like the cyclic antidepressants, starting doses of these drugs should be low (half of the dose given younger adults), and doseage increments should be small, and guided by clinical response, toxicity and the degree of platelet MAO inhibition.

## Electroconvulsive Therapy

Electroconvulsive therapy is a safe and clinically effective treatment for the elderly depressed patient who has a sever depressive disorder, and is an appropriate choice for the older patient who either has not responded to antidepressants or has developed sever side effects from them. ECT can be life-saving for the frail, malnourished, depressed, suicidal elderly patient. Although controlled research studies in the elderly are lacking, clinical experience has strongly suggested that ECT is particularly helpful for the elderly depressed patient who is severely agitated or withdrawn, and who may be delusional (Salzman, 1982; Weiner, 1982; Salzman and van der Kolk, 1984). Symptoms of severe guilt, loss of interest, early morning insomnia, and anorexia predict good response to ECT.

The primary side effect of ECT in patients of all ages is impairment of recent memory. This is particularly undesirable in elderly patients who may be more susceptible to this side effect, especially if they already have memory impairment. Pettinati and Bonner (1984) have shown that older patients develop more cognitive dysfunction following ECT as measured by the Trail making test. There are no research reports that discuss the clinical or toxic effect of ECT in patients with dementia who are also depressed. In mild cases of dementia, however, clinical experience suggests that successful antidepressant response to ECT improves the older patient's subjective sense of memory function, and has been associated with small increases in Wechsler memory scores (Salzman, 1970, unpublished data).

Older patients who have not received ECT often respond to fewer treatments than do younger patients. However, those elderly patients who have had several prior courses of electroconvulsive therapy sometimes appear to be resistant to the usual course of ECT, and may require more treatments than the average younger patient (i.e., > 12). The mechanism for this apparent tolerance is not understood.

Unilateral nondominant electrode placement in the elderly produce less post-ictal confusion and a shorter awakening time than bilateral electrode placement (Fraser and Glass, 1978). Electroconvulsive therapy is contraindicated in patients of all ages who have increased intracranial pressure (Salzman, et al., 1975) but has been successfully administered to depressed elderly patients who have suffered a stroke with residual neurologic deficits (Karliner, 1978). ECT has also been successfully administered to elderly patients with aortic aneurysms, to those who have had myocardial infarctions (Karliner, 1978) and to those who have implanted pacemakers (Abiuso et al., 1975; Jauher et al., 1979).

Administration of electroconvulsive therapy to the elderly depressed patient should routinely include a thorough pretreatment physical examination with particular emphasis on cardiovascular, neurologic and mental status functioning. Adequate pretreatment oxygenation and administration of oxygen during and after the treatment, as well as thorough muscle relaxation are also necessary. Cardiac monitoring is advised during the first one or two treatments for the very old, or very frail elderly patients with normal cardiac functioning; elderly patients with cardiovascular disease should be monitored during all treatments.

## Treatment Resistant Depressions

In most clinical circumstances when an older depressed patient fails to respond to an adequate trial of a cyclic antidepressant, treatment strategies shift to the use of a monoamine oxidase inhibitor, or electroconvulsive therapy. Recent data in younger patients have suggested that the use of adjuvant T3 or lithium carbonate may be added to enhance therapeutic efficacy (Salzman and van der Kolk, 1984; Jenike, 1985; Borson and Raskind, 1986; Goff and Jenike, 1986). However, there have been no antidepressants and adjuvant therapy for treatment resistant patients. The arrhythmias (Salzman and van der Kolk, 1984), and the use of lithium may exacerbate cognitive dysfunction in the older depressed patient as well as lead to cardiovascular and renal toxicity (Liptzin, 1984). In the absence of controlled studies, therefore, adjuvant therapy should be employed with caution in the elderly.

## Patients with Cardiovascular Disease

Treatment of the depressed elderly patient who also has hypertension is a delicate and difficult task. Antihypertensives may cause depression or aggravate a preexisting depression. They may also interact with antidepressants in three ways potentially harmful to the older patient. First, volume-depleting diuretics may exacerbate orthostatic hypotension caused by antidepressants and necessitate a reduction in the diuretic dosage (Kanter and Glassman, 1980). Second, the uptake of guanethidine, bethanidine, and debrisoquin into presynaptic adrenergic synapses is inhibited by most cyclic antidepressants, thus interfering with the action of these drugs (Salzman and van der Kolk, 1984). The antihypertensive effect of clonidine is also blocked, and clonidine given in combination with imipramine has produced a hypertensive crisis in an elderly patient (Hui, 1983). Third, because all antidepressants, especially tertiary amines, produce orthostatic hypotension, blood pressure may be rapidly reduced to dangerous levels when the older patient who is receiving both anti-depressants and antihypertensives stands up quickly (Gerner, 1984; Salzman, 1985a, 1985b). If antidepressant drugs cannot be given because of these effects, then the older depressed patient should be treated with ECT.

## Patients with Cerebrovascular Disease

Antidepressant drugs, in carefully selected patients may also be a safe and effective treatment for the poststroke patient. Although specific studies of depressed poststroke patients who are elderly have not been conducted, Lipsey et al., (1984) and Robinson, et al., (1983) have demonstrated the effectiveness of these drugs in the treatment of depression. As noted, ECT is also safe and effective, and may be used when antidepressant drugs are contraindicated.

## Depression and Cognitive Disorder

Memory, concentration, and other cognitive functions are dependent, to some degree, on adequate CNS acetylcholine functioning. In older patients, acetylcholine neurotransmission is reduced, and in patients with senile dementia of the Alzheimer's type, it is virtually absent (Salzman, 1984a). For these reasons, older patients are more susceptible to the anticholinergic effects of antidepressants, especially the tertiary amine cyclic antidepressants (Salzman and van der Kolk, 1984). Cole et al., (1983), reviewing the literature concluded that these drugs can cause both confusional states, as well as speech and memory problems and measurable deficits in recall of learned information. Branconnier and Cole (1981), comparing amitriptyline, a strongly anticholinergic cyclic antidepressant with trazodone, a drug with no anticholinergic properties, demonstrated that recall of recently acquired information was superior with the non-anticholinergic drug.

These data suggest that antidepressants with anticholinergic properties may be especially toxic to older people, especially if they already have memory impairment. With the exception of trazodone and fluoxetine, all antidepressants, including the monoamine oxidase inhibitors, are anticholinergic and thus may be used cautiously in depressed elderly patients who may also have observable signs of dementia. ECT should be employed in cases of severe depression when antidepressant drugs cannot be used.

## Conclusion

Depression in the elderly is a frequent, crippling and sometimes life threatening illness. In milder forms, treatment may be limited to supportive measures, psychotherapy or brief use of psychostimulant drugs. For more severe depressions, cyclic antidepressants, and to a lesser extent, monoamine oxidase inhibitors are usually employed, and for the most severe depression, electroconvulsive therapy is usually indicated. In order to minimize potential drug toxicity, all elderly patients should have a careful pretreatment physical examination including an ECG. The older patient is more susceptible to antidepressant side effects because of age-related pharmacokinetic alterations as well as increased CNS drug sensitivity. For most (but not all) older patients, doses may need to be lower than those used for the average younger adult patient, but must be sufficient to produce adequate blood levels for therapeutic effect. Serious medical illness, including cardiovascular or cerebrovascular disease are not contraindications to treatment with antidepressant drugs or ECT. The treatment of the cognitively impaired, depressed elderly patient is difficult because drug and ECT toxicity may further compromise memory, concentration, and other cognitive functions. However, when antidepressants are cautiously administered, the therapeutic antidepressant effect may outweigh anticholinergic toxicity, especially in the mild or moderately demented depressed patient.

It should be remembered that in most cases, depression in the elderly is a treatable illness; the hopelessness of the older depressed patient should not be allowed to influence the physician's decision to treat or not to treat.

REFERENCES

Abernathy, D.R., Kerzner, L., 1984, Age effects on alpha-1-acid glycoprotein Concentration and imipramine plasma protein binding, J. Am. Geriat.Soc., 32:705.
Abiuso, P., Dunkleman, R., Proper, M., 1975, Electroconvulsive therapy in patients with pacemakers, J. Am. Med. Assoc., 240:2459.
Ahles, S., Gwirtsman, H., Halaris, A., Shah, P., Schwarcz, G., Hill, M.A., 1984, Comparative cardiac effects of matprortiline and doxepin, J. Clin. Psychiatry, 45:460.

Ashford, W., Ford, C.V., 1976, Use of monoamine oxidase inhibitors in elderly patients, Am. J. Psychiatry, 136:1466.

Bertilsson, L., Mellstrom, B., Sjoqvist, P., 1979, Pronounced inhibition of noradrenaline uptake by 10-hydroxy metabolites of nortriptyline, Life Sci, 25:285.

Borson, S., Raskind, M., 1986, Antidepressant resistant depression in the elderly, J. Am. Geriat. Soc., 34:245.

Branconnier, R.J., Cole, J.O., 1981, Effects of acute administration of trazodone and amitriptyline on cognition, cardiovascular function and salivation in the normal geriatric patient, J. Clin. Psychopharmacol., 1:2.

Brown, R.P., Kocsis, J.H., Glick, I.D., 1984, Efficacy and feasibility of high dose tricyclic antidepressant treatment in elderly delusional depressives, J. Clin. Psychopharmacol., 4:315.

Cole, J.O., Branconnier, R., Saloman, M., Dessain, E., 1983, Tricyclic use in the cognitively impaired elderly, J. Clin. Psychiatry, 44:14.

Charatan, F.B., 1985, Depression and the elderly: Diagnosis and treatment, Psych. Ann., 15:313.

Cutler, N.R., Zavendil, A.P. III, Eisdorfer, C., Ross, R.J., Potter, W.Z., 1981, Concentrations of desipramine in elderly females are not elevated, Am. J. Psychiatry, 138:1235.

Feighner, J.P., Cohn, J.B., 1985, Double-blind comparative trials of fluoxetine and doxepin in geriatric patients with major depressive disorder, J. Clin. Psychiatry, 46:20.

Fraser, R.M., Glass, I.B., 1978, Recovery from ECT in elderly patients, Br. J. Psychiatry, 133:524.

Friedel, R.O., 1975, Relationship of blood levels of Sinequan to clinical effects in the treatment of depression in aged patients, in: "A Monograph of Recent Clinical Studies," J. Mendels, ed., Excerpta Medical. 1975.

Gallagher, D.E., Thompson, S.W., 1983, Effectiveness of psychotherapy for both endogenous and nonendogenous depression in older adult out-patients, J. Gerontol., 38:707.

Gerner, R.H., 1984, Antidepressant selection in the elderly, Psychosomatics, 25:528.

Georgotas, A., Fridman, E., McCarthy, M., 1983, Resistant geriatric depressions and therapeutic response to monoamine oxidase inhibitors, Biol. Psychiatry, 18:195.

Goff, D.C., Jenike, M.A., 1986, Treatment-resistant depression in the elderly, J. Am. Geriat. Soc., 34:63.

Hrdina, P.D., Rovei, V., Henry, J.F., 1980, Comparison of single dose pharmacokinetics of imipramine and maprotiline in the elderly, Psycho-pharmacology, 70:29.

Hui, K.K., 1983, Hypertensive crisis induced by interaction of clonidine with imipramine, J. Am. Geriat. Soc., 31:164.

Jarvik, L.F., Mintz, J., Steuer, J., 1982, Treating geriatric depression: A 26-week interim analysis, J. Am. Geriat. Soc., 30:713.

Jauer, P., Weller, M., Hirsch, S.R., 1979, Electroconvulsive therapy for a patient with a cardiac pacemaker, Br. Med. J., 1:90.

Javaid, J.I., Hendricks, K., Davis, J.M., 1983, Alpha-1-acid glycoprotein involvement in high affinity binding of tricyclic antidepressants to human plasma, Biochem. Pharmacol., 32:1149.

Jenike, M.A., 1984, Use of monoamine oxidase inhibitors in elderly depressed patients, J. Am. Geriat. Soc., 32:571.

Jenike, M.A.,1985, "Handbook of Geriatric Psychopharmacology",PSG Publishing, Littleton, N.J.

Kantor, S.J., Glassman, A.H., 1980, The use of tricyclic antidepressant drugs in geriatric patients, in: "Psychopharmacology of Aging, " C. Eisdorfer, W.E. Fann, eds., Spectrum, New York.

Kaplitz, S.E., 1975, Withdrawn apathetic geriatric patients responsive to methylphenidate, J. Am. Geriat. Soc., 23:271.

Karliner, W., 1978, Cardiovascular disease and ECT, Psychosomatics, 19:238.
Karliner, W., 1978, ECT for patients with CNS disease, Psychosomatics, 19:781.
Kayton, W., Raskind, M., 1986, Treatment of depression in the medically ill elderly with methylphenidate, Am. J. Psychiatry, 137:963.
Lemberger, L., Bergstrom, R.F., Woten, R.L., Farid, N.A., Enas, G.G., Aronoff, G.R., 1985, Fluoxetine: Clinical pharmacology and physiologic disposition, J. Clin. Psychiatry, 46:14.
Lipsey, J.R., Pearlson, G.D., Robinson, R.G., 1984, Nortriptyline treatment of post-stroke depression: A double-blind study, Lancet, i:297.
Lipzin, B., 1984, Treatment of mania, in: "Clinical Geriatric Psycho-pharmacology," C. Salzman, ed., McGraw-Hill, New York.
Nelson, J.C., Jatlow, P.I., Block, J., Quinlan, D.M., Bowers, M.B., 1982, Major adverse reaction during desipramine treatment, Arch. Gen. Psychiatry, 39: 1419.
Nelson, J.C., Jatlow, P.I., Quinlan, D.N., Bowers, M.B., 1982, Desipramine plasma concentration and antidepressant response, Arch. Gen. Psychiatry, 39:1419.
Nelson, J.C., Jatlow, P.I., Mazure, C., 1985, Desipramine plasma levels and response in elderly melancholic patients, J. Clin. Psychopharmacol., 5:217.
Pettinati, H.M., Bonner, K.M., 1984, Cognitive functioning in depressed geriatric patients with a history of ECT, Am. J. Psychiatry, 141:49.
Preskorn, S.H., Mac, D.S., 1985, Plasma levels of amitriptyline: Effect of age and sex, J. Clin. Psychiatry, 46:276.
Robinson, D.S., 1981, Monoamine oxidase inhibitors and the elderly, in: "Age and the Pharmacology of Psychoactive Drugs,", A. Raskin, S.A. Robinson, J. Levine, eds., Elsevier, New York.
Robinson, R.G., Lipsey, J.R., Price, T.R., 1985, Diagnosis and clinical management of post-stroke depression, Psychosomatics, 26:769.
Salzman, C., 1981, Stimulants in the elderly, in: "Age and the Pharmacology of Psychoactive Drugs,", A. Raskin, D.S. Robinson, J. Levine, eds., Elsevier, New York.
Salzman, C., 1982, Key concepts in geriatric psychopharmacology-Altered pharmacokinetics and polypharmacy, Psychiat. Clin. N. Amer., 5:181.
Salzman, C., 1982, Electroconvulsive therapy in the elderly patient, Psychiat. Clin. N. Amer., 5:191.
Salzman, C., 1984, Neurotransmission in the aging central nervous system, in: "Clinical Geriatric Psychopharmacology,", C. Salzman, ed., McGraw-Hill, New York.
Salzman, C., 1985, Clinical guidelines for the use of antidepressant drugs in geriatric patients, J. Clin. Psychiatry, 46:46.
Salzman, C., 1985, Geriatric Psychopharmacology, Ann. Rev. Med., 36:217.
Salzman, C. 1985, Clinical use of antidepressant blood levels and the electrocardiogram, New Eng. J. Med., 313:512.
Salzman, C., 1986, Caution urged in using MAOI's with the elderly (letter to the editor), Am. J. Psychiatry, 143:118.
Salzman, C., van der kolk, B.A., Shader, R.I., 1975, Psychopharmacology and the geriatric patient, in: "Manual of Psychiatric Therapeutics," R.I. Shader, ed., Little Brown, Boston.
Salzman, C. van der Kolk, B.A., 1984, Treatment of depression, in: "Clinical Geriatric Psychopharmacology," C. Salzman, ed., McGraw-Hill, New York.
Smith, R.C., Reed, K., Leelavathi, D.E., 1980, Pharmacokinetics and the effects of nortriptyline in geriatric depressed patients, Psychopharm. Bull., 16:54.
Steuer, J K., 1982, Psychotherapy for depressed elders, in: "Depression in Late Life," D.G. Blazer, ed., Mosby, St. Louis.
Ward, N.G., Bloom, V.L., Wilson, L., Raskind, M., Raisys, V.A., 1982, Doxepin plasma levels and the therapeutic response in depression: preliminary finding, J. Clin. Psychiatry, 2:126.

Weiner, R.D., 1982, The role of ECT in the treatment of depression in the elderly, J. Am. Geriat. Soc., 30:710.
Ziegler, V.E., Biggs, J.T., 1977, Tricyclic plasma levels:  Effect of age, race, sex, and smoking, J. Am. Med. Assoc., 238:2167.

STATUS OF ALZHEIMER DISEASE RESEARCH

Zaven S. Khachaturian

National Institute on Aging
Physiology of Aging Branch

Since its inception in 1974, the National Institute on Aging (NIA), the Federal agency with the prime responsibility for conducting and supporting research on the biomedical and behavioral processes of aging and the diseases of aging, has targeted Alzheimer's disease (AD) as one of the most important research priorities and challenges. Within the Public Health Service (PHS) of the Department of Health and Human Services (HHS), the NIA shares an interest and responsibility for this research with its sister institutes, the National Institute of Allergy and Infectious Diseases; and the National Institute of Mental Health, ADAMHA.

Among the many debilitating disorders of old age, the most frustrating include those that lead to a partial or complete loss in cognitive functioning. Alzheimer's disease is one of the most persistent and devastating dementing disorders of old age, eventually leading to a complete loss of memory and ability to learn. Alzheimer's disease presents enormous problems to the families of victims and raises complex social and economic issues for the public. At the same time, the disease offers unusual scientific challenges.

Alzheimer's disease is no longer regarded as a natural consequence of aging, as it was only a few years ago. It affects a substantial proportion of the aged. Although the exact number of people affected is not known because of the difficulties involved in accurate diagnosis it is estimated that between 2.5 and 3.0 million people have this disease in its various stages. Many of the families of AD patients are now well organized to provide support and share information through such organizations as Alzheimer's Disease and Related Disorders Association, Inc. (ADRDA).

The general public is better informed about the disease through the efforts of the NIA Public Information Office and the media. Congress and the Federal Government have begun to formulate public policy concerning services and research, and several agencies within the PHS have designated AD as a high-priority public health issue. A growing number of scientists have begun to study a broad spectrum of problems associated with the disease. In a relatively short period we have learned a considerable amount, but AD today still presents some challenging scientific opportunities for neuroscience. In the following account, I will attempt to provide an overview of the magnitude of the problem presented by AD and the remarkable scientific achievements that have already been made.

The number and proportion of elderly in the United States are rapidly increasing and are already having profound influences on American economic, social, and political thinking and behavior. Biomedical research and its applied technologies have made it possible for an increasing number of people to survive until their 70s or 80s. Perhaps the most significant impact will prove to be economic: the costs of needed health care, clinical medicine, and biomedical research. Persons aged 65 years and older are at greatest risk for disease and, consequently, have the greatest need for medical services. Many age-related disabilities tend to be chronic, rather than acute, requiring long-term care. Such care is expensive, and the costs are expected to rise rapidly due to increased numbers of elderly and the growing cost health care. Long-term care costs of AD patients and other aged persons will be considered in the Department's ongoing study of catastrophic illness due to the President by the end of the year.

The following are some of the most dramatic demographic changes of this century: 1) the number of people over 65 years has risen from 3 million in 1900 to 27 million today and is projected to reach 43 million by 2020. At the same time, the proportion of those over 65 has risen from 4.1 percent in 1900 to 11 percent in 1980; 2) the greatest increases are among those over age 85 years who are likely to require special care. This segment of the population is expected to grow rapidly over the next 15 years and to reach over 5 million by 2000; 3) although nearly 68 percent of older people consider themselves healthy and 90 percent live independently, nearly 86 percent have one or more chronic health conditions or disabilities; and 4) the elderly account for 15 percent of all visits to physicians, 34 percent of all days spent in short-stay hospitals, 89 percent of all nursing home occupancy, and 29 percent of all money spent on personal health care. In 1988, the total cost of health care services to the elderly will reach nearly 200 billion dollars.

Among the many age-related disabilities, those related to changes in the central nervous system or brain functioning have important implications for both public policy relating to health care services and national priorities for biomedical research. Failure in cognitive functioning is one of the principal indicators for institutionalization of the elderly on long-term care facilities. Long-term custodial care in an institutional setting is extremely expensive, often impersonal, and can contribute to further deterioration of health.

Approximately 10 percent of the elderly population show clinically significant cognitive deficits. The frequency of intellectual impairment is considerably higher among those living in nursing homes, where an estimated 50 percent or more have some form of mental impairment. A significant number of these are now recognized to have AD. In 1986, the annual national expenditure for nursing home care is projected to be approximately $40 billion. It is estimated that during the next few years this expenditure will become a staggering $80 billion in constant dollars. The current estimated all direct and indirect costs for AD alone, including nursing home care, is $38 billion per year. This, also, will grow over the next 10 years.

An important issue associated with AD is that of accurate diagnosis. There are as yet no specific studies identifying the frequency and cause of reversible cognitive impairments in the elderly, but it is estimated that up to 20 percent of persons aged 65 and over who have been labeled "demented" have reversible brain disorders that require evaluation and treatment. Misdiagnosis is extremely costly and a tragic waste when it leads to long-term institutionalization. There is clearly an urgent need to continue the quest for scientific knowledge concerning diagnosis and treatment possibilities for dementia and the biological mechanisms of aging and of such dementing disorder as AD. In 1983, the NIA, in collaboration with the American Association of Retired Persons (AARP), sponsored a research planning workshop on the Diagnosis of Alzheimer's Disease. This workshop identified some crucial scientific opportunities for further research on diagnosis. Now, in 1986, this meeting has begun to bear fruit.

The first finding concerns a protein present in nerve cells involved in the formation of the two types of brain lesions (neuritic plagues and neurofibrillary tangles) that are hallmark of AD. The significance of this finding is that this abnormal protein is unique to the brains of AD patients, it is not found in normal brain, also it is found only in very specific regions of the AD brain that have significant cell loss. This is a crucial finding because it provides the medical scientist a potential tool of clear cut diagnosis of this disease; and also it opens the door for finding out the mechanism by which the abnormal lesions develop in the brain of AD patients.

The second important discovery concerns another protein called "tau", a protein in the normal nerve cell, but shown to be the major component of paired helical filaments (the neurofibrillary tangles). the abnormal protein associated with AD. Tau is known to promote the assembly of microtubules (ingredient parts inside of a nerve cell) which are involved in the transport of biological molecules between the nerve body and its terminals. The significance of finding that a normal protein, such as tau, is associated with a major lesion in AD raises the possibility that, in selected nerve cells in this disease, certain chemical modifications of tau might occur which will allow the nerve cell to form tangles. This finding now will allow scientists another avenue to explore the exact mechanism by which this lesion in AD is caused.

The dimensions of the health problems posed by age-related changes in the central nervous system are vast. Basic research into the neurobiology of aging as the route to resolving these problems has been demonstrably successful in advancing knowledge of the human brain and providing the first real insights into some of the more baffling neurological disorders. The treatment of Parkinson's disease patients with L-dopa to replace the loss of a vital brain chemical, dopamine, and the discovery of the enkephalins and endorpohins-the brain's own "opiate" drugs--are important examples.

These advances have come about because of a critical combination of talent and technology in neuroscience. It is now possible to obtain a detailed picture of what happens at the molecular level of a nerve cell as well as a clearer idea of how large clusters of nerve cells and systems operate in elaborating complex human behaviors. Enthusiasm in the field of neuroscience is running high, and areas of investigation, convergent approaches are focusing on key issues of neurobiology. In order to move toward the fundamental goal of prevention of nervous system disorders, develop effective treatments for those presently afflicted, and ensure the rapid transfer of research advances to clinical applications, it is essential to capitalize on this new momentum in biological models, and the necessary technology--the methods and tools to make the observations fruitful. The neurosciences can now command all three of these elements. There has never been a lack of good ideas or experimental models, but only in the past 20 or 30 years have there been significant gains in technological progress. These achievements in technology are expected to continue making a substantial difference in the rate of advancement of knowledge in neuroscience.

Although systematic studies of age-related changes in the human brain have a 100-year history, strong interest in this subject is recent. During the last decade a growing community of neuroscientists, spurred partly by the availability of Federal funds for research, has begun to study a broad range of topics in the neurobiology of aging. These range from basic molecular to clinical issues, and from the physical chemistry of membrane transport mechanisms to the neuropsychiatric assessment of the aging brain. Not long ago, little was known about "senility," and AD was considered a hopeless affliction of the aged. Now we know that chemical and physical changes in the brain can account for some of the memory deficits in AD and the benign forgetfulness of the aged. The remarkable pace of scientific progress in this area of research increases the likelihood that some forms of dementia will be treatable by pharmacological agents.

Research supported by the PHS has also made it possible to start formulating a coherent scientific story on the pathogenesis of AD and to identify a number of exciting scientific opportunities that are ready to be exploited. Of even greater importance is that it is now possible to propose testable hypotheses that can provide a framework for interrelating some of the observations reported by scientists working in this area of research.

During the past few years, it has been clearly established that the hallmark of AD is a serious defect in the cholinergic system (one of the many chemicals used by nerve cells for cell to cell communication). This finding has stimulated considerable scientific activity aimed at identifying the exact nature of this neurochemical defect and finding a pharmacological means of ameliorating the disease. This type of research has been driven by the assumption that the neurochemical deficits in AD result primarily from biochemical abnormalities in the synthesis or release of the neurotransmitter acetylcholine; it is assumed that the affected brain cells would function normally if these biochemical abnormalities could be corrected. Thus, the search for treatment has focused on pharmacological manipulations aimed at 1) increasing the supply of the substrate necessary for the synthesis of the neurotransmitter such as use of choline or lecithin, 2) increasing the amount of the neurotransmitter released, 3) prolonging the availability of the neurotransmitter at the synaptic junction by blocking its breakdown, and 4) manipulating the sensitivity of receptors at the postsynaptic membrane.

Despite some promising initial results in treatment of AD with agents such as choline, lecithin, and physostigmine, this effort in cholinergic pharmacology has not produced any consistent or long-lasting treatment for AD. Several theories attempt to explain this lack of success. First, it is unlikely that AD results from a deficit in a single neurotransmitter system. There is mounting evidence that multiple neurotransmitter systems and neuropeptides are involved. Second, the observed neurochemical changes in AD might be epiphenomena associated with or a consequence of cell death. In AD cell death occurs in specific regions of the brain, particularly in areas richly innervated with cholinergic cells. Third, the neurochemical deficits might be a consequence of other changes within the cell, such as abnormal oxidative or glucose metabolism.

Investigators have yet to determine why brain cells die in AD and whether or not such cell death can be averted by pharmacological means. There are several working hypotheses concerning the possible mechanisms of cell death. One of the most active areas of study focuses on the chemistry of neurofibrillary tangles within nerve cells that are the classic pathological markers of AD. It is now known that these filaments are composed of highly insoluble protein formed by unknown chemical reaction. These insoluble protein masses might form a physical blockage that interferes with axoplasmic transport mechanisms, thus leading to cell death. It is essential that future research focus on the biochemistry of beta-pleated proteins, cross-linking reactions and the enzymology of such reactions.

Another important area of study concerns the role of modulators (chemicals that modify the effects of a neurotransmitter) and neurotrophic factors affecting the functioning and viability of cells. There is some evidence that the function and viability of the nerve cell is compromised when there is no chemical feedback or neurotrophic factor from a target cell. The role of neuropeptides such as somatostatin and the mechanisms by which they modulate neuronal activity are not well understood. Whether or not such neuromodulators also serve as trophic factors is not known. The chemistry of neuromodulators and the neurotrophic factors is an area that needs greater emphasis.

A third area of needed study concerns the biochemistry of metabolism within the cytosol (inside the nerve cell), especially oxidative metabolism and glucose utilization. It is important to have a better understanding of changes in such metabolic pathways associated with aging and disease states.

A fourth cluster of essential studies looks at membrane biophysics and how membrane changes influence transport and homeostasis of essential ions such as calcium. There is some evidence that aging, as well as certain diseases, causes changes in the transport mechanisms that regulate cytosol-free calcium concentration. We need to learn more about the biophysics of ion channels, pumps, and transport systems associated with cell and organelle membranes.

Finally, we need to know more about such environmental toxins as aluminum and infectious agents such as the slow-acting viruses or virus-like particles that have been associated with cell death in AD. The chemistry of how such agents interfere with cell functioning is still not well understood. Also, we do not know why there appears to be selective vulnerability; the role of genetic factors in such selectivity is an area needing greater study.

All of these results are extremely important, because they provide a crucial beginning for piecing together the AD puzzle. It is now possible to formulate testable hypotheses that can provide a common framework for interrelating a number of the discrete findings discussed here. For example, in study after study we are seeing the importance of calcium levels within the cell in terms of cell-to-cell communication and even the viability of the cell itself. Time after time, findings in AD brains point to a disruption in the delicately balanced homeostatic system of transporting calcium across the cell membrane. Such a disruption of the system could be a consequence of exposure to a neurotoxin, such as aluminum, pathogenic agents involving either genes or infectious agents, other insults, or even aging. Further study should allow us to develop integrated theories of aging and better understand the biological mechanism of diseases such as AD.

The NIA is concerned with furthering knowledge on multiple aspects of AD. Efforts in this area include studies of family stress problems relating to the care of AD victims and the development of family care and service delivery models.

Dr. Marcia Ory, of the NIA Behavioral and Social Research Program, recently has reported that research is just beginning to focus systematically on how families and other social supports affect and are affected by AD and related disorders. Additional studies are needed on the social and psychological aspects of AD to help advise family members and professionals who are currently caring for older persons with AD. Identification of the range of informal and formal services is especially important for understanding how to balance familial and professional support in a cost-effective and humane way.

The majority of persons with AD live at home and receive care from a relative or friend. Family members are shown in study after study to be the primary caregivers of the elderly patients. However, few studies have systematically documented actual caregiving behaviors, with large numbers of AD patients, with varying levels of impairment representing the full spectrum of the disease. We need to know who is giving what kind of care to what types of patients with what results. We also need to know how changing social and demographic trends (such as the increasing participation of women in the paid work force) will affect informal caregivers' availability and willingness to care for AD patients in the future.

The role of families and informal caregivers in the perception of and response to AD symptoms is another area that merits investigation in greater detail. Beliefs about the causes and treatments of a particular illness have been shown to affect whether - and in what ways - the family responds to illness symptoms. Little is known about how families and other informal caregivers seek professional advice and treatment. Such research should include studies of familial, psychosocial, or environmental factors that are associated with the early recognition of AD symptoms, with denial of serious symptoms, with the decision to seek professional advice and treatment, and the different approaches to management at home.

Relevant to AD, substantial literature is being accumulated on the role that the family and other informal supports play in the onset, course, and outcome of a variety of chronic diseases and disabilities. There is some evidence that familial attitudes, behaviors and interactions can either aggravate or lessen the occurrence of the cognitive and behavioral deficits associated with AD. Research is needed to explore how social and behavioral factors, interacting with biological processes, affect the onset and/or exacerbation of symptoms associated with AD.

Families and informal caregivers of persons with dementing disorders experience a variety of physical, psychological, social and financial difficulties. More research is needed on the antecedents and consequences of these different types of burdens. Characteristics of both the caregiver and the patient, as well as the caregiver context need to be further delineated. We need to know, for example, how family members of different ages, sexes, socioeconomic and cultural backgrounds, or levels of responsibility are affected by having a relative with AD. We also need to know what factors contribute to stress and why families reach a breaking point.

There are several key family resources for helping AD patients remain at home, including: 1) competent health care; 2) Alzheimer support groups; and, 3) respite care. Additional research may find ways to help informal caregivers understand and cope with the symptoms of AD and the burdens of caregiving. Little attention has been given to the ways in which families use - or fail to use - both informal and formal support services to care for AD patients. Further research is needed on ways to assist those who are trying to care for AD patients at home.

The use of formal supports does not consistently reduce the burdens on caregivers. Carefully planned clinical trials are needed to evaluate the effectiveness of different types of health and social services. Additional research is also needed on how families, health professionals, and AD patients relate to each other, particularly in institutional settings. Contrary to popular stereotypes, families do not typically abandon older relatives who have been institutionalized but continue to be involved.

In her report Dr. Ory concludes that the burden of AD on patients, informal cargivers and the health care system is enormous. Identification of the range of informal and formal services is especially important for understanding how to balance familial and professional support in a cost-effective and human way.

In summary, the systematic study of AD was begun only within the last decade, despite the fact that the disease was first described nearly three-quarters of a century ago. In this brief period, our knowledge of this disease has advanced from nearly total ignorance to a level at which it is possible to begin testing potential treatments and to formulate viable hypotheses to explain its causes.

The scientific community now has the tools, the knowledge base, and the means to solve the problem of AD within the next decade. This remarkable progress in dementia research has been made because the availability of scientific knowledge, technology, and methods--the bricks and mortar to start building a structure--has been more than equalled by increased interest and enthusiasm in the medical community and among the general public.

The PHS, of which the National Institute of Aging is a part, has supported a significant portion of basic biomedical research in this country during the last 30 years. A tremendous amount of this work has had direct and indirect bearing on our understanding of the basic mechanism of cell function, including that of neurons. Using knowledge gained from such areas of science as biochemistry, cellular and molecular biology, bioengineering, physics, genetics, recombinant DNA, and cloning technology, it is now feasible to make rapid progress in understanding the cause or causes of AD as well as other disabling disorders of the aged.

There is no reason to doubt that progress and scientific achievements will be any less spectacular during the next few years as they have been recently, provided that we are able and willing to maintain the enthusiasm of the scientific community and provide the necessary resources. The challenges of understanding AD and finding a cure will require national resolve to maintain the momentum we have begun.

GATEKEEPERS: CHANGING ROLES AND RESPONSIBILITIES FOR PRIMARY CARE

PHYSICIANS WITH AGING FAMILY SYSTEMS

Richard L. Douglass

Departments of Family Medicine and Community Medicine
School of Medicine, Wayne State University
Detroit, MI  48201

INTRODUCTION

For primary care physicians to adjust to the dramatic challenges brought about by an aging society, it is first necessary for them to recognize that many traditional aspects of "front line" medical practice are in a state of virtual revolution.  Although modern medical history has been frequently changed due to technical or scientific progress, the demographic consequences of such incremental events are now confronting us with the most fundamental changes since the advent of antibiotics. This demographic imperative, as stated by Califano in 1978, has sweeping implications for primary care medical practice in terms of which patients are to be served, which disease processes will dominate our attention, and even what attitudes we bring to our work regarding the ultimate objectives of medical practice.  Such professional objectives as prevention of death and extension of life are in conflict with more appropriate geriatric objectives of quality of life and quality of terminal care.  As the practice of primary care medicine becomes increasingly geriatric, the inevitability of death will become a more constant theme in all aspects of daily practice.

Most of us are acutely aware that by the year 2020 almost 20% of the total U.S. population will be over age 60 (Califano, 1978).  This population explosion in the last quarter of the lifespan is altering all aspects of society, and particularly medical practice and medical care organization.  An estimated 2.5 to 3 million victims of Alzheimer's Disease in the country in 1984 will expand to an estimated prevalence of over 4 million by the turn of the century (Secretary's Task Force on Alzheimer's Disease, 1984); this is an increase of at least one million new cases within the next fourteen years.  Needless to say this should be a sobering realization when this rapid increase in morbidity is of a disease for which there are poor diagnostic and proven treatment methods, and an unknown etiology.

The following discussion will examine the gatekeeping role of primary care medicine as a traditionally sound and currently appropriate response to the medical fallout of increased longevity and the growing geriatric emphasis in primary care (Kane and Kane, 1980; Vorhees, 1983; Catlin, Bradbury and Catlin, 1983).  Specific reference will be given to Alzheimer's Disease at the individual and family levels and the response alternatives for family practice.

THE PRACTICE ENVIRONMENT

Since the creation of Medicare, health care costs, largely hospital costs, have risen constantly (Special Committee on Aging, 1985). The economic aspects of medical care have become dominant forces in the practice environment. Although a gatekeeper role has always been a distinguishing feature of primary care medicine, the economic environment has drawn new attention to this role due to new organizational forms of medical care delivery. Prepaid health care in all of its mutations and experimental combinations is rapidly replacing traditional fee for service practice. As a result the "intake-disposition-referral" elements of primary care medicine, as implied by the term "gatekeeper," have become of central importance to all of the more specialized components of practice systems of ambulatory care (Gillette, 1984).

The cost-effectiveness of primary care physicians as gatekeepers in prepaid health care plans is still uncertain. To an extent such an assessment will be confounded by the changing demographic profile of all patient populations where at least half of all primary care patients in all settings will be over age 60 by the year 2000. Costs associated with care are known to be directly related to the age composition of the patient population, a fact that will influence the cost-basis outcome of any attempt to determine if gatekeepers in prepaid practices actually reduce the total cost of service delivery (Cohen, 1977).

Another element of the practice environment is the important role of the family of geriatric patients. The majority of all personal health care for frail elderly patients is not provided by physicians, nurses, or trained health care providers; over two-thirds is provided by adult family members. All outcomes of clinical medicine for the frail elderly are influenced by the knowledge, skills, physical ability and motivation of family caregivers. This is especially true when the index patient is afflicted with Alzheimer's Disease. In such situations the index patients' care brings with it primary care concern for adult, frequently mature, family caregivers whose emotions and physical health can be significantly affected by the weighty burden of home care for a demented adult (Hedley, Ebrahim and Sheldon, 1986).

Of the frail elderly, at least 20% can be expected to have Alzheimer's Disease after the age of 70. Two-thirds of these patients are in the care of family members whose first course of medical care is with a primary care physician. The remaining third of the frail elderly, as defined by Medicare, are currently residents of long-term care facilities and over 70% of this group were admitted under the orders of a primary care physician. Thus the central role of primary care medicine in geriatrics is apparent. Not apparent, however, is the degree to which geriatric medicine, gerontology, and other aspects of the new demographic profiles of the patient population are taught and appropriately implemented in the field.

THE PRACTICE SETTING

Just as the environment for medical care is changing in economic and demographic leaps, so also is the setting of primary care itself. Instead of a largely self-contained practice, primary care providers are finding themselves as team members, with a host of specialists for referral. The gatekeeper role, while traditional, is now more clearly essential to both primary care and specialty practices. The advanced ability in physical diagnosis and patient interviewing which should distinguish primary care physicians is now the pivotal process from which several other physicians and other professionals derive their patients and clients.  As the patient population becomes largely geriatric it is important for primary care physicians to be well versed in community services for the elderly, in-home or institutional respite care, self-help and advocacy groups, as well as neurologists and other specialists for medical referral or diagnostic assistance.  With the Alzheimer's Disease patient, it should be assumed that a family is "in treatment" rather than just a patient; this requires a large repertoire of referral services for the primary care physician.

THE CONTROVERSY

While primary care physicians are generally considered to be the most appropriate professionals to serve as gatekeepers for large and complex health care systems, this presumption is not without a degree of controversy.  Issues of cost, quality of care, appropriateness of training and accessability have been raised regarding the planned use of physicians as system gatekeepers.  Social "case managers," health care advocates and other conceptualized models have been suggested as alternatives to primary care physicians.  Some of the central elements in the debate are presented below.

Proponents of medical gatekeepers argue:

1.  In all recent studies of preferences of the elderly, medical sources are the first choice for health care services, advice and management;

2.  Primary care physicians have traditionally served as medical gatekeepers and are appropriately trained for the role;

3.  Medical gatekeepers are more credible and conversant with the medical specialists;

4.  Long-term, continuous physician-patient relationships are known to be associated with the best medical care.  High quality physical diagnosis and interview skills, hallmarks of primary care medicine in general, are essential elements in geriatric medicine too.

Opponents of medical gatekeepers, however, might argue that:

1.  Compared to non-physician gatekeepers, medical gatekeepers are expensive and can afford less time for each patient or family unit;

2.  Medical training fails to network physicians with allied health, social services, community services and income maintenance programs that are key elements of successful geriatric services;

3.  The current state of readiness, the level of training and relevant experience of primary care physicians, in general, are poor as a basis for largely geriatric gatekeeper roles.  This generalization is most acutely true when the presenting complaints are Alzheimer's Disease or related disorders.  A consequence of the poor state of geriatric training is premature nursing home placements, ill-advised guardianship decisions, and unnecessary burdens to patients and their families.

RECOMMENDATIONS

On the basic assumption that both the proponents and opponents of

primary care medical gatekeepers have valid points,
the following recommendations are proposed as a means of speeding
the development of more adequate and efficient services to the
elderly and, especially, the families who are afflicted by
Alzheimer's disease.

1.  Because it is unlikely that medical training (including
    continuing medical education) will soon encompass non-
    medical curricula, primary care gatekeepers should not
    attempt to be general purpose referral sources for their
    elderly patients.  Instead, medical gatekeepers should
    learn to utilize a broad network of other community
    service by use of non-medical care managers who may
    practice within the medical practice or in a local
    service agency.  Medical gatekeepers should actively
    support the development of geriatric case management
    system in places where none exist.  In this way, both
    medical and non-medical primary care and continuity of
    are will be in the hands of experts.  Routine
    consultation and conferences between primary care
    physicians and non-medical case managers are essential;

2.  Geriatric and primary care career recruitment should commence
    during the first and second years of medical training.  Only in
    this way will adequate numbers of new physicians be available
    for geriatric medical services in the near future;

3.  Specialized geriatric and geriatric neurological training
    should be standard in all medical training and in all primary
    care specialty resident training;

4.  Gatekeeper systems should be evaluated on the basis of quality
    of care outcomes and not as instruments of cost containment.

These recommendations, although limited, are consistent with the
medical care manpower needs of the near future.  Better primary care of
the elderly should result in fewer hospitalizations, better home care,
delayed institutionalizations, and higher quality of care for patients and
families alike.  These are lofty objectives yet they are ones that the
primary care specialties can hardly afford to ignore.

REFERENCES

Califano, J.A. Jr., 1978, The aging of America:  Questions for the four-
   generation society, The Annuals of the American Academy, 438: 96-107.
Secretary's Task Force on Alzheimer's disease, 1984, "Alzheimer's
   Disease," Final report, U.S. Department of Health and Human Services,
   U.S.G.P.O., Washington, D.C.
Kane R.L. and Kane, R.A.,1980, Alternatives to institutional care of the
   elderly:  Beyond the dichotomy, The gerontologist, 20: 249-259.
Vorhees, J., 1983, The Family physician as gatekeeper, Continuing Education,
   July, 619-621.
Catlin, R.F., Bradbury, R.C. and Catlin, R.J.O., 1983, Primary care
   gatekeepers in HMO's, The Journal of Family Practice, 17, 4: 673-678.
Special Committee on Aging, United States Senate, 1984, "Developments in
   Aging, U.S.G.P.O., Washington D.C., Report 99-5, Volume 1, 1985.
Gillette, R.D., 1984, Are family physicians ready to be gatekeepers?, The
   Journal of Family Practice, 18, 5: 679-680.

Cohen, D, 1977, Approach to the geriatric patient, <u>Medical Clinics of North America</u>, 61: 855-866.

Hedley, R., Ebrahim, S. and Sheldon, M., 1986, Opportunities for anticipatory care with the elderly, <u>The Journal of family practice</u>, 22, 2: 141-145.

ADRDA AND THE PHYSICIAN


Mary Martinen

Chairperson of the Advisory Board - Detroit Chapter


The diagnosis of Alzheimer's Disease or other irreversible memory loss is as devastating as is a diagnosis of any terminal disease. Concerns are raised about the future, what will happen next, what plans must be made, what can be done to make the diagnosis easier to deal with?

Unlike many other serious illnesses such as cancer, the natural course of dementia is not well defined. Breast cancer patients with positive lymph nodes can be given adjuvant therapy with a documented improvement in survival. Patients with oat cell cancer can expect a four to ten month increase in life expectancy if treated. Staging of the illness can be performed as a guide to therapy and to provide prognostic information. Tumor markers like CEA and acid phosphatase may be used to monitor response to treatment. For persons not yet afflicted with the illness, diagnostic screening to detect it in its early stage or preventive measures may be offered. As death approaches in the terminal stages, hospice care may help both patient and family through the terminal stage.

Alzheimer's Disease however is a disease of unknown etiology with no means of prevention. Treatment of the disease is in a very early stage. The work of the research teams approaching the problem from multiple directions offers hope of new approaches in the future, but little can be done now to halt its progression or reverse the decline in cognitive functioning. The complications of the illness can be treated however. Persons with day/night sleep reversal can be given tranquilizers at bedtime. Hallucination and paranoia can be helped with major tranquilizers. Certainly a concurrent illness which can precipitate a deterioration in function can also be treated. At present one of the most effective treatments for the patient with Alzheimer's Disease is helping the care giver cope more effectively with their care. Learning to deal with a person whose illness is progressive is an important factor in relieving stress for the care giver and helping the demented patient retain as much of a normal life as possible.

The day to day care of a patient with memory loss presents unique problems for those who care for them. Dementia does not immediately deprive its victims of their physical vigor but of the rational and emotional processes that make him or her a unique personality. It is as if the care giver is slowly losing a person who has meant a great deal to them, and must adjust to new demands in the context of their own grief. One daughter whose mother was gradually forgetting her children was relying on brothers and sisters to relieve her of some of the care. Realizing that this was causing a strain for all of them, she stated "I hope I don't run out of brothers and sisters". I informed her that she was. Not because they were unwilling to aid her in their mother's care but because her mother was forgetting them so quickly it was as if her care was being assumed by strangers.

As the illness progresses, new roles are assumed and old ones are lost. Spouses and children become wardens looking out for the safety of someone who wanders or parents cleaning the body of someone incontinent. The control of finances must be taken from the former head of a household. Spouses lose their helpmate, consoler, lover, confidant.

If the care giver is a child, earlier problems related to their upbringing may surface. It is hard to be teacher to a previously abusive parent. The children are also more quickly forgotten than the spouse.

Unlike someone who is physically ill, the person with dementia may become abusive, hostile, or withdrawn. They are unable to say in return for their care "I appreciate all you are doing. I love you."

The gradually increasing demands build up until the care giver burns out feeling guiltily inadequate. It is not uncommon for care givers to be afflicted with pneumonia, heart attacks, ulcer disease or depression as their energies become exhausted. It is the guilt of burn out that adds to the difficulty of making a decision for the demented person to be cared for in an alternate setting such as a nursing home. It is a great support to families to understand what is happening and what to expect next. The Alzheimer's Disease and Related Disorders Association is an important resource to which both physician and family can turn for help with the next steps.

RESOURCES FOR THE PHYSICIAN

Not all physicians are comfortable with the work-up and long term follow-up of the patient with memory loss. The Alzheimer's Association provides a list of physicians experienced in treating the illness who may be available for consultation or continuing care. A physician who is comfortable with demented patients may become part of the referral network. Those who are not may learn of physician colleagues in their area who may assist them. Many educational programs are sponsored by ADRDA. Most are for families or other health care workers, but some are targeted to physicians themselves.

Legitimate research is occurring throughout the country to uncover new solutions for the problems of dementia. Juxtaposed is a proliferation of articles on quack or semi-scientific treatments. Families have read as much as they can about new or potential breakthroughs in treatment and often bring articles to the physician's office for advice and guidance. ADRDA on the national level and on many local levels provide advisory boards to answer questions about the validity of research, the proximity of a research project to clinical application, or the lack of scientific value of a specific entity.

In a time of shrinking research dollars National ADRDA provides funding for research projects. This allows physicians with scientific expertise to obtain needed financial support or to participate in the evaluation of applications from other researchers.

RESOURCES FOR PHYSICIAN AND FAMILY

No one person can provide care twenty-four hours per day without relief. The Alzheimer's Disease and Related Disorders Association provides the names of referral sources to physicians and families that provide alternative care. Day care with structured activities for impaired adults and respite care on a full time basis are important adjuncts to care in the home. The Detroit Chapter is fortunate to have received a grant through the Department of Mental Health which provides funding for partial respite care in the person's home. It is important for physicians to realize that there are alternatives to nursing home placement since the latter is not a desirable option for many families. Experience with alternatives that prove inadequate for the care of a particular person can help families cope with some of the guilt associated with nursing home placement if this is the best option for them. Because of its organizational structure, ADRDA is a channel for funding of multiple projects. Fund raisers provide avenues by which families and concerned physicians can become involved in providing support to others and for donating time and money to conquer the disease.

RESOURCES FOR THE FAMILY

The diagnosis of Alzheimer's Disease or other irreversible dementia produces a grieving process. Many families benefit from support groups - voluntary meetings of families who meet to gain information or to ventilate about specific concerns. Knowing that others are dealing with similar problems helps families feel less alone and gives helpful advice from someone who has shared the same experience. The newsletter provides support in a written form for people unable to attend a support group and provides information about new research and the possibility of future treatments.

Legal and financial issues are a great concern. At this time there is almost no public funding to provide for the financial burden of a demented person's care. The loss of rational powers produces other concerns. At what time should a relative assume power of attorney or legal guardianship? What financial arrangements need to be considered if long-term care must be provided in a nursing home? What is the financial impact of a divorce? The Alzheimer's Disease and Related Disorders Association provides important information and directs families to knowledgable resources.

If emotional issues are a major concern, the help line is available to provide advice and emotional support. The Detroit Chapter also provides on-site counseling sessions. Using the talents of qualified volunteers, family counseling for up to three visits is provided free of charge and referrals made after this time if so chosen.

ADRDA is an organization with which every physician providing care to persons with memory loss should become familiar. It may be a referral source for patients, an avenue by which knowledge is exchanged, and a tremendous help to the families of the patients.

# HOME HEALTH CARE FOR VICTIMS OF ALZHEIMER'S DISEASE

Susan Hicks in consultation with Karen Linell
and Mary Jane Curle

Renaissance Health Care
20700 Greenfield, Suite 320
Detroit, Michigan  48237

## INTRODUCTION

"As a home health care professional I was dedicated to care in the home as an alternative to institutionalization. What has been called the `Best kept secret in health care' was no secret to me.  I had spent ten years as a resource specialist at one of the best Home Health Agencies in the state of Michigan.  But when the time came to make arrangements for my own father, newly diagnosed with Alzheimer's I knew he, like most Alzheimer's patients, would not qualify for home health care under the Medicare program.  Dad was well in Stage II when his diagnosis was provisionally made.  He was one of those rare Alzheimer's patients who was very combative.  I knew he would have been unmanageable at home without a great deal of assistance.  He also had no other medical problems - leaving him ineligible for home health care. The decision to institutionalize him came very hard for me as a home health professional.  But it was the only option available amid resources and services that I knew were beyond his qualification, and unsuitable for his condition."

## CERTIFIED HOME HEALTH CARE

Home health care is available for patients of all ages and in many different forms, but each program carries its own qualifications, limitations and payment mechanisms.  Because Alzheimer's disease is primarily a chronic, progressive disease, most people suffering from Alzheimer's disease are not eligible for service under the Medicare program. For those qualifying, care may be provided under the Medicare program and other third party reimbursable insurances such as Medicaid, Blue Cross and other private insurances.  Care may also be provided in the home under various aging programs or special volunteer or grant programs funded in different locations.  Home care may be delivered from a private duty nursing agency for patients or their families with the ability to pay for service. Familiarity with the resource network which changes frequently as programs begin or dissolve and familiarity with the criteria for qualification for each discrete program often requires assistance of a professional.

In most cases, hospital discharge planning departments have access to information about the most common of these programs.  Information may also be obtained from senior citizen information and referral departments or from the local Alzheimer's foundation.

The decision to care for the Alzheimer's patient at home requires more than family commitment. It is most helpful for the family to have access to someone with medical expertise, a realistic assessment of the care options and the professional distance to make an unbiased recommendation. The private physician may be looked to by the family in crisis when such a decision must be made. Unfortunately, a lack of knowledge of available resources often makes the physician's easiest recommendation that of a nursing home.

In the introductory case mentioned above home, health care was impossible. For others it is a far wiser solution, and with the appropriate mix of services, can be managed at home with family support for many years. Care in the home provides the familiar surroundings that provide a security to the Alzheimer's patient. Maintenance of the patient's independence and ability to care for themselves for as long as possible is critical. Also, being a part of the routine that the patient is accustomed to, and experiening the love that only family can provide can make a difference in the life expectancy of an Alzheimer's patient. Dr. Joseph Gadbaugh, a Detroit area Geriatrician, states that in his experience Alzheimer's patients have a life expectancy of about three years in a nursing home. Alzheimer's is the most frequent reason for institutionalization according to the March 1986 publication, Coordinator. They also state that for every Alzheimer's patient in the nursing home there are three more at home. If the funding by Medicare for home health care programs expanded to include chronically ill patients, like those with Alzheimer's, many more could avoid premature institutionalization. They would live longer in the presence of those they love. Their loved ones would be able to manage the patient at home with significantly reduced stress if home care resources could be provided for them.

The physician with a better understanding of home health care can guide the family through the difficult decision of where to provide care. Under the Medicare program, a certified home health care agency may directly bill the Medicare program for services provided to patients meeting the program qualifications. In general, patients who are under the care of a physician, considered medically homebound and in need of skilled care meet program criteria for service. An occasional Alzheimer's patient, having the `fortune' of an additional qualifying skilled diagnosis meets Medicare's regulations. One such qualifying Alzheimer's patient was Renaissance Health Care's William S., case #4329.

William was admitted to Renaissance after hospitalization for pneumonia. A Stage II Alzheimer's patient, he was fairly easy for his family to manage with assistance at home. Under the Medicare program, William qualified as homebound due to his confusion and extreme shortness of breath on ambulation. However as mentioned before, his Alzheimer's alone would not have met the skilled care provision. Because William also had a diagnosis of Pernicious Anemia requiring monthly B-12 injections, he met the qualifications. Only Alzheimer's patients who are currently under treatment in the hospital for primary diagnosis of unstable hypertension or diabetes, for stroke or hip fracture or a host of other `skilled' diagnoses would qualify.

Qualifying patients may receive, under the physician's orders, an array of appropriate services which could include Skilled Nursing, Home Health Aide, Physical Therapist, Speech Pathologist, Occupational Therapist, Medical Social Worker, or Nutritionist. Medicare defines the program as an intermittent' service, so for most patients care is provided several times per week. Nurses have the opportunity to provide assessment and treatment. They also have the opportunity to teach the patient and most importantly -

their family.  The nurse will carry out the care plan as ordered by the physician and will coordinate the other home health care services on the case.

The discharge planning unit at the hospital where William was an in-
patient conferred with his attending physician about the appropriateness of
home health care.  Renaissance Health Care, a certified home health agency,
was contacted and care was begun the day after discharge.  With shorter
hospital stays, good discharge planning is crucial for Alzheimer's patients.
A plan of nursing care for the B-12 injection, and for home health aide
service twice weekly for family respite was drawn up.  No other services
were deemed necessary for this patient.  By qualifying, patients, such as a
stroke victim, might need every one of the services available.

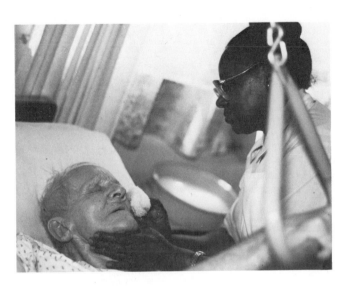

Renaissance's aide, Carrie, provides personal care
under the Medicare home health program.

The home health agency may continue to provide care as long as the
patient meets the program qualifications.  Once the need for skilled nursing
care and treatment are no longer present, the agency must initiate the
discharge.  For most patients, this is within the first month or two of
care.  At Renaissance, the average length of stay for all patients is
approximately 36 days.  For patients with continued skilled care needs and
homebound status, such as William's monthly B-12 injections or catheter
care, home health care may continue for a longer period.

William has had two hospitalizations for recurrent pneumonia.  A recommendation from the home care nurse was a change in his diet.  His difficulty
in swallowing regular foods due to a former stroke made him a good candidate
for pneumonia.  The nurse, Kay, suggested a diet of pureed food which
greatly improved his health status.  She also taught the family safety
techniques in feeding the patient.  Obvious tips such as feeding the patient
only when awake and fully sitting up, and not giving the patient foods that
could cause choking, were reinforced by the nurse.

Wheelchair bound William could still be taught positional changes - the
`wheelchair push-ups' - that help avoid skin breakdown.  His family was
taught to encourage the position changes and turning while in bed, as well
as given information about stimulation and reorientation.  The nurse, Kay,
encouraged his wife and daughter to allow William to do as much as possible

for himself. She made suggestions for home activities to encourage visual and auditory stimulation such as placing his wheelchair near a window with activity, watching television or listening to the radio, and encouraging friends and family to talk and visit with the patient.

Their nurse also provided information about the Alzheimer's Association in William's area - their support groups and a hot line services for families in distress. Kay made arrangements for durable medical equipment that the patient would need at home. A hospital bed and bedside commode were obtained under the doctor's orders from a local medical supply company. While in the hospital, William had received an egg crate mattress to help prevent skin breakdown and this continued to be used at home. The home care nurse also provided the medical supplies required for the treatments she would be performing at home. If lab work was required, she could draw blood for iron binding or other tests as ordered by the physician. The results would be both phoned to the attending physician and mailed to their office.

The home health nurse is responsible for maintaining an open line of communication between the homebound patient and their physician. By phone contact to inform the doctor of significant changes in the patient's condition, and by mailing the physician updates in the patient's care plan, the community health nurse functions as an extension for the doctor. The physician's responsibility in utilizing a certified home health care agency is to be available for phone communication from the home health team member, and to sign and return physician's order confirmations in a timely manner. Changes in reimbursement mechanisms have made prompt return of the physician's orders a matter of fiscal survival for a home health agency.

When assisting the family in the decision for home health care or institutionalization, the physician should be aware that in most locations, there are many players in the certified home health care market who can provide widely varying standards and services. When Renaissance Health Care was incorporated in 1976, there were only two other agencies providing community health care service. In 1986, that number has grown to over 60 agencies. For-profit and not-for-profit agencies may now participate in the Medicare program. Free-standing, privately owned agencies now compete with large national chains. Department stores, pharmacy chains and large conglomerates are also a part of the home health industry. Also, hospitals have continued the trend of either acquisition, joint venturing, or forming their own home care agencies.

Again, the discharge planners in hospitals should be familiar with the differences in agencies and their hospital's position. For many hospitals, a close working relationship with only a few of the many agencies competing for patient referrals has enabled them to both develop joint programs that meet physician needs and to acquire a depth of knowledge about the quality of care provided. A large, private, non-profit home health care agency such as Renaissance Health Care is able to provide program development services to physicians requesting specific protocols be followed to patients with high tech needs. Renaissance is also affiliated in a joint venture with the hospitals of the Detroit Medical Center and has a commitment to meeting the post-discharge needs of the specific patients they serve.

The physician should consider several areas in making an independent selection of home health care agencies. In addition to good community reputation, an agency should be approved for all forms of home health care. New agencies do not, for example qualify for the Blue Cross home health program. Home health care agencies providing medical supplies may be an important service to the Alzheimer's family who is often homebound too. It is also important that an agency is able to provide all of the various medical disciplines under the Medicare home health program.

204

For patients in an inner city environment like Detroit, a physician should be aware of whether the agency will be able to provide service to a patient who would otherwise qualify for the program but are without insurance coverage. An agency's affiliation with teaching institutions is another indicator of credibility and community standing. Renaissance, for example, is affiliated with three schools of nursing and provides their community health experience. The agency is also affiliated with Wayne State University's School of Medicine and gives third and fourth year medical students a first hand look at the benefits and complexity of care in the home. Other considerations for selection that the doctor may look for might be availability for 24-hour answering service, other special grants and programs that the agency can offer its patients alone, and an effective response time. A final consideration might be the most telling: asking other physicians about their experience with the agency under consideration, or checking with patients themselves who have used the service. Renaissance Health Care asks all patients for an anonymous evaluation of service, and from their ratings shows a 95% overall service ranking as good or excellent. Patients and family are quick to both praise and complain if the level of professional service and personal caring is or is not acceptable.

PRIVATE DUTY NURSING SERVICES

All patients qualify for private duty nursing care. All patients who can afford to pay, that is. Of course, not all Alzheimer's patients are candidates for home care. Family decisions about private duty must consider the primary caregiver's health status, financial resources, other dependents, and the progression and characteristics of the disease. For many Alzheimer's and other chronically ill persons who are ineligible for skilled nursing care under the home health program, a good private duty service can make the difference between maintaining their loved one at home or making the decision to institutionalize. For a fee, the private duty agency can provide registered nurses, LPNs, aides, sitters or companions. Some can also provide therapists upon request.

Patients may find these services listed under the nursing section of the yellow pages. In making the decision for care, cost and quality of care would be the first consideration. Prices do vary considerably, even in the same geographical area - at times up to as much as 60% difference. While cost shopping can be checked by family members, the physician could advice them to ask about minimum time required in the home by the nursing service. If the caregiver needs help in getting the patient our of bed and dressed in the morning, and help again at bedtime, four hour minimums would require payment for eight hours daily. Renaissance Health Care is affiliated with a private duty agency, Royal Home Care. They chose to make available special services which waive the large minimum blocks of time. Royal's ˋwake-up/tuck-in' care allows families to have a break in their constant care of Alzheimer's patient without over-extending their financial resources.

Again, word of mouth is a good indicator for the type of service and satisfaction with a private duty agency. Patients should be able to expect prompt, courteous service that is dependable. Caregivers should be bonded, referenced and should be working under the supervision of a staff nurse at the agency. The physician may again be asked to help in the choice between the need for a registered nurse or and LPN. The doctor's knowledge of the medical needs of the Alzheimer's patient should be valuable in selection of the educational level needed by the home care professional employed.

Families should explain the patient's condition fully to the intake nurse to help in the assignment of a caregiver who will be experienced and able to work with the Alzheimer's patient.

Dissatisfaction with a private duty agency or one of their employees need not occur more than once. Proliferation of these agencies and the fact that the patient is the paying customer usually yields prompt response to any difficulties.

The problem for even the most affluent of families becomes the long term expense of private duty care. For those needing 24 hour service, several months of care can run into many thousands of dollars. Therefore, this cannot be the long term solution for most patients. Some families are able to manage by using private duty care as a respite when the primary caregiver is exhausted.

ADDITIONAL HOME CARE RESOURCES

Various other programs for which the Alzheimer's patient may qualify are available on a limited basis and may be of assistance in maintaining the patient in their own home. Renaissance, for example, is affiliated with two volunteer respite programs for which an Alzheimer's patient would be eligible. Funded through the Senior Companion program and Retired Senior Volunteer Programs, senior volunteers are available to provide family relief for up to 20 hours weekly. Other programs of respite are available on a limited basis to help the family cope with the demands of constant patient care.

In some communities, Alzheimer's patients who are over the age of 60 would qualify for programs funded by the Older Americans Act. These can be helpful supplementary services to families without other resources. Again, Renaissance, has a grant from the Detroit Area Agency on Aging for a specific catchment area in northeast Detroit. Under this grant, homemaker and minor chore services may be provided free of charge for seniors unable to perform these tasks for themselves any longer. An elderly spouse taking care of an Alzheimer's patient would certainly meet qualifications for these programs. Other Older Americans Act programs which may be available include senior day care, home repair, information and referral, meals at home, some transportation services, and personal care. The physician could also recommend that the family contact the local senior citizen department for more information.

FINAL RECOMMENDATIONS

While this chapter has primarily dealt with home care resources as they exist for Alzheimer's patients, a few words are appropriate regarding what should be. For skilled care patients, home health care has been proven to be a cost effective mode of health care delivery. Congress has been slow to fund any extension of home health into the chronic care segment. But pressure has begun to mount for long term care funding for senior citizens, which would certainly also benefit the elderly Alzheimer's patient.

The first recommendation would be to advocate for the expansion of home health benefit to include coverage for long term care needs, such as those of the Alzheimer's patient. Keeping Alzheimer's patients in their home will maintain their independence, their dignity and their security among the familiar things and routines of home for as long as possible. It would be a more humane alternative to the institutionalization of an Alzheimer's patient which often means restraint and heavy medication. It would definitely help the family through teaching and home medical support. Renaissance Health Care is able to provide skilled home health care at a cost of approximately $17 per day-far less than the cost of hospitalization or nursing home placement.

A second recommendation would be to extend funding for Older Americans Act services to include personal care and home health aid. Not all Agencies on Aging choose to fund these components of their programs. But as health care costs and needs continue to escalate with our graying population, the need for emphasis on the priority services of food and medical care must be recognized.

Another suggestion to assist in the home care of Alzheimer's patients would be to begin additional respite care programs. Volunteer and staff programs of respite care enable family members to survive the constant care requirements of the Alzheimer's patient. If more agencies were able to provide the respite care that Renaissance provides for its patients, more families would be able to avoid premature nursing care placement based on their exhaustion.

As well, a final recommendation would be to provide a home health care educational component to all schools of medicine. Students in the Wayne States's Medical School home health experience relate that the experience was valuable in understanding the role of the home care team in relation to the physician and in seeing how much of an opportunity the home care staff has to really help the patient. A frequent criticism of medical school curriculums has been the dearth of education on gerontological topics and community health is rarely included. The well-informed physician is best able to help their patients and families through the crises that are often a part of Alzheimer's disease. Physicians with a good understanding of the provision and limitations of home health care and the resources available to aid in home care of the Alzheimer's patient will be invaluable.

# UNDERSTANDING PROGRESSIVE DEMENTIA:

## MAKING A CASE FOR THE CASE HISTORY

Dorothy Booth

College of Nursing
Wayne State University
Detroit, MI   48202

Ann Whall

School of Nursing
University of Michigan
Box 0482, 400 N. Ingalls
Ann Arbor, MI    48109

Some very relevant information about Alzheimer's disease and other progressive dementias has surfaced through the endeavors of health care professionals who painstakenly compiled case histories and noted observations over time of patients who presented with cognitive disorders.  For example, during the first decade of this century, Alois Alzheimer, a neuropathologist, used a case study approach with historical dimensions to describe behavioral and mental changes in a patient with a progressive and irreversible form of dementia (Wolstenholme & O'Conner, 1970).  Today, this condition is referred to as Alzheimer's disease (AD or senile dementia of the Alzheimer's type (SDAT).  The information obtained by using the case history approach and clinical observations served as the impetus for Dr. Alzheimer's post—mortem exploration of brain cells to identify changes associated with the dementia (Reisberg, 1981).  This report is divided into two sections, the first section focuses upon the use of case histories to describe the onset and progression of AD, and the second portion describes a program of research which has developed a health history profile to discriminate between AD and other disorders.

From the discovery that characteristic brain changes were seen in persons who had displayed similar changes in memory and behavior, researchers were able to reach the conclusion that AD is a primary dementia, not a dementia secondary to other conditions.  It has been the hope that in vivo biological markers could be identified and used in making the diagnosis with a high degree of accuracy.  However, this has not yet happened (LaRue, Dessonville & Jarvik, 1985).  LaRue et al., have pointed out that few longitudinal studies have been conducted to provide the data needed to understand the development of mental dysfunctions in the latter half of the life span, and no data are available from cohort or cross sequential studies to help us distinguish between changes that accompany aging and changes from other influences at the time of measurement.

The recommendation for comprehensive case histories by Gurland & Toner (1983), and others, therefore, remains very timely and important.  Gurland and Toner (1983), concerned with the dilemmas encountered in making an accurate diagnosis, have discussed the need to establish a timetable of the appearance of cognitive deficits and changes in the patient's ability to handle instrumental tasks such as the activities of daily living. Relationships between the data on this timetable and the appearance of other signs associated with progressive dementia can then be identified.  This information is needed to make a differential diagnosis between "pseudo dementias", acute conditions, or progressive dementias that present with memory change, decreased ability to make good judgments, or language difficulties. Gurland & Toner make it very clear that it is not a safe practice to formulate the diagnosis of progressive dementia solely on the results from psychological tests, clinical observations and other procedures without considering the chronological events and their relationship to the disabilities evidenced in the patient. It would be difficult to construct a chronological timetable such as the one suggested by Gurland et al. (1985), without eliciting historical information from persons who have been closely associated with the patent over time.

Rosen (1983) also supports the use of the case history approach. He has suggested that in making the diagnosis of AD, one of the first components of the patient's evaluation includes taking "a detailed history from a reliable informant, usually a spouse or offspring" (p. 51). The informant needs to be asked questions that will provide information about the "nature and history of the symptomatology, including the initially observed symptoms, the emergence of new symptoms, the nature of the onset, and the course of functional decline: (Rosen, 1983, p.51). From Rosen's experiences, informants are not able to give definitive information about the time of onset of the disorder, but they are able to recall the progressive deterioration in the patient's functional abilities.

Barry (1984) has concurred with Gurland & Toner, Rosen and others stating that it is important to ask about the length of time that has elapsed since the demented patient's mind was functioning normally, and over what time span the disorientation developed. A reliable relative or friend who knew the patient well can be invaluable in establishing these facts, according to Barry.

Other support for the case history approach comes from the criteria developed for diagnosing dementias that is delineated in the most recent edition of the Diagnostic and Statistical Manual of Mental Disorders (DSM III) published by the American Psychiatric Association (1980). For example, the first criterion focuses on loss of intellectual ability that is severe enough to interfere with social or occupational function, and one of the components of the third criterion for making a diagnosis focuses on changes in personality, such as alterations or accentuation of premorbid characteristics. Evidence that could only be obtained from the patient's case history, then, provides information that is vital in making the diagnosis of dementia. The guidelines provided in the DSM III manual recommend that historical information along with data obtained from the physical exam, psychological and mental status, and neurodiagnostic tests and procedures be used to provide the evidence needed to rule out other disorders and make a diagnosis of primary dementia. Other diagnostic procedures (i.e. CAT scans to determine cortical atrophy, and electro-physiological measures to determine whether EEG slowing is present) also are recommended because there are no known neurological procedures available to unequivocally confirm the diagnosis of a primary degenerative brain disorder.

Compiling substantive historical and observational information is an intricate matter that requires the use of a systematic approach if the information obtained is to be accurate and comprehensive in nature. Skills in interviewing and making relevant observations are needed. This is especially true because persons afflicted with AD or related disorders most often are not able to give reliable information about themselves, and family members who are considered for use as surrogate informants for patients with dementia may or may not be able to provide detailed, reliable historical information. According to some of the literature, those chosen as surrogate informants need to be selected using the following guidelines: (a) high frequency of contact (i.e., at least two contacts per week with the patient); (b) having known the patient for at least ten years prior to the onset of the dementia; (c) reporting an interactive and congenial relationship with the patient (i.e., has taken part in activities and enjoyed good times together and shared information, feelings, etc., with the patient) and (d) have good cognitive abilities.

Whenever possible, more than one surrogate informant should be interviewed on behalf of the patient with dementia, and comparisons made to determine the amount of congruence between the information received from each informant. This will serve as a safeguard against the inclusion of data that are not reliable or that has been colored by emotions stirred in informants who have assumed the caregiver role. Use of some open ended questions as well as structured questions in the interview process will provide the surrogate informants the opportunity to reflect on the timetable of events that took place prior to the premorbid stage of the disorder. It also encourages the informants to describe factors that they believe are associated with the development of dementia in the patient.

## Examination of Alzheimer's Disease (AD) Case Histories

Using the case history method as an approach to describe the onset and progression of AD has been identified as important. Therefore, the use of case histories as a tool to chronicle the person's life experience as well as to focus upon risk factors that have been theoretically and empirically related to the onset of AD is important. Toulmin (1976) and others have discussed the importance of the use of health histories to identify and describe risk factors. An overview of a series of studies in a program of research is presented in the section. An AD case history, the Life Factor Profile, which was developed and examined in terms of ability to discriminate between persons with AD versus non AD is also described. This tool is seen as having potential utility for clinical practice as well as research. The program of research is currently in the third phase of study.

The initial Life Factor Profile was developed using two approaches: empirical findings which had described factors believed to be related to the onset and progression of AD were compiled and placed in a questionnaire format and then data provided by first degree relatives of persons who were diagnosed with Alzheimer's disease were used to extend the questionnaire. This latter data were collected in open ended interviews and focused upon health and life style practices which the family member believed to be related to the onset and progression of AD. These data were combined with empirical findings and examined by a panel of experts in AD on onset and progression to address, to some extent, construct and face validity. Areas of the case history included hereditary/familial factors such as the occurrence of Down's Syndrome or Parkinson's Disease, social factors such as isolation, disease and disease treatment history such as head injury and metabolic disorders, nutritional/dietary factors, as well as degree of physical activity. Demographic data such as employment, educational level, and places of residence were also examined.

In the first study a convenience sample of twenty persons with AD and twenty without this condition from a nursing home population were examined. That is, the Life Factor Profile was completed using data provided by first degree relatives (e.g., spouses and children) who had daily contact with the person with AD. The diagnostic protocols for diagnosis of AD were examined using criteria identified as necessary for the presumptive diagnosis of AD. Those without the condition had also been examined to determine that AD was not present.

In the second study thirty subjects with AD were randomly selected through relatives participating in AD support groups. A senior citizens comparison group of thirty of similar age, gender, and race was also randomly selected for comparison on the Life Factor Profile. The senior citizens were examined for mental clarity prior to inclusion in the study and the AD diagnostic protocol was again examined for the AD group. In addition, consistency between the responses of relatives were examined and found to be significantly correlated in the majority of items on the case history. In both studies the case histories which were related to empirical findings and life experience as reported by relatives was significantly different from the AD group versus those without this condition.

The third phase or study in this program of research, will be a double blind study in which 200 persons with cognitive dysfunction, but without a final diagnosis, will be divided into AD versus non-AD on the basis of the case history presented on the Life Factor Profile. Thus, the discriminant validity of this case history instrument will be examined; test-retest reliability and internal consistency will also be examined.

In summary, case histories have been identified as important clinical tools in the identification of many health conditions such as lung cancer, breast cancer, and heart disease. Case histories have thus reduced important clinical data which were found to have important research implications. Case histories of those with AD and the development of an instrument to examine these case histories are thus seen as important clinical and research effort. Beyond the discriminant validity study, one which examines the case histories of those who on post mortem examination were found to have AD, is also seen as important.

ACKNOWLEDGEMENTS

This program of research has been supported by the following grants:
Division of Nursing, HRA, HHS, R21-NU00831
Division of Nursing, PHS, HHS, R01-Nu01003-01

REFERENCES

American Psychiatric Association, 1980, "Diagnostic and Statistical Manual of Mental Disorders," American Psychiatric Association, Washington, D.C.

Barry, P.B., 1984, Confusion when it's Alzheimer's and when it isn't, Transition, 1:47-55.

Gurland, B., and Toner, J., 1983, Differentiating dementia from nondementing conditions, in: "Advances in Neurology, The Dementias," R. Mayeux and W.G. Rosen, eds., Raven Press, New York.

LaRue, A., Dessonville, C., and Jarvik, L.F., 1975, Aging and mental health, in: "Handbook of the Psychology of Aging," J.E. Birren and K.W. Schaie, eds., Van Nostrand Reinhold Co., New York.

Reisberg, B., 1981, "A Guide to Alzheimer's Disease", Free Press, New York.

Rosen, W.G., 1980, Clinical and neuropsychological assessment of Alzheimer's disease, in: "Advances in Neurology, The Dementias," R. Mayeux and W.G., Rosen, eds., Raven Press, New York.

Toulmin, S., 1976, On the nature of physician's understanding, Journal of Medicine and Philosophy, 1:32-50.

Wolstenholme, G.E., and O'Conner, N., 1970, "Alzheimer's Disease and Related Conditions," Churchill, London.

# EXERCISE TREATMENT FOR WANDERING BEHAVIOR

Susanne S. Robb

Associate Chief, Nursing  and  Associate Professor
Service for Research                School of Nursing
VA Medical Center                   University of Pittsburgh
Pittsburgh, PA 15240                Pittsburgh, PA  15261

## BACKGROUND

Persons who experience confusion and disorientation pose a variety of management problems for caregivers.  One such problem is wandering behavior that leads people to walk out of their residences and become injured or lost.

The role of physiologic and anatomic changes in causing cognitive impairment and, in turn, wandering behavior, is not known.  Ruling out treatable dementias which may be caused by drug toxicity, depression, vitamin B-12 deficiencies, and numerous other factors (Blumenthal, 1979; Solomon, 1979; Steel and Feldman, 1979; Wolanin and Phillips, 1981), there are at least two types of true dementia, neither of which presently can be cured (The Aged brain, 1982).  The first type is arteriosclerotic, or multiple infarct dementia; the second is Alzheimer's disease.

Mitigating against a biophysiological explanation of wandering behavior is the fact that given similar levels of cognitive impairment, ability to move about, ages, and kinds of dementia diagnoses, some elderly people wander while others do not (Monsour and Robb, 1982).  Thus, some people believe that wandering behavior is the product of a functional relationship between a person and a specific social environment (Earnest, et al., 1978; Perez, 1980).  When the behavior is deficient, or the individual or the environment or both factors can be altered to restore behavior, management has focused on treating the individual and assumed that there were deficiencies in the environment.  Interventions used have included vitamins; sedatives; tranquilizers; oxygen; physical restraint; placement on locked units; and alarm systems.  Individuals who wander are usually placed in long term care institutions where custodial care is the rule.  Little or no emphasis is placed on attempting to restore or improve behavioral efficiency via environmental changes.  The institutional environment often creates dependent behavior that requires less management effort from staff (Perez, 1980, p.94).

Environmental factors that have been suggested as causes for wandering behavior include:  (1) relocating and becoming lost or seeking to learn a new environment (Hiatt, 1980; Mace and Rabins, 1981; Monsour and Robb, 1982), and (2) factors that restrict opportunities to communicate needs or feelings (Hiatt, 1980; Mace and Rabins, 1981; Monsour and Robb, 1982).

Given that there is no specific curative treatment for most of the dementias, evaluation of the adequacy of management strategies depends on "quality of life" criteria (for example, morale, interpersonal relationships, functional status, and so forth) (Cross, Gurland and Mann, 1983). Benefits for demented people using one management strategy versus another have not been determined, although many such strategies have been used or suggested.

## PURPOSE AND HYPOTHESES

The overall objective of this study was to evaluate on intervention for wandering behavior; namely changes in elderly, male clients' wandering and wandering-related behaviors as a result of participation in a physical exercise program. Hypotheses concerned the effect of exercise on both daytime and nighttime behaviors. Expected daytime behavior changers were: (1) less wandering behavior (changes in intra-unit location, more time spent in each location, and less motor activity), (2) less energy expenditure (decreased voluntary limb and head movement), and (3) fewer bizarre or ritualistic verbalizations. Predicted nighttime behavior changes were: (1) less wandering behavior, (2) increased bed occupancy, (3) increased sleeping, and (4) fewer bizarre or ritualistic verbalizations.

## DEFINITION OF WANDERING

Care was taken in developing an operational definition of "wandering" to differentiate this behavior from deliberate escaped/runaway or generally acceptable/ "normal" movement. Thus, a wanderer was defined as a person who moved, under his or her own volition, into unsafe and/or inappropriate situations while experiencing impaired cognitive status. Operationally, impairment on both the Mini-Mental State (MMS) (Folstein et al., 1975) and Mental Status (MSQ) (Kahn et al., 1960) questionnaires; that is , an $MMS < 23$ points and $MSQ < 28$ points. Movement was defined by three measures: the number of changes in location within the resident's unit, time spent in each location, and time the resident spent moving his entire body through space. Institutional policies precluded verification of current tendencies to enter unsafe/inappropriate situations. Predefined criteria and retrospective record review were used to document subjects' manifestations of this component of the definition.

## METHODOLOGY

### Design

This quasi-experimental study involved a multiple pre- and post-test design, consisting of a single group of subjects, to measure effectiveness of a single treatment, exercise. Dependent variables were measured three times, at four-week intervals, before the exercise intervention; eight weeks after the twelve-week long exercise program began; and six weeks after the program ended.

### Subjects

Criteria for subject selection were (1) current status as a wanderer; (2) male; (3) age > 50 years; (4) expected to stay through all sex observation periods; (5) physician permission, based on absence of selected acute illness; (6) ability to walk or move about by wheelchair; (7) ability to communicate and follow simple instructions; and (8) evidence of cognitive impairment.

## Dependent Variables

Study hypotheses required comparisons of the following variables across six daytime observations periods: (1) changes in intraunit location, (2) time spent in each location, (3) motor activity, (4) limb and head movement, (5) initiative in limb and head movement, and (6) bizarre or ritualistic verbalizations. Data from six nighttime observation periods were compared for the following variables: (1) changes in intraunit location, (2) time spent in the bedroom, (3) motor activity, (4) bed occupance, (5) sleeping, (6) bizarre or ritualistic verbalization, and (7) silence.

All data were collected using behavior mapping., Data collectors were trained initially to meet an interrater reliability standard of 95% or higher. Adherence to this standard was reevaluated in each phase of the design. Daytime behaviors were recorded on each subject for 10 minutes per hour for a total of six hours per day, per two-day observation period. Nighttime behaviors were observed once each hour for eight hours per night for two nights per observation period. Multiple measures, recommended by Sackett (1978), were used to summarize behavioral observations. However, results with the various measures were quite similar. Thus, only one measure was reported for each variable. The measures chosen were those that seemed conceptually appropriate. For example, total behavioral changes per session was chosen for changes in location, mean duration per behavioral change was chosen for the time spent in each location, and estimates of duration was chosen for all other daytime variables. Nighttime variable measures selected were total behavior changes per session for changes in location and percent of possible frequency, for all other variables.

## Independent Variable

The exercise program was conducted according to a detailed protocol. In brief, each subject received 12 weeks of exercise over a 13 week period. Thirteen weeks were required to compensate for five holidays when exercise were not held. Any sessions missed by subjects due to exercise leader absences were made up on Saturdays. Sessions were usually held five days per week, Monday through Friday, for two hours each, in outdoor locations. The program was provided from September through mid-December, 1983. Graduate student assistance from the masters degree program in Exercise Physiology at University of Pittsburgh served as leaders. The following goals served to structure the exercise program: (1) avoid physical harm from excess effort, (2) minimize stress assumed to occur when obtrusive monitoring devices are employed, (3) deliver enough exercise to satisfy assumed needs for energy expenditure, and (4) allow for individual levels of ability and motivation.

Initial fitness testing was done by the exercise leaders to place subjects in on of three exercise regimens described in The Fitness Challenge, (1968). Fitness testing included the amount of time that subjects could (1) walk and (2) stand on one leg without undue difficulty; a controlled pace/distance test; grip strength, measured with a dynamometer; and range of motion, measured with a goniometer, Exercise regimens were modified, based on fitness testing, to substitute walking for activities that involved balancing or jogging.

Pulse checks, close observation for signs of cardiorespiratory distress, and cardiopulmonary resuscitation training for exercise leaders were the main strategies used to avoid effort-induced physical harm.. Subjects were encouraged by praise and other rewards to remain in motion from the start of the exercise period until they had expended enough energy that they were "too tired" to want to continue moving. This end point was operationally defined as "failure of task performance despite verbal and nonverbal effort." Typical rewards were arrival at destinations that offered contact with pet animals, and opportunity to observe building construction, or a small smack "to go."


RESULTS

The exercise intervention had no impact on daytime wandering behaviors, but did seem to produce changes in nighttime behaviors. No significant differences ($p > 0.1$) were observed within the subject group (N=20) across the six observation periods for any of the three dependent variables used to indicate daytime wandering behavior, nor were trends in values in the expected direction. Wandering-related behaviors that included extraneous energy expenditure and various kinds of verbalizations, also remained unchanged by the exercise program.

Three variables were considered to indicate wandering behavior at night: (1) number of location changes, (2) time spent in the bedroom, and (3) time spent in motion. A significant difference ($p < 0.05$) was observed for two of the three indicators: number of location changes and time spent in motion. The number of locations visited per ten minutes was stable between 2.0 and 3.1 locations before and during the exercise program, declined to 1.7 immediately following the program, and then increased to 2.5 locations six weeks after the program ended (F= 2.43; df = 5,90; p = 0.04). The time spent in motion decreased form the baseline period (13 to 22% of the time) to 8% of the time by the eighth week and 7% of the time by the thirteenth week of the exercise program, and increased toward baseline levels six weeks after the program ended (11% of the time) ( F=4.19; df =5,90; p = 0.002). Changes in values for time spent in the bedroom were on the expected direction, but were not statistically significant ($p > 0.05$).

Immediately following the exercise program, the percent of time subjects were silent at night increased significantly ($p < 0.05$) from 1.4 to 1.6 percent while the percent of time spent in social/personal conversation declined from 1.6 to 0.0 percent ($p < 0.05$). The amount of bizarre/ritualistic verbalization was not significantly changed. F-values were as follows: no interaction/ silent (F = 4.41; df = 5,90; p = 0.001), social/personal conversation (F = 3.45; df = 5,90 p = 0.007), and bizarre/ritualistic remarks (F = 1.34; df = 5,90; p = 0.253).

Serendipitous findings form this study, apart from the impact of exercise on wandering behavior, can be summarized as follows:
1. Subjectively, a majority of the men enjoyed the program as evidenced by their regular and willing attendance, improved facial expressions and verbalized comments.
2. The program objective, energy expenditure, to a point where desire to move about was satisfied, was achieved for most subjects in 60 minutes or less. Subjects improved significantly (p =0.001) in the mean amount of time they needed to exercise before becoming "too tired, " from 16 minutes in the first week to 34 minutes in the last week. Three subjects progressed to the point where they needed to jog, rather than walk to achieve this goal.
3. Range of motion improved significantly, for 87 to 96 points (p = 0.007), probably as a result of the flexibility exercises provided within the warm-up, stimulus, and cool-down phases of each session.
4. Based on exercise program content, changes in the following attributes were not expected an did not occur: muscle strength, cardiovascular fitness, and balance.

5. Cognitive status did not change for the time of pre- to post-program testing.

6. The terms, wandering behavior and wanderer, were defined differently within and across health disciplines, despite the fact that both terms were used to label substantial numbers of elderly people and, in turn, to guide treatment plans.

## SIGNIFICANCE

Subjects in this study were among the oldest (50-87 years, $\overline{X}$ = 69.5, S.D. $\pm$ 8.7) and most impaired (cognitively and physically) males to be subjected to a regular, vigorous, exercise regimen. It is noteworthy that, given preventive measures, no injuries or fatalities occurred and most subjects did not object to exercising.

This study was not designed to evaluate costs in relation to benefits. However, to facilitate such evaluation in future studies, records of program costs were maintained. Costs for project personnel to dress (and additional task necessitated by the exercise program) and exercise subjects, as well as for fitness testing and exercise supplies and equipment, totaled $39,102.42. Due to subjects' short term memory deficits, one-to-one exercise leader to subject ratios remained the rule, rather than the exception. Assuming that elderly wanderers require constant, close supervision when exercising and can require over an hour to achieve goals, exercise as a treatment for wandering may prove to be expensive.

In view of the partial support for the study hypotheses that developed despite considerable institutional resistance to the exercise program, further study of exercise as an intervention for wandering behavior in elderly people is warranted.

## SUGGESTIONS FOR FUTURE RESEARCH

Recommendations to guide future studies of this treatment are as follows:

1. Test exercise with wanderers who are truly free to wander (free of chemical or physical restraints), for example, people living at home or attending day care centers and who may have just started to demonstrate the behavior. Alternatively, an institutionalized group could serve as subjects if management policies and procedures did not restrict the behavior.

2. Timing of exercise effects needs to be considered, and possibly categorized as short term (first 8 hours after exercise), intermediate (second 8 hours), and long term (third 8 hours).

3. Attention must be given to possible energizing effects of exercise as well as energy-depleting effects. Impacts of exercise on subjects' ability to perform activities of daily living, affect, and social behavior, in addition to the target behavior wandering need to be determined.

4. Given some evidence that females may manifest different patterns of wandering behavior than males, continued attention to sex differences in designing future studies is required.

## ACKNOWLEDGEMENTS

This research was funded by the Division of Nursing, United States Public Health Service, Department of Health and Human Services, grant # R01 NU00957-01, 1983-August 31, 1984.

REFERENCES

The Aged Brain, 1982, Why does dementia occur despite viable brain
    function?, The NIH Record, 34:7.
Blumenthal, M.D., 1979, Psychosocial factors irreversible and irreversible
    brain failure, Journal of Clinical and Experimental Gerontology,
    1:39-55.
Cross, P.S., Gurland, B.J., and Mann, A.J., 1983, Long-Term institutional
    care of demented elderly people in New York and London, Bulletin of the
    New York Academy of Medicine, 59:267-275.
Ernst, P., Beran, B., Safford, F., and Kleinhauz, M., 1978, Isolation and
    symptoms of chronic brain syndrome, The Gerontologist, 18:468-74.
"The fitness challenge... in the later years, an exercise program for
    older Americans," (DHEW Publication No.. (OHD) 75-20802), Government
    Printing Office, Washington, D.C.
Folstein, M.F., Folstein, S.E., and McHugh, P.R., 1975, Mini-Mental State:
    A practical method for grading the cognitive state of patients for the
    clinician, Journal of Psychiatric Research, 12:189-98.
Hiatt, L.G., 1980, The happy wanderer, Nursing Homes, 29:27-31.
Kahn, R.L., Goldfarb, A.I., Pollack, M., and Peck, A., 1960, Brief objective
    measure for the determination of mental status in the aged, American
    Journal of Psychiatry, 117:326-28.
Mace, N.L., and Rabins, P.V., 1981, "The 36-Hour Day," The John Hopkins
    University Press, Baltimore.
Perez, J.I., 1980, Behavioral studies of dementia: Methods of investigation
    and analysis, in: "Psychopathology of the aged," O. Cole and J.E.
    Barrett, eds., Raven Press, New York.
Sackett, G.P., 1978, "Observing behavior, Volume II: Data collection and
    analysis methods," University Park Press, Baltimore.
Solomon, J.G., 1979, Remediable causes of dementia, Virginia Medicine,
    106:459-62.
Steel, K., and Feldman, R.G., 1979, Diagnosing dementia and its treatable
    causes, Geriatrics, 34:79-83.
Wolanin, M.W., and Phillips, L., 1981, "Confusion: Prevention and care,"
    C.V. Mosby, St. Louis.

# THE RELATIONSHIP BETWEEN CONFUSION AND ABUSE

Linda R. Phillips

University of Arizona, College of Nursing
Tucson, Arizona   85721

Under the best of circumstances, caring for a confused or demented elderly person is difficult, because the behaviors associated with confusion are so disruptive. Acute confusion, for example, is characterized by behaviors such as restlessness; purposeless activity; anxiety, fright and apprehension; agitation; verbosity; confabulation; rambling, repetitive speech; dependent and demanding attention getting behavior; withdrawal; belligerence; and combativeness (Gebbie and Lavin, 1975). The characteristics of early dementia include forgetfulness, declining interest, difficulty focusing attention, indifference, uncertainty and hesitancy (Quayhagen, 1977). As dementia progresses, behaviors such as confusing night and day; complaining about the neglect and interference of other people (particularly significant others); inattention to health, hygiene and safety; losing possessions and accusing significant others of taking them; and inability to retain or follow simple directions are manifested (Wolanin and Phillips, 1981; Quayhagen, 1977). Whereas health professionals working in institutional settings for eight hour periods of time find these kinds of behaviors frustrating, challenging and difficult, family members caring for elders twenty-four hours a day in the home setting can find these kinds of unpredictable behaviors to be nearly impossible to manage. The purpose of this paper is to explore some of the ways in which an elder's confusional state affects the family caregiving dynamics and, consequently, the quality of family caregiving, to examine the factors associated with confusion that increase the likelihood of the elderly person being exposed to abuse and to identify the clinical implications of these relationships.

## FAMILY CAREGIVING DYNAMICS AND
## THE QUALITY OF FAMILY CAREGIVING

Although the existence of the family caregiving role for the frail elderly is well documented in this country (Brody, Poulshock and Masciocci, 1978; Kohen, 1983; Shanas, 1979; Stoller and Earl, 1983, Archbold, 1980; Archbold, 1983; Cantor, 1983), little research has sought to describe the dynamics and the quality of family caregiving. In an effort to generate a theoretical model which described the dynamics of family caregiving, Veronica Rempusheski and I (Phillips and Rempusheski, In Press) undertook an inductive study using the grounded theory method (Glaser and Straus, 1967, Glaser, 1978). The sample, which was drawn from individuals who responded to one of two newspaper advertisements, consisted of 39 family caregivers (14 who had answered an ad for "good" relationships and 25 who answered an ad for "abusive" relationships). Nineteen of the subjects resided in the midwestern United States and 20 subjects resided in the southwestern United States. These 39 subjects described a total of 36 elders who had physical and mental disabilities and care needs that ranged from mild to acute. All the subjects were caucasian and related to the elder by consanguinal or acquired kinship ties. In both locations, the majority of caregivers lived with the elders they described. By analyzing the tape recorded comments of the caregivers, we generated and empirically induced theoretical models to describe the dynamics of family caregiving from the caregiver's perspective. Some of the concepts identified in that investigation provided a framework for understanding the possible relationship between confusional states and elder abuse. These concepts included the caregiver's (1) Image of the Elder, (2) Image of Caregiving, (3) Intrapersonal Responses to Images and (4) Role Beliefs.

## Image of the Elder

Image of the Elder is the mental picture that the caregiver has of the elderly individual which is derived from past associations, present observations, and the reconciliation of past with present images. According to Goffman (1963), as individuals interact over time, each develops a constantly evolving "dossier" about the other which contains, among other things, a history of events, impressions, normative role expectations and evaluations which uniquely identify the one person to the other. This "dossier" is used by each individual as the basis for their on-going interactions with the other person. One of the mental tasks that caregivers constantly perform is reconciling the past image of the elder with the present image of the elder. Reconciliation can result in "spoiling of the elder's image either when the elder's present image is less positive than the past image or when the elderly one is viewed negatively both in the past and present. A spoiled identity can be used by the caregiver as a righteous excuse for extreme negative behavior management strategies some of which, such as hitting or locking up, fit the definition of elder abuse found in the literature.

Characteristics of confusion place the confused elderly person in double jeopardy. Because the elderly person is mentally impaired, he or she is stigmatized and already "less than human". In addition, the behavior of the confused person may be so alien and repugnant to the caregiver that the person becomes additionally stigmatized and "spoiled". This attitude is particularly pronounced if the caregiver has not connected the confused behavior with a sanctioned, acknowledged, health-related problem such as Alzheimer's disease.

## Image of Caregiving

The second concept from the framework of relevance to this discussion is Image of Caregiving which is defined as the degree to which the caregiver's personal imperatives, standards and values are realized by the caregiving situation. From the data collected in this study, it appears that caregivers come to the caregiving situation with an implicit set of standards regarding their behavior, the behavior of other people and life in general. These standards or proscriptions constitute an ideal against which observations and perceptions of "reality" are judged. During the process of providing care, caregivers continually attempt to reconcile their proscriptions about caregiving with the perceived reality of caregiving that they face every day. The results of this reconciliation process can have profound implications for the behaviors that they display in the course of caregiving.

The behaviors displayed by confused people can have a profound impact on the reconciliation of proscriptions with the perceived reality of caregiving. When confused elders are seen by the caregiver as being "well" or only sporadically confused, behaviors that violate established standards of behavior can be interpreted by the caregiver as intentional and provocative. This effect can be particularly profound when the caregiver views the elder as the original source of the family's standards and cannot identify a plausible reason for the elder's behavior.

## Intrapersonal Responses to Images

Intrapersonal Responses to Images is the third concept induced in the study that has relevance for understanding the relationships between confusion and abuse. Intrapersonal Responses to Images are the intrapsychic, affective responses that the caregiver has to the results of reconciling the past with present images and reconciling proscriptions with the realities of caregiving. Anger, frustration, and embarrassment are examples of the types of responses that caregivers of the confused elderly have toward their images. Anger and frustration seem to be related to power conflicts in which the caregiver views the confused elder's behavior as a deliberate challenge to the caregiver's standards or efforts, or as a deliberate attempt to be aggravating.

Anger in response to confused behavior is also associated with a personal characteristic displayed by some caregivers which we identified as caregiving dogmatism. Following Rokeach (1963, p. 195), caregiving dogmatism is defined as a relatively closed cognitive organization of beliefs and disbeliefs about caregiving organized around a central set of beliefs about absolute authority which, in turn, provide a framework for patterns of intolerance and qualified tolerance toward the elder. Caregiving dogmatism is demonstrated as strong, unyielding opinions about how elders and caregivers should be and should behave, closed-mindedness in considering alternative beliefs or behaviors and a personal projection of right and justice in actions and thoughts. The unpredictable behavior of a confused elder can provide a dogmatic caregiver with multiple reasons for retaliation.

Embarrassment seems to be associated with three types of situations each of which is supported by the work of Goffman (1956) and associated with the behavior of confused elders. In the first, the caregiver views the elder and himself as an inseparable unit, a partner in an intertwined, reciprocal role relationship. Therefore, the credibility of the entire team is threatened and embarrassment results. In the second situation, the caregiver assumes the role of observer and experiences vicarious embarrassment _for_ the elder. In the third type of situation the caregiver becomes embarrassed because the elder reveals a dark secret about the caregiver or the caregiver's family. Caregivers who respond with embarrassment are likely to use caregiving management strategies that will control the source of the discomfort. At least among the caregivers interviewed for this study, some of the strategies that are used are negative, abusive and denigrating to the older person.

## Role Beliefs

The last concept discovered for the study of relevance for this discussion is Role Beliefs which is the dominant interpretation that the caregiver has for the purpose of the caregiving role. At least three conceptual dimensions underlie the caregiver's Role Beliefs. These are related to the overall purpose that the caregiver ascribes to caregiving, including

(a) Assessing/Nurturing, a positive role expression, (b) Monitoring, and (c) Testing, both negative role expressions.

The confused elderly are particularly at risk for having caregivers whose Role Beliefs include Monitoring and Testing because of the nature of confusion. A confused elder is frequently disruptive and unpredictable. As a result, a caregiver seeking to control chaotic behavior through whatever means is at hand is a logical prediction under these circumstances.

CLINICAL IMPLICATIONS

This paper has explored some of the factors that indicate a theoretical relationship between the presence of a confused elder in the family setting and the presence of elder abuse. Before proceeding with the clinical implications of these observations, it would be wise to exercise a word of caution. Although there is theoretical evidence and some empirical evidence that some confused elders receive abusive treatment for their family caregivers, the evidence does not suggest that every confused elder is the victim of abuse. In fact, there are so few studies on elder abuse, in general, and on the abuse of confused elders, in particular, that drawing any kind of inference about the incidence or prevalence of this phenomenon is impossible. Most of the caregivers of confused elders who I interviewed reported that, on occasion, they resorted to the use of an isolated abusive act in order to cope with the elder's behavior. The range of these abusive acts included occasional verbal assault, threats, embarrassments, withholding food or drink, slapping and confining to bed, chair, room or locking out of the house. Because of the sampling technique used, the caregivers I interviewed, however, cannot be viewed in any way as representative of the total population (of family caregivers). In addition, the few tests of the relationships between confusion and abuse that have been conducted have produced conflicting results. Nevertheless, I believe that because of the strong theoretical support, clinicians cannot ignore the possibility that caregivers who are burdened with the care of a confused elder may abuse the elder. This may be true for professional care providers working in nursing homes, as well as for family and other care providers in the community. As a result, I believe that as clinicians, we must increase our sensitivity to the problem but not increase our levels of suspicion to the point that we see an abused elder behind every caregiving situation. In addition, there are other types of interventions that we, as clinicians, can use to prevent, identify and ameliorate this problem.

1.) Provide the caregiver with a logical, disease-based explanation for the behavior that the elder is displaying.

2.) Provide the caregiver with the opportunity to verbalize his/her images. This may help to neutralize some high risk situations.

3.) Caregivers need to begin to find normality in the situation they are facing.

4.) In-home, community based nursing services can help to ameliorate the potential for abuse by providing on-going monitoring for the situation, a social watchdog which is extremely important in cases of potential abuse, as well as ongoing support and instruction in providing caregiving for a confused elder.

5.) Caregivers need to understand that there is more than one way to fulfill filial or spousal responsibility.

6.) Provide respite care.

## CONCLUSION

Although the empirical evidence supporting a relationship between elder confusion and elder abuse is scant, there is sufficient theoretical support that the possibility of an individual confused elder being abused by his or her caregiver cannot be ignored. Confusion appears to alter the dynamics of caregiving in such a way that the responses of caregivers are difficult to predict. As clinicians, we have the responsibility of remaining sensitive to the special problems of families who provide care to confused elders. Sensitive support and astute assessment may be key to improving the quality of care for confused elders at home and in preventing the possibility of a difficult situation turning to abuse.

## REFERENCES

Archbold, P.G., 1980, Impact of parent-caring on middle aged offspring, Journal of Gerontological Nursing, 6:78-85.

Archbold, P.G., 1983, Impact of parent-caring on women, Family Relations, 32:39-45.

Brody, S., Pulshock, S.W., and Masciocci, C.F., 1978, The family caring unit: A major consideration in the long-term support system, Gerontologist, 18:556-61.

Cantor, M., 1983, Strain among caregivers: A study of experience in the United States, Gerontologist, 23:597-604.

Gebbie, K.M., and Lavin, M.A., 1975, "Classification of Nursing Diagnosis," C.V. Mosby Company, St. Louis.

Gelles, R.J., 1972, "The Violent Home," Sage Publishing Co., Beverly Hills.

Glaser, B., 1978, "Theoretical Sensitivity," Sociology Press, Mill Valley.

Goffman, E., 1956, "The Presentation of Self in Everyday Life," Prentice-Hall, Inc., Englewood Cliffs.

Kohen, J.A., 1983, Old but not alone: Informal social supports among the elderly by marital status and sex, Gerontologist, 23:57-63.

Phillips, L.R., and Rempusheski, V.F., Caring for the frail elderly at home: Toward a theoretical explanation of the dynamics of poor quality family caregiving, Journal of Advanced Nursing, In press.

Quayhagen, M.P., 1977, Confusion in the elderly, Workshop presented at Vail, Colorado.

Rokeach, M., 1954, The nature and meaning of dogmatism, Psychological Review, 61:194-204.

Shanas, E., 1979, The family as a social support system in old age, Gerontologist, 23:64-70.

Stoller, E.P., and Earl, L.L., 1983, Help with activities of every day life: Sources of support for the noninstitutionalized elderly, Geronotologist, 23:64-70.

Wolanin, M.O., and Phillips, L.W., 1961, "Confusion: Prevention and Care," V.C. Mosby Company, St. Louis.

A SYSTEMATIC APPROACH TO THE NURSING CARE OF

ACUTELY ILL GERIATRIC PATIENTS WITH COGNITIVE IMPAIRMENT

Donna Lenore Wells

Sunnybrook Medical Centre - University of Toronto
Toronto, Ontario, Canada

This afternoon I am going to discuss two examples of clinical nursing research related to the care of geriatric patients who suffer both an acute illness and irreversible cognitive impairment. Cognitive impairment refers to alteration in orientation, memory, language, insight, judgment, attention, perception, and thought content.

The first study provides an example of the inductive research process. It is designed to expand nursing knowledge via a systematic investigation of observations made in clinical practice, and thereby develop precise definitions of problems. The second project is more deductive in nature in that the study hypothesis and tentative nursing protocol are derived from theoretical and related research findings. In this study, substantive nursing knowledge is being sought regarding solutions to a clinical practice problem.

Cognitive impairment in elderly patients is one of my main clinical interests. I am overwhelmed continually by the multitude of problems related to the care of these patients which require investigation. However, two major issues have emerged from my clinical and consulting work during the last three years that demand systematic inquiry. The first is the early and often premature discontinuance of rehabilitation in elderly, orthopaedic patients with Alzheimers disease, a type of therapeutic nihilism. The second problem relates to the probability that the hospital setting exacerbates symptoms of helplessness in cognitively impaired, elderly patients. I call this phenomenon the frying pan/fire syndrome. Problem one is the subject of the first part of the presentation.


THERAPEUTIC NIHILISM

Each year I am involved in the care of approximately 80 to 90 elderly orthopaedic patients who have suffered hip fracture. A percentage of these patients also have cognitive impairment as a result of Alzheimers dementia. I have made certain observations regarding these patients:
1. They do not respond to usual therapeutic and rehabilitation techniques (e.g. early mobilization and progressive rehabilitation).
2. As a result they are being discharged from active or acute treatment programs by physiotherapy, occupational therapy, nursing and medicine-- a form of therapeutic nihilism. This compromises the patient's opportunity for complete recovery from the orthopaedic trauma and

impedes the return to the pretrauma functioning level. It follows then that this decreases the patient's chance to return to the community in his/her previous capacity.

3. Despite good intentions, staff often lack specific knowledge relating to the special care needs of elderly, cognitively impaired patients.

Because of the significance of these problems in relation to rehabilitation and outcome, I decided to identify the predominant issues surrounding care of these patients as they are described by orthopaedic staff nurses. My assumption was that knowledge of the major issues would lead to the precise definition of specific clinical problems so that directions for nursing care could be established. Consistent with Linker's Theory of Planned Change (Havelock, 1976), I felt it was crucial to articulate the perceptions of the problems as held by staff nurses. Then I could expect the nurses to consider alternative guidelines for giving care, and to be committed to the implementation of these guidelines. Another assumption I made before pursuing this study was that these patients were not "placement problems" and therefore could be rehabilitated actively and discharged back to the community.

The study I conducted subsequently was basic and descriptive in nature, and has been reported in ten orthopaedic patients who had been admitted during a one-year period with a secondary diagnosis of Alzheimer's disease. All were over 65 years of age.

The patients' records were reviewed retrospectively to answer the following questions:

1. What are the most common pre- and postoperative problems of elderly orthopaedic patients with Alzheimer's disease?

2. How do orthopaedic nurses describe these problems?

3. What interventions do orthopaedic nurses use most commonly with respect to these problems?

(Common was defined as those problems or interventions that were recorded for more than one-half of patients.)

The data revealed the following problems and related nursing interventions commonly recorded by nurses during the preoperative period: 1) confusion—described as forgetful, unsure of location, unable to relate events leading to hospitalization, and incoherence—necessitating frequent reality orientation and physical restraint; 2) restlessness and agitation—described as attempts to leave unit, climbing over side rails, removing bed and night clothes, and noisy—necessitating physical and chemical restraints.

The most common postoperative problems recorded by nurses also included restlessness and agitation, and confusion. These two problems were similarly described and managed. However, additional descriptors of restlessness and agitation in the postoperative period included refusal of therapies and such rehabilitation techniques as transfers and ambulation, and the inability to complete standard postoperative assessment protocols (e.g. active dorsi-plantar flexion to test for nerve intactness).

A third common postoperative problem, not noted in the preoperative period, was sadness. Patients were described as "weepy", "cries frequently", "feels isolated", "refuses to take food and fluids", and "withdrawn". The most common nursing interventions were frequent reassurance and assistance with meals.

Five issues for nursing practice were identified from these data:
1. Care of these patients is complicated and rehabilitation is delayed or discontinued when there are multiple, complex problems.
2. Orthopaedic nursing interventions are not specific enough to compensate for cognitive deficits.
3. Confusional behaviours are not precisely defined; therefore, nursing interventions tend to be limited when it comes to the cognitively impaired patient.
4. The data revealed the presence of an acute on chronic confusional state. Restlessness and agitation decreased after the tenth postoperative day. This is evidence that these behaviours may not be part of the irreversible disease process, but rather may be signs of an underlying treatable cause.
5. The last issue identified is that the total patient is affected. Using Myra Levine's model of nursing (Levine, 1983), the ill, hospitalized patient is the focus. Disruption has occurred in the four areas of conservation. The patient's energy is depleted as a result of the orthopaedic trauma and restlessness; his structural integrity is compromised as a result of surgery and non-compliance with positioning and exercises; his personal integrity is compromised related to impaired communication and sadness; his social integrity is compromised related to separation from family and friends, and impaired communication.

With this knowledge of the major issues, precise problem statements can be made and related nursing interventions selected, again using Levine's model as a guide. The assumptions underlying these interventions are:
1. Cognitive and behavioural disorders associated with Alzheimers disease and exacerbated by orthopaedic injury can be managed with specific deliberate nursing interventions. The nurse provides individualized, skilled, and knowledgeable care.
2. The patient has competencies which can be optimized. The patient should be involved in care. The focus is on abilities not on disabilities or impaired function; in this way conservation of a proper balance between nursing intervention and patient participation is maintained.
3. The environment can be prosthetic. It can be manipulated to assist the patient in adjusting to the situation and prevent decompensation. The nurse then participates actively in the patient's environment.
4. Optimum rehabilitation potential and return to pre-admission functional level can be achieved if the conditions described above are met. This concept of health constitutes a broader definition of the end of acute care treatment away from a medical to a nursing model. In other words, the end of treatment includes recovery from the fractured hip plus a recovery of function.

Levine also states that the nursing diagnosis provides direction and influences interventions. Therefore, the diagnosis should be specific. Table 1 summarizes the exact nursing diagnoses (Kim & Moritz, 1982, and Jones, 1982), their defining characteristics, and relevant nursing interventions.

The nursing goals are to provide a structured and familiar routine through which the environment is explained or interpreted to the patient by a consistent caregiver. Another goal is to minimize the effect of the patient's impairment and related feelings of depression in order to facilitate care and rehabilitation. In the same way, the patient's energy is conserved; structural integrity is restored; the need to interact is satisfied. Therefore personal and social integrity are maintained.

As a result of this basic research project, nursing diagnoses were precisely defined. Nursing interventions specific to these diagnoses were then selected, resulting in the successful rehabilitation of these patients.

TABLE 1. The Orthopaedic Patient with Alzheimers Disease--Nursing Diagnoses,
Defining Characteristics, and Relevant Nursing Interventions

| Diagnoses | Characteristics | Interventions |
|---|---|---|
| 1. Alteration in thought processes | - loss of memory<br>- disorientation | - consistent caregiver<br>- simple, frequent orientation<br>- minimize potential confusion precipitators (e.g. sleep deprivation) |
| 2. Thought processes impaired | - impaired communication | - clear & simple communication (approach directly, gain eye contact, refer to patient by proper name, identify self, speak slowly, do not shout, use short sentences, allow patient time to respond, repeat self exactly)<br>- use touch<br>- reduce personal space |
| 3. Thought processes impaired | - inability to follow instructions<br>- minimal capacity for learning | - clear & simple communication (as above)<br>- teach one skill at a time<br>- encourage participation in care<br>- use demonstration & gesture |
| 4. Consciousness alteration (delerium) | - restlessness<br>- agitation | - identify cause<br>- treat cause (may need to consult physician)<br>- coopt family for consistency<br>- use touch to calm, comfort patient<br>- manipulate the environment (avoid restraint, ↓ stimuli, provide consistent caregiver, early mobility) |
| 5. Depression | - weepy<br>- sad<br>- reduced intake | - consistent caregiver<br>- offer support (use touch, personal belongings, dress in street clothes)<br>- encourage independence |

THE FRYING PAN/FIRE SYNDROME

Of course, one thing always leads to another. Linked to the first
problem, that is the early discontinuance of therapy to elderly, hip fracture patients with Alzheimers disease, is the second problem that I am going
to discuss. This related to the probability that the hospital setting
exacerbates symptoms of helplessness in elderly patients, especially those
with irreversible cognitive impairment. In other words, admitting these
persons from the community, where they were functioning satisfactorily in
the premorbid condition to the acute care hospital is like taking them from
the frying pan and placing them in the fire.

The frying pan symbolizes the premorbid state in which the patient is
vulnerable to helplessness by virtue of age and the cognitive impairment,

but manages in a familiar environment. The fire represents the hospital which, by its very organization and unfamiliar environment, increases vulnerability to helplessness in these patients. Helplessness is defined as:

"a state that is associated with an external orientation towards control and power. The central notion is that the self is vulnerable and unable to affect the outcome of the situation, no matter what the action..." (Wolanin & Phillips, 1981)

From personal observations, the frying pan/fire syndrome impedes the rehabilitation process. The clinical question is: What is an appropriate treatment and management protocol for the hospitalized elderly with cognitive impairment? This question led to the goal of this study, which is to select and test the effectiveness of specific nursing interventions in reducing helplessness and improving patient outcomes in this target population. Presently, the study is at the design stage.

A review of the literature revealed an absence of research examining either the effects of hospitalization on the cognitively impaired elderly or the efficacy of particular interventions on outcomes. However, certain social and psychological theories and related research findings regarding the phenomenon of helplessness have provided direction to both the formulation of my study hypothesis and the selection of the nursing protocol. This is the focus of the discussion.

There are many ways to conceptualize the frying pan/fire syndrome. Goldfarb (1969), for example, summarizes the psychodynamic process underlying old-age helplessness in this way. The loss of resources concomitant with normal aging results in decreased competence or ability to determine and satisfy personal needs; hence, there is an increase in vulnerability to feelings of helplessness which is reflected in behaviours such as passivity and dependence; absence of initiative to make decisions or choices; fear and anger.

The model of normal aging, described by Kuypers & Bengston (1973), explains loss of competence in old age as a function of social system changes. With aging, we experience loss of role (and with this, loss of knowledge and productivity), loss of referent or peer group, and an absence of norms or guidelines for our behaviours. As a result, the older person is forced to depend on the feedback of others to evaluate his performance. Unfortunately, in our society this feedback tends to be negative. Lacking support for alternate ways of viewing his performance, the older person buys into this negative feedback, behaves and is treated accordingly. Eventually external feedback and negative expectations become internalized to the point where the elderly individual's coping skills atrophy and he labels himself as incompetent. According to Kuypers & Bengston, this completes the cycle. To alleviate the problem or break the cycle, they suggest encouraging an internal locus of evaluation and control which in turn fosters self-labelling as able and increases ability to cope. Research focussing on the institutionized, cognitively intact elderly lends support to this assertion. Schultz (1976), for example, demonstrated that increasing choice and control over life events within the institution counteracts physical, psychological and social decline. Although theoretically and empirically appropriate, however, such interventions are not applicable to the population under study. The cognitively impaired by virtue of their impairment have lost insight and problem solving abilities. As a result, they have lost the capacity to develop and maintain an internal locus of control and must depend on others to help satisfy their needs.

To avoid feelings of despair (which is similar to helplessness) and achieve a sense of integrity, personality theorists describe specific life-span, developmental tasks that need to be accomplished. Tasks applicable to the geriatric population as outlined by Peck (1956) include: the establishment of new roles and activities, a focus on comforts, enjoyments and mental tasks, and an emphasis on past successes to de-emphasize body discomforts. I would argue that it is a formidable undertaking for the aged to complete these tasks, given the physiological and sociopsychological contingencies of normal aging as shown in Table 2 (Steffl, 1984).

All of the changes involve losses; therefore the aged are vulnerable to feelings of helplessness and may demonstrate dependency behaviours. It may be impossible for the cognitively impaired to accomplish the tasks of aging without assistance, since they suffer abnormal intellectual losses as well as the other insults of aging.

Moving from the frying pan into the fire, the hospital exacerbates helplessness behaviours related to explicit characteristics of its organization, well described in Goffman's model of institutional totality (Goffman, 1961). The following characteristics are included.

Overprotectiveness of staff. Staff perform routine tasks even when the clinical situation improves, and often without an assessment of the patient's capabilities.

Infantilization of patients. This is the tendency to treat the elderly as children, not mature adults. It occurs through the use of bedrails, restraints, bows in hair, and by staff performing total care.

Depersonalization associated with hospitalization. This involves the removal of personal belongings and reference to patients without the use of their proper names (e.g. "chronics" in Room 202).

Staff expectations of older patients (especially those with dementia). The expectation is that these patients will not recover and that they need help. The result is that the expectation of disability becomes the disability itself.

The medical model of cure. This model continues to dominate the acute-care environment. The focus is on disease and the physical history almost to the exclusion of a psychosocial and premorbid functional history. Therefore recovery from illness becomes the measure of successful outcome, while recovery of function, which requires more time and a particular approach, is ignored. Subsequently, the patient may be labelled "chronic" and/or "placement problem" and further acute care is discontinued.

Acute care environment. This environment is unfamiliar and fast paced. Elderly patients simply cannot keep up. As well, in this environment, communication in understandable terms, especially for demented patients, is

TABLE 2. Physiological, Social and Psychological
         Contingencies of Aging

Losses accompanying aging:

1. Physiological   -   decline in vigor & strength
2. Psychological   -   "looks", body image
3. Personal        -   spouse, friends
4. Social          -   position, leadership
5. Philosophical   -   purpose in living
6. Religious       -   unable to attend church

limited if not totally absent. Yet effective communication is essential to the administration of nursing care (King, 1981).

These adverse features of hospital organization reinforce feelings of helplessness and dependency behaviours, and reflect attitudes of health professionals toward these patients as incompetent and dependent.

The key conclusions from this review of the psychosocial dynamics of helplessness are:
1. Aging and cognitive impairment result in personal and interpersonal perceptions of decreased competence to solve problems and satisfy personal needs, leading to feelings of helplessness;
2. Specific behaviours associated with helplessness are passivity and dependency on others;
3. The hospital environment reinforces the above perceptions and behaviours;
4. Attempts to reverse the helplessness phenomenon by increasing personal choice and control are not relevant to the population under study, given the nature of both cognitive impairment and hospital structure.

These conclusions can be used to identify a nursing protocol, aimed at reducing helplessness and improving outcomes, that is more specific to the hospitalized elderly with cognitive impairment. As previously noted this is the objective of the present research.

There are two basic features of the selected nursing protocol. One feature is the personalization of communication. The aim is to provide individualized, therefore meaningful, communication through the use of techniques specific to the cognitively impaired. The rationale underpinning this approach is compensation for decline in competencies and therefore facilitation of care and rehabilitation. As noted by King (1981), communication is fundamental to nurse-patient interactions and to goal attainment.

The second feature of the protocol is the repatterning of the environment. The goal is to make the environment prosthetic for the cognitively impaired elderly. The rationale is to reduce dependency behaviour and thereby promote rehabilitation and recovery from illness. According to King (1981), the external environment can be altered so that it is conducive to the promotion of health.

The protocol outlined in Table 3 will be tested using a "small n" research approach (Robinson & Foster, 1979). Briefly, it involves:
1. establishing a baseline for the behaviours of interest, by observing the patient for a period of time (the dependent variable);
2. administering the proposed interventions (the independent variable) and continuing to record the measures of the dependent variable noting any changes;
3. removing the independent variable (the reversal phase) and continuing to monitor the dependent behaviour for a specified time.
The main hypothesis to be tested is that specific nursing interventions designed to personalize communication and provide environmental repatterning will improve the physical and psychological level of function in elderly patients with cognitive impairment.

The small sample methodology is an appropriate choice as the goal of this project is to conduct an in-depth analysis of the efficacy of a specific intervention protocol in an applied situation, that is, rehabilitation of the cognitively impaired, hospitalized elderly person. It is hoped that this approach will result also in the production of additional hypotheses and the demonstration that this is an effective clinical protocol. Both could be the subject of more rigorous testing.

231

TABLE 3. A nursing Protocol Designed to Reduce Helplessness and improve
Outcome in hospitalized Elderly Patient with Cognitive
Impairment.

| PERSONALIZED COMMUNICATION (Bartol, 1979) | REPATTERNED ENVIRONMENT (Wolanin & Phillips, 1981) |
|---|---|
| IDENTITY<br>-use of proper name<br>-eye contact<br><br>TOUCH<br>-gentle; to hands, arms<br> shoulders, back<br><br>INFORMATION<br>-concise, clear, simple, slowly<br> spoken using words to patient<br> understands<br>-keep voice calm, low and<br> reasonably modulated<br>-use gestures to augment<br> words (e.g. smile)<br>-present information one<br> step at a time<br>-give time to respond to<br> verbalizations | STRUCTURE<br>-quiet setting<br>-head of bed slightly elevated<br>-doors, curtain, drapes open<br> (except during care)<br>-night light<br><br>CUES<br> -clock, calendar<br>-personal articles (e.g. clothes,<br> toiletries, family pictures)<br>-personal aids in place (e.g. eye<br> glasses)<br>-instruction card<br><br>CONSISTENCY<br>-same caregiver<br>-same room<br>-similar daily routine, including<br> responsibility for self-care as<br> able |

SUMMARY

In summary, these two projects demonstrate the inter-relationship
between clinical practice and nursing research. In the first study presented, observations in clinical practice led to an investigation and
formulation of the precise problems encountered in the care of elderly,
orthopaedic patients with Alzheimer's disease. This is a form of inductive
research process. The second study is more deductive in nature. Based on
general knowledge of theoretical and empirical findings about the phenomenon of helplessness, specific nursing interventions are hypothesized as
practical impact on patient care, and offer a more substantive base for
nursing practice in relation to care of the hospitalized elderly with
irreversible cognitive impairment.

REFERENCES

Bartol, M., 1979, Dialogue with dementia: Nonverbal communication in
patients with Alzheimer's disease, J. Gerontol. Nurs., 5:21.
Goffman, E., 1951, "Asylums," Doubleday, Garden City, New York.
Goldfarb, A.I., 1969, The psychodynamics of dependency and the search for
aid, in: "The Dependencies of Old People," R.A. Kalish, ed., Institute
of Gerontology, The University of Michigan - Wayne State University,
Ann Arbor.
Jones, P.E., and Jakob, D.F., 1980, "The Definition of Nursing Diagnoses:
Report of Phase 2," University of Toronto, Faculty of Nursing,
Toronto.
Kim, M.J., and Moritz, D.A., 1982, "Classification of Nursing Diagnoses,"
McGraw-Hill Book Company, New York.
King, I.M., 1981, "A Theory for Nursing," John Wiley & Sons, Inc., New York.

Kuypers, J.A., and Benston, V.L., 1973, Social breakdown and competence a
    model of normal aging, Human Develop., 16:181-201.
Levine, M.E., 1983, Introduction to Clinical Nursing, in: "Conceptual
    Models of Nursing," Robert J. Brady Co., Bowie.
Peck, R.C., 1956, Psychological developments in the second half of late
    life, in: "Psychological Aspects of Aging," J.E. Anderson, ed.,
    American Psychological Association, Washington, D.C.
Robinson, P.W., and Foster, D.F., 1979, "Experimental Psychology: A Small-n
    Approach," Harper & Row, New York.
Schultz, R., 1976, Effects of control and predictability on the physical and
    psychological well-being of the institutionalized aged, J. Per. Soc.
    Psychol., 33:563-573.
Steffl, B.M., 1984, "Handbook of Gerontological Nursing," Ban Nostrand
    Reinhold Company Inc., New York.
Wells, D.L., 1985, The elderly orthopaedic patient with Alzheimer's disease,
    Ortho. Nurs., 4:6, 16-23.
Wolanin, M.O., and Phillips, L.R.F., 1981, "Confusion Prevention and Care,"
    The C.V. Mosby Company, St. Louis.

URINE CONTROL IN PATIENTS WITH CHRONIC DEGENERATIVE BRAIN DISEASE

Mary Marmoll Jirovec

Wayne State University
Detroit, Michigan

Normative influences have determined that in Western culture
people will empty their bladders at designated toileting facilities and
in private.  The ability to control the flow of urine is taken for
granted by individuals and expected by society.  Urine control, however, is a complex phenomenon.  It may be defined as the ability to
inhibit the passage of urine until a culturally determined time.  This
requires the presence of an adequate stimulus to initiate the
micturition reflex, neuromuscular and structural integrity of the
genitourinary system, the cognitive ability to adequately interpret and
know how to respond to the sensation of a full bladder, and the mo-
tivational basis to want to inhibit the passage of urine.  At the same
time, the individual must be mobile enough to be able to react to a
full bladder before the urge to urinate overwhelms inhibiting ability.
Finally, the person must attend to body sensations and environmental
cues in order to know when and how the flow of urine should be controlled.

TYPES OF URINARY INCONTINENCE

Urinary incontinence can generally be classified as acute or
chronic.  Acute incontinence is generally sudden in onset and limited
in duration to the acute condition with which it is associated
(Ouslander, et al., 1985).  Examples of these are illnesses that limit
mobility or impair cognitive functioning, acute urinary tract infections, fecal impactions, or drug therapies.

Chronic incontinence is a more persistent form of incontinence
involving repeated, involuntary instances of urine loss.  This type of
incontinence may be one of five types:  stress, urge, overflow, functional, or mixed incontinence.  Stress incontinence is associated with
leakage of small amounts of urine at times when intraabdominal pressure
increases,such as sneezing, laughing, coughing, rising, etc.  It is
found most frequently in women and is related to a weakening of the
urethral sphincter musculature and surrounding tissues.  Urge
incontinence involves the loss of varying amounts of urine because of
an inability to inhibit bladder contractions until the toilet is
reached.  It is accompanied by a feeling of urgency, a felt need to get
to the bathroom almost immediately.  This can result from a variety of

central nervous system changes anywhere along the nerve pathways to and from the bladder.

Overflow incontinence is associated with the loss of small amounts of urine when the bladder is excessively full. Because the bladder is not being emptied properly, small amounts are leaked in order to compensate for the excessively high intravesicular pressure. Overflow incontinence can happen in spinal cord injury, as a complication of diabetes, or because of drugs that inhibit bladder contractions. More frequently it occurs in combination with a mechanical obstruction that constricts the urethra such as prostatic hypertrophy.

A fourth type of incontinence is termed functional incontinence (Ouslander, et al., 1985, Williams, et al., 1982). This involves the inability to reach the toilet before urine is lost. Functional incontinence is a broad classification that encompasses individuals with any number of impairments related to mobility, cognitive functioning, self-care abilities, motivation, or environmental factors. The origin of the incontinence lies outside the genitourinary system. Mixed incontinence is a situation involving more than one of the four basic types.


URINE CONTROL IN ALZHEIMER'S DISEASE

Urinary incontinence is commonly encountered when caring for patients with Alzheimer's disease. There is little empirical data, however, on the incidence of urinary incontinence in Alzheimer's disease. Data available indicates the incidence is disproportionately higher than that in the general elderly population. One of the earliest studies found two-thirds of patients with low scores on a test of verbal learning were incontinent of urine (Isaacs, 1962). The incontinent patients had moderate to severe cognitive impairment (Isaacs, 1963). Others have also found a strong association between impaired mental status and urinary incontinence (Brocklehurst and Dillane, 1966b; Isaacs and Walkey, 1964a). Hodkinson (1973) found a highly significant correlation between mental test scores and urinary incontinence with incontinence being associated with lower cognitive scores. Of more recent studies, one found 70 percent of patients with some type of senile dementia were incontinent of urine (McLaren, et al., 1981). In another, patients 80 years and older with dementia were three and a half times more likely to be incontinent (Campbell et al., 1985).

Causes of Urinary Incontinence in Alzheimer's Disease

While it is generally accepted that urinary incontinence is a frequent occurrence in Alzheimer's disease, the cause of the incontinence is not know. Only profound dementia is a cause in itself of urinary incontinence (Newman, 1962). Patients with Alzheimer's disease can be expected to experience incontinence related to known etiologies in the same proportion as other elderly. Yalla et al. (1985) found that of their sample of 48 incontinent, institutionalized elderly, urological diagnoses did not differ according to cognitive impairment. Cognitively impaired subjects evidence urological diagnoses similar to those without cognitive impairment. There is no evidence that Alzheimer patients are less likely to have difficulties with sphincter weakness, detrusor instability, prostatic hypertrophy, etc. Alzheimer patients, however, will be less able to compensate for the various types of incontinence. For instance, an Alzheimer patient may not remember to keep their bladder empty. Rather, they must respond

quickly as they sense that urine is leaking or that they feel an
urgency to urinate.

Patients with Alzheimer disease will also evidence changes in the
lower urinary tract associated with normal aging.  Again, the changes
in themselves do not cause loss of urine control.  In combination with
other factors, however, age related changes may contribute to an
eventual loss of urine control.  Brocklehurst and Dillane (1966a)
concluded that almost all of their sample of 40 continent elderly women
had abnormal bladders.  Forty-three percent had bladder capacities of
250 ml or less.  Half had residual urine after voiding of 50 ml or more
and almost three quarters did not empty their bladders completely.  The
majority did not evidence a desire to void until their bladders were at
capacity and many evidenced uninhibited detrusor contractions.

In addition to normal age related changes, several studies have
established an abrupt increase in the incidence of urinary tract
infections with age (Goldman, 1977).  Brocklehurst et al. (1968) found
that 17% of a large sample (n=557) of elderly had infected urine.  In
addition, the female urethra is hormone-dependent and susceptible to
menopausal changes.  The prevalence of postmenopausal tissue atrophy,
previous trauma during childbirth, and gravitational forces over time
(Wells & Brink, 1981) make these changes in women almost a normal age
related occurrence.  The changes make maintaining urine control an
emerging issue for all elderly.  For persons with Alzheimer's disease
the problem is even greater.

## Functional Incontinence in Alzheimer's Disease

A key to incontinence in Alzheimer's disease may be functional
incontinence.  Functional incontinence can be related to cognitive
ability, mobility, self-care abilities, or environmental factors.  In
Alzheimer's disease any one of these may be a factor in the genesis of
urinary incontinence.  For instance, incontinence is likely to be at
least partly the result of a cognitive disorder.  As impulses reach the
cerebral cortex from the bladder, the person becomes aware of the need
to urinate.  At that moment the individual must be able to adequately
interpret the meaning of the impulse from the bladder in order to
consciously inhibit urination.  Problems can arise if the patient does
not understand the meaning of the sensations he or she is experiencing,
what the proper response to the sensations should be, where to go in
response to a full bladder, or how to remove clothing and assume the
position needed to maintain urine control.  These are learned behaviors
which are subject to the memory losses associated with Alzheimer's
disease.  It seems very likely that urinary incontinence in Alzheimer's
disease is at least in part due to a memory defect.

Similarly, mobility is often impaired in Alzheimer's disease.
Patients must be able to physically get to the bathroom if they are to
maintain continence.  When the patient has Alzheimer's disease, they
often are faced with the problem of not being able to remember sanitary
routines.  If they have additional physical limitations impairing their
ability to reach the toilet, their difficulties with urine control are
greatly expanded.  Many of the urological changes that occur with
increased frequency as a person ages result in some type of urgency.
Impaired mobility further decreases the likelihood the patient will be
able to maintain continence.

While cognitive ability is always impaired in Alzheimer's disease
and mobility may be decreased, self-care ability may further compromise
the patient's ability to maintain urine control.  As cognitive ability

decreases, the patient's ability to remove clothing and handle hygienic needs is often lessened. This adds a third factor that may contribute to functional incontinence in Alzheimer's disease.

A fourth and equally potent factor contributing to functional incontinence are environmental cues and consequences. Much of the incontinence seen in Alzheimer's disease occurs in nursing homes. The incontinence may be in part a function of what the patient learns from the nursing home environment. The nursing home staff sometimes approach the problem of incontinence with resignation. They do not indicate to the Alzheimer patient that urine control is an expected behavior. In fact, methods to handle the consequences of incontinence such as diapering are quickly instituted. Seldom does the solution for incontinence include some mechanism for compensating for the cognitive deficit while still maintaining continence. Since removing a diaper is often difficult, what is meant to be a solution to the problem often makes it more difficult for the patient to use the toilet. In fact, the Alzheimer patient may learn that further attempts to control urine are futile. The environment is often unintentionally structured to manage the incontinence rather than maximize continence.

Loss of urine control frequently occurs when an elderly Alzheimer patient first enters a nursing home. It is not unusual for the elderly to experience some incontinence under physical or psychological stress. The incontinence may be related to some physiological state (fever, infection, diuretic medication, etc), emotional upset (loss of a loved one, feelings of abandonment, etc.) or confused states (temporary disorientation to new surroundings, confusion due to dehydration, etc.). If the nursing home staff label the patient as "incontinent" from the outset, the patient will be treated differently than one labeled as "continent." If memory problems resulted in episodes of incontinence at home, the staff will treat the patient as if they expect incontinence at admission. Eventually, the patient will "learn" to be incontinent.

The behavioral deficits often seen in nursing home residents are partly a function of the nursing home environment and its concomitant experiences (Hoyer, 1973). McClannahan (1973) identified a number of environmental characteristics within nursing home settings that influence motor activity, verbal behavior, and self-care ability. A review of several studies demonstrated the importance of environmental factors in influencing resident's behavior (Hoyer, 1973). Lester and Baltes (1978) studied nurse's verbal responses to various patient behaviors and found dependent behaviors were most often reinforced with a positive verbal response by the nurse, while independent behaviors were usually followed by no response. Other studies have shown that changing environmental contingencies can alter behavior of elderly nursing home residents in areas related to self-care (Gottfried & Verdicchio, 1974), eating behavior (Baltes & Lascomb, 1975; Baltes & Zerbe, 1976a; Baltes & Zerbe, 1976b, Geiger & Johnson, 1974), activity level (MacDonald & Butler, 1974, McClannahan & Risley, 1975), socialization (MacDonald, 1978), and memory (Langer, et al., 1979).

## Research on Intervention Strategies for Incontinence with Alzheimer Patients

Little research has been done specifically on urine control in Alzheimer's disease. Several researchers, however, have demonstrated the impact of environmental manipulations on the toileting behavior of cognitively impaired elderly. Sanavio (1981) used a repeated treatment design with two elderly men with senile dementia in long-term care.

Environmental contingencies were related to soiling versus toileting. These were alternated with consequences not contingent on toileting behavior. Both patients improved when the consequences were contingent on their behavior. Pollack and Liberman (1974) did a similar study with six geriatric patients with chronic brain failure. However, reinforcements and punishments were given irregularly. The result was no improvement in any of the patients. Two of the patients worsened.

Schnelle, et al. (1983) studied 21 incontinent geriatric nursing home residents with some type of physical limitation. Using randomly assigned experimental and control groups, all patients were checked for wetness on a regular basis. The experimental group was prompted to toilet at each check and was given social approval or disapproval at the check depending on their wetness or dryness. Patients were not toileted unless they requested help when prompted. This required the patient's involvement in the toileting procedure. At the end of the 21 days of treatment, the experimental group was significantly less incontinent and requested toileting more frequently than the control group. Clay (1978) also attempted to reverse incontinence with four elderly with some type of dementia. Habit training was used with social reinforcement and self-reinforcement. Two of the four patients improved, one was completely continent with reminders; and one did not improve.

Other researchers have studied the effect of environment on urine control using psychogeriatric patients. Grosicki (1968) studied the effect of social and material rewards using nonrandom control and experimental groups. There was no improvement for the experimental group, while the control group decreased incontinence. The appropriateness of the experimental manipulation could be questioned. Improvement in the control group would seem to demonstrate the impact of regular checks for wetness. Hartie and Black (1975) focused on nighttime toileting with social and material rewards if the bed was dry. Using five long-term psychogeriatric patients, bed wetting was decreased by almost 50 percent. King (1980) also used psychogeriatric patients to study urine control. Fifteen patients selected from various wards were moved to a new trial ward where regular toileting was initiated with a variety of other interventions. Urinary incontinence was decreased for all but one of the subjects.

Carpenter and Simon (1960) used 4 groups of long-term psychiatric patients to study incontinence. The three experimental groups were given habit training, habit training with social reinforcements, and habit training with material reinforcements respectively. The fourth group was used as the control group and given the usual care. The two habit training groups with reinforcements decreased in urinary incontinence. The control group's incontinence increased, demonstrating further the impact of environment on urine control. Wagner and Paul (1970) studied 35 chronic psychiatric patients. After baseline data was collected, material and social rewards and long-term incentives to maintain continence were given. Thirteen of the patients became continent during the baseline period when they were being checked regularly for wetness. The other subjects demonstrated significantly less incontinence when compared to their baseline incontinence levels.


METHODS

A study was conducted in order to explore factors associated with urine control in elderly nursing home residents with chronic memory problems* (Jirovec & Wells, 1985a, 1985b). The sample consisted of 61 elderly residents of a combined long-term care and retirement facility in a rural Michigan town. The subjects were patients who had been identified by the charge nurse on the day shift as having chronic memory problems that made it necessary for the staff to make allowances or plan nursing care to compensate for the patient's memory difficulties. Patient diagnoses could not be used to identify potential subjects because of the unreliability of the medical diagnoses. Only 16 subjects had specific diagnoses related to some type of chronic degenerative brain disease. Of the 61 subjects, 42 had some mention of organic brain syndrome, senile dementia, dementia, or memory problems in the histories; however, specific diagnoses were not made. The subjects were all white, with 8 men and 53 women. They ranged in age from 66 to 105 years with a mean age of 87 years.

The study examined the impact of cognitive ability, mobility, and environmental factors on urine control in nursing home patients with chronic memory problems. Specifically, the independent variables thought to affect urine control were scores on three cognitive ability measures [a shortened version of the Philadelphia Geriatric Center Mental Status Questionnaire (Fishback, 1972), the visual counting test (Fishback, 1977), and the set test (Isaacs & Akhtar, 1972)], scores on an upper limb mobility test, the distance subjects were able to walk, speed of walking, balance scores and a variety of environmental measures such as toilet visibility, toilet distances, and nursing care factors.

Once permission was obtained according to an approved human subjects protocol, the data were collected in three phases. In the first phase participant observation techniques were used. Each patient was observed by two researchers on different days and when different nurse aides were caring for the patient. After the observation period, the nurse aid was asked to indicate if the patient was reminded to toilet, if the patient used an adult diaper, if restraints were usually used, and the patient's degree of urine control. After the researchers had compiled their impressions independently and obtained independent feedback from different nurse aides, questions on the questionnaire related to environmental factors, clothing, and urine control were answered.

Phase two consisted of direct interviews with the patients. During this time the mental status questionnaire, the visual counting test, and the set test were administered. Upper limb mobility was measured by having patients complete a total of 25 movements involving the arms and hands and counting the number of movements successfully performed. The total distance the patient could walk was measured using a measure wheel and a stop watch was used to determine the time taken to walk and the patient's ability to stand in one place without holding on.

During the third phase of data collection environmental factors such as toilet distances were measured and the patient's chart was reviewed for findings on the most recent physical examination and medications being used. Finally, the nurse aides were asked to keep a record of patients' fluid intake on two separate nonconsecutive day shifts. For the nine patients residing in the retirement section of the home where care was minimal, the intake record was kept for one day.

---

*The research was supported by a grant from the Alzheimer's Disease and Related Disorders Association

FINDINGS

Subjects were divided into two groups — continent and incontinent. Differences between the groups on findings of the most recent physical examination were explored using Chi square analysis. No significant findings were found with the exception of the diagnosis of depression/psychoses, primarily depression. More continent patients were diagnosed as depressed when compared to incontinent patients. None of these diagnoses were made by a psychiatrist. An explanation for the differences may be related to the fact that depression is less likely to be overlooked by a general practitioners in continent patients because they are less impaired. A review of the medication records also showed no differences between continent and incontinent patients in medications being taken.

Fluid intake was also examined in relation to urine control group (see Table 1). It was expected that incontinent patients would have a lower intake than continent patients. However, the two groups did not differ significantly on daily fluid intake measures. This was a surprising finding, as the literature suggests an association between inadequate fluid intake and incontinence. The lack of intake differences may have been related to measurement inaccuracy. The nurse aides who measured intake were also the ones who fed many of the patients and, therefore, determined in part the amount of fluid taken.

Cognitive ability scores were compared using three urine control groups continent, sometimes incontinent, and completely incontinent. Incontinent patients scored significantly lower on all measures of cognitive ability (Jirovec & Wells, 1985b). In general, cognitive ability scores decreased as urine control decreased.

Mobility was also examined in relation to membership in one of the three urine control groups described above. Patients' mobility differed significantly according to urine control (Jirovec and Wells, 1985b). That is, continent patients could walk faster, walk farther, and balance longer than incontinent patients. Continent patients needed less help in walking and were better able to get out of a chair alone when compared to incontinent patients. When patient variables were used to predict if the patient would be continent or incontinent, mobility emerged as the first predictor of the ability to control urine. If the patient could get to the bathroom alone, the patient was likely to be continent. If the patient needed help getting to the bathroom, the patient was most likely to be incontinent.

Environmental factors were also examined. Continent and incontinent patients differed significantly on the types of cues provided by the nursing home (see Table 2) (Jirovec & Wells, 1985a). Incontinent patients lived in areas of the home where the toilet facilities were less visible. Restraints were also used much more frequently with incontinent patients. More than two-thirds of the incontinent patients

Table 1. Fluid intake according to urine control group

| Group | Minimum | Maximum | Mean | Standard Dev. |
|---|---|---|---|---|
| Incontinent | 345ml | 1635ml | 771ml | 274ml |
| Continent | 315ml | 1298ml | 787ml | 261ml |

Table 2. Frequency of environmental cues according to urine control group.

| Environmental Cue | Continent Group | Incontinent Group |
|---|---|---|
| Sign on or near toilet* | 16 | 3 |
| Color contrast on or around door* | 14 | 3 |
| Lighted sign signifying location* | 10 | 1 |
| Toileting reminders* | 3 | 21 |
| Use of protective sheet on bed* | 14 | 26 |
| Use of restraints* | 1 | 21 |
| Use of adult diaper* | 0 | 25 |

*p < 0.01

were tied into chairs. Almost all were diapered. The use of re-straints and diapers were not accompanied by regular toileting remind-ers and removal of the restraints so that the patient could get to the bathroom. Only three incontinent patients were reminded regularly to use the toilet. Most were reminded only on an irregular basis.

RECOMMENDATIONS

Environmental factors are associated with urine control in pa-tients with Alzheimer's disease. The impact of environmental manipu-lations on urine control has been demonstrated by other researchers. Changing environmental contingencies, however, may not be enough. Proper care must involve evaluation of the incontinence, assessment of the patient and environment, and an individualized plan of care.

The most neglected aspect of care for patients with Alzheimer's disease who have urine control problems is a thorough evaluation by an urologist or urological nurse practitioner. It is imperative that treatable urological disease be ruled out. None of the incontinent patients in the present study were evaluated by a urologist. If the incontinence occurs during some acute episode, an astute family practi-tioner will recognize the possibility that the incontinence will be reversed. If, however, the incontinence becomes more established, evaluation of the cause will greatly aid in planning care and may serve to relieve the incontinence with medical treatment.

If medical treatment does not relieve the incontinence, caretakers should assess the patient and the environment for information that will maximize the likelihood the patient can be helped to maintain continence. It is important to try to establish when the incontinence started and how caretakers responded to the incontinent episodes. The assessment should focus on the person's cognitive ability, mobility, and self-care ability. Many factors will provide clues in relation to appropriate intervention strategies (see Table 3).

In addition to patient assessment, the environment should be evaluated. Often environmental characteristics exacerbate problems identified during the patient assessment. If the patient is having difficulty finding the toilet, is the toilet readily visible? If the patient has difficulty with mobility, is the patient being exercised regularly in order to maximize mobility? If the patient has difficulty

Table 3.  Assessment of urine control in Alzheimer's disease

| Assessment area | Indications |
|---|---|
| Does patient take a long time to find the toilet?<br>Does the patient know where the bathroom is located?<br>Does the person evidence restlessness before an incontinent episode?<br>Is confusion increased before an incontinent episode? | Provides information regarding memory problems that may contribute to incontinence. |
| Is the patient able to get to the bathroom alone?<br>How quickly is the patient able to get to the bathroom?<br>Can the patient balance alone while standing?<br>Is the patient generally mobile?<br>Is the patient free to move around at will? | Provides information regarding mobility problems that may contribute to incontinence. |
| Is patient able to manipulate clothing?<br>Is patient able to button and zipper clothing?<br>Can patient dress self alone? with help?<br>Does patient perform hygiene activities for self? | Provides information regarding self-care abilities used to self-toilet. |
| Does the patient ask to go to the bathroom?<br>If placed on a toilet, does the patient urinate?<br>Is the patient concerned after incontinent episodes?<br>How does the patient react to incontinence? | Provides information of patient's potential ability to control urine if toileted. |
| What amounts of urine does the patient lose?<br>What are the usual times the patient urinates?<br>Does the person drink adequate amounts fluid?<br>Is fluid intake regular? | Provides information useful for planning care to promote continence. |

manipulating buttons, can velcro closures be provided?  If the patient
is being diapered, is help provided for removal to toilet?  Greater
attention should be given to environmental factors that promote rather
than inhibit urine control.

An individualized plan of care is an important component of
continence care.  Generally, care plans to promote continence have
utilized scheduled toileting, habit training, or behavior modification.
Scheduled toilet involves toileting the patient at times, usually two
hour intervals for the convenience of staff.  Habit training refers to
encouraging patients to toilet according to their bladder patterns.  As
accidents occur, patients are encouraged to toilet sooner until they
are able to maintain continence.  Behavior modification involves a
program of rewards and punishments to promote continence and extinguish
incontinence.  Behavior modification programs assume the incontinence
is not due to cognitive impairment or mobility difficulties.

None of these plans of care is entirely appropriate for patients
with Alzheimer's disease.  The appropriate approach is what will be

called <u>individualized scheduled toileting behavior</u> (ISTB), a synthesized application of scheduled toileting, habit training, and behavior modification.  Specifically, the patient's usual voiding patterns
should be determined.  In addition, fluid intake should be addressed.
Patients should be offered adequate amounts of fluid at regular times
in order to insure a regular pattern of urination.  Once voiding
patterns have been established, the patient should be helped to toilet
at these individualized times.  A toileting schedule will help to
compensate for the cognitive deficit.  Toileting behavior should be
encouraged with an overall approach that emphasizes the appropriateness
of continence.  If an adult diaper is used to control for accidents, it
should be easily and readily removed.  Toilets should be visible and
accessible.

     Mobility, also, should be addressed.  If patients do not walk
around alone, they should be helped to ambulate regularly.  Nursing
homes should avoid the use of restraints.  If their use is deemed
necessary, they should be removed on a regular basis to allow the
patient to walk and toilet.  Patients needing help with ambulation,
should be provided help regularly and religiously.  Mobility skills
must not be allowed to atrophy.

     An Alzheimer patient with urine control problems should be provid-
ed with these three care directives - medical evaluation, assessment
and ISTB - before the incontinence is approached with only urine
containment procedures.  Medical evaluation should insure no treatable
urological condition contributes to the incontinence.  Patient and
environment assessment should identify areas amenable to intervention.
Lastly, an <u>individualized scheduled toileting behavior</u> program should
be instituted in an attempt to reverse the incontinence.  Implementation of all three strategies will result in an overall approach that
attempts to reverse the incontinence rather than merely managing the
urine control problem.


CONCLUSIONS

     Urinary incontinence in Alzheimer's disease is inevitable in the
late stages of the disease.  The pervasive acceptance of the incontinence earlier in the disease, especially in nursing homes, is inappropriate.  Alzheimer patients often experience functional incontinence
alone or in combination with another urological problem.  They develop
urological conditions to the same extent as the general population.
What begins as a simple case of stress, urge or overflow incontinence
for the Alzheimer patient, however, quickly develops into a mixed
incontinence - functional incontinence in combination with another
urine control problems.

     Of primary importance in caring for Alzheimer patients with
incontinence is a recognition that the incontinence may be related not
only to an urological problem, but to a cognitive deficit, mobility
limitation, and/or environmental factor.  The limited research that has
been done with Alzheimer patients included in the sample has established the association between these factors and urine control.
Caretakers should structure care of incontinent Alzheimer patients with
this knowledge in mind.

     Alzheimer researchers, also, must not be complacent regarding
urine control in Alzheimer's disease.  The costs of incontinence are
staggering in terms of its adverse effects on the health, social
functioning, and psychological well-being of the patient, its effects

on the workload and stress endured by caretakers, and its cost burden related to laundry and supplies. The cost to society is even greater when one considers the fact that incontinence often contributes to the decision to place a patient in a nursing home (Ouslander, 1985). New strategies of intervention that are specifically developed for patients with some type of chronic degenerative brain disease need to be tested so caretakers can be provided better guidelines for decreasing incontinence in Alzheimer's disease. These strategies should be tested at home as well as in institutions so that family members and agency staff can work together to prevent loss of urine control as a patient's condition worsens.

We need not be resigned to urinary incontinence in Alzheimer's disease. The problem should be handled aggressively by both caretakers and researchers. The potential for improving the quality of life for these patients, their families, and professional caretakers warrants efforts to address and conquer this all too common problem.

REFERENCES

Baltes, M.M. and Lascomb, S.L., 1975, Creating a healthy institutional environment for the elderly via behavior management. The nurse as a change agent. International Journal of Nursing Studies, 12: 5-12.

Baltes, M.M. and Zerbe, M.B., 1976a, Independence training in nursing home residents. Gerontologist, 16: 428-432.

Baltes, M.M. and Zerbe, M.B., 1976b, Reestablishing self-feeding in a nursing home resident. Nursing Research, 25: 24-26.

Brocklehurst, J.C. and Dillane, J.B., 1966a, Studies of the female bladder in old age. Part 1. Cystometrograms in 100 incontinent women. Gerontological Clinics, 8: 285-305.

Blocklehurst, J.C. and Dillane, J.B., 1966b, Studies of the female bladder in old age. Part 2. Cystometrograms in 100 incontinent women. Gerontological Clinics, 8: 306-319.

Brocklehurst, J.C., Dillane, J.B., Griffiths, L. and Fry, J., 1968. The prevalence and symptomatology of urinary infection in an aged population. Gerontological Clinics, 10: 242-253.

Campbell, A.J., Reinken, J. and Mclash, L., 1985, Incontinence in the elderly: Prevalence and prognosis. Aged and Aging, 14: 65-70.

Carpenter, H.A. and Simon, R., 1960, The effect of several methods of training on long-term, incontinent, behaviorally regressed hospitalized psychiatric patients. Nursing Research, 9: 17-22.

Clay, E.C., 1978, Incontinence of urine: A regime for retraining. Nursing Mirror, 146: 23-24.

Fishback, D.B., 1977, Mental status questionnaire for organic brain syndrome with a new visual counting test. Journal of American Geriatric Society, 25: 167-170.

Geiger, O.G. and Johnson, L.A., 1974, Positive education of elderly persons: Correct eating through reinforcement. Gerontologist, 14: 432-436.

Goldman, R., 1977, Aging on the excretory system. Kidney and bladder, in: "Handbook of the biology of aging, C.E. Finch and L. Hayflick, eds., New York, Van Nostrand Reinhold.

Gottfried, A.W. and Verdiocchio, R.G., 1974, Modifications of hygienic behaviors using reinforcement therapy. American journal of Psychotherapy, 28: 122-128.

Grosicki, J.P., 1968, Effect of operant conditioning on modification of incontinence in neuropsychiatric geriatric patients. Nursing research, 17: 304-311.

Hartie, A. and Black, D., 1975, A dry bed is the objective. Nursing Times, 71: 1874-1876.

Hodkinson, H.M., 1973, Mental impairment in the elderly. Journal of the Royal College of Physicians in London, 4: 305-317.

Hoyer, W.J. 1973, Application of operant techniques to the modification of elderly behavior. Gerontologist, 13: 18-22.

Isaacs, B., 1962, A preliminary evaluation of a paired-associate verbal learning test in geriatric practice. Gerontological Clinics, 4: 43-55.

Isaacs, B., 1963, The diagnostic value of tests with toys in old people. Gerontological Clinics, 5: 8-22.

Isaacs, B. and Akhtar, A.J., 1972, The set test: A rapid test of mental function in old people. Age and Aging, 1: 222-226.

Isaacs, B and Walkey, F.A., 1964, A survey of incontinence in elderly hospital patients. Gerontologic Clinics, 6: 367-376.

Jirovec, M.M. and Wells, T.J., 1985a, April. Determinants of Urinary Incontinence in Elderly with Memory Problems, Paper presented at the meeting of the Midwest Nursing Research Society, Chicago, Illinois.

Jirovec, M.M. and Wells, T.J., 1985b, November. Factors associated With Chronic Degenerative Brain Disease. Paper presented at the meeting of the Gerontological Society of America, New Orleans, LA.

King, M.R., 1979, A study of incontinence in a psychiatric hospital, Nursing Times, 75: 113-1135.

Langer, E.J., Rodin, J., Beck, P., Weinman, C. and Spitzer, L., 1979, Environmental determinants of memory improvement in late adulthood. Journal of Personality and Social Psychology, 37: 2003-2013.

Lester, P.B. and Baltes, M.M., 1978, Functional interdependence of the social environment and the behavior of the institutionalized aged. Journal of Gerontological Nursing, 4: 23-27.

MacDonald, M.L., 1978, Environmental programming for the socially isolated aging. Gerontologist, 18: 350-354.

MacDonald, M.L. and Butler, A.K., 1974, Reversal of helplessness: Producing walking behavior in nursing home wheelchair residents using behavior modification procedures. Journal of Gerontology, 29: 97-101.

McClannahan, L.E., 1973, Therapeutic and prosthetic living environments for nursing home residents. Gerontologist, 13: 424-429.

McClannahan, L.E. and Risley, T.R., 1975, Design of living environments for nursing home residents: Increasing participation in recreation activities. Journal of Applied Behavior Analysis, 8: 261-268.

McLaren, S.M., McPherson, F.M., Sinclair, R. and Ballinger, G.R., 1981, Prevalence and severity of incontinence among hospitalized female psychogeriatric patients. Health Bulletin, 39: 157-161.

Newman, J.L., 1962, Old folk in wet beds. British Medical Journal, 1: 1824-1828.

Ouslander, J., Kane, R., Vollmer, S. and Menezes, M., July 1985, Technologies for managing urinary incontinence. (Health Technology Case Study 33), OTA-HCS-33, Washington, D.C.: U.S. Congress, Office of Technology Assessment.

Pollack, D.D, and Liberman, R.P., 1974, Behavior therapy of incontinence in demented inpatients. Gerontologist, 14: 488-491.

Sanavio, E., 1981, Toilet retraining psychogeriatric residents. Behavior Modification, 5: 417-427.

Schnelle, J.F., Traughber, B., Morgan, D.B. Embry, J.E., Binion, A.F. and Coleman, A., 1983, Management of geriatric incontinence in nursing homes. Journal of Applied Behavior Analysis, 16: 235-241.

Wagner, B.R. and Paul, G.L., 1970, Reduction of incontinence in chronic mental patients: A pilot project. Journal of Behavior Therapy and and Experimental Psychiatry, 1: 29-38.

Wells, T.J. and Brink, C.A., 1981, Urinary continence: Assessment and management. in: "Nursing and the aged," J.M. Burnside, ed., New York, McGraw-Hill.

Williams, M.E. and Pannill, F.C., 1982, Urinary incontinence in the elderly. Annals of Internal Medicine, 97: 895-907.

Yalla, S., Resnick, N. and Reilly, C., November 1985, <u>Causes and Correlates of Urinary Incontinence in Extremely Aged Patients: New Findings.</u>  Paper presented at the Annual Meeting of the Gerontological Society of America, New Orleans, LA.

COGNITIVE PSYCHOPATHOLOGY AND THE PHENOMENON OF WANDERING:

RESEARCH AND CLINICAL NURSING APPROACHES

Pam Dawson

Sunnybrook Medical Centre
Toronto, Ontario, Canada

The increasing population of those over the age of eighty years and the concomitant increase in the incidence of Alzheimer's disease and dementia pose caregiving challenges for both health care professionals and family members providing support in the community. It is realistic to expect the discipline of nursing as a caregiving discipline to provide leadership and guidance to non-profesional and family caregivers. However to transit knowledge and skill, it is necessary to clearly define the knowledge about Alzheimer's disease and dementia which is relevant to caregiving and how application of this knowledge influences caregiving. Where gaps exist in knowledge relevant or applicable to caregiving then efforts to contribute to knowledge are required. The intent of this paper is to focus on the practice of research. Through the inter-relationship of research in practice caregiving, leadership can be developed which is enabling to both caregivers and recipients of care. I hope to illustrate the inter-relationship between research and practice and its potential through first sharing specific studies about Alzheimer's disease and dementia which have influenced my practice and secondly, through the presentation of a clinical problem encountered in practice for which research was required in order to develop caregiving approaches.

The objective of caregiving may be questioned when diagnoses such as Alzheimer's disease and dementia are known to be progressive and irreversible. However, because of previous work of individuals such as Kahn (1966) and Brody and her colleagues (1971, 1974), the prevention and reversal of Excess Disability can be seen as an appropriate caregiving objective for those suffering from Alzheimer's disease and dementia. Because of the common inability to articulate and describe status and needs accompanying illnesses such dementia, such afflicted individuals are at high risk of developing excess disability. Excess disability exists when "the magnitude of the disturbance is greater than what can be accounted for by physical or cerebral pathology" (Kahn, 1966). Wandering is of particular concern with in the context of excess disability. Excess disability can be acquired through preventable injury which is a possibility as a consequence of wandering. On the other hand, excess disability in the form of contracture can be induced by enforced immobility when increasing rigidity accompanies an illness as in the case of Alzheimer's disease.

One method of preventing and reversing excess disability is the systematic identification and promotion of existing abilities. The identification of remaining abilities has been the objective of an evolving assessment which I am currently using in my practice of individuals suffering from intellectual psychopathology. Through ability assessment the role of enhancement or compensation by nursing can be determined. This assessment is based on several studies and the combined experience of colleagues in nursing and other health disciplines. Three of the studies which have been used in the development of the assessment will be presented from the following perspectives: (1) their purpose, method and findings; (2) their potential relevance for clinical nursing decision making and action; and (3) the findings relevant to these studies through my assessment of twenty patients with intellectual psychopathology, nine of whom are considered wanderers and eleven who are non-wanderers. The first study examined a relationship between wandering behaviour and parietal signs in patients with Senile Dementia of the Alzheimer's type. While the overall intent of this study was of interest, it was the methods used which seemed to have potential for ability assessment and enhancement. In this study twenty-one patients, of whom five were wanderers, with a provisional diagnosis of Senile Dementia of the Alzheimer's type, were evaluated to test the hypothesis that: "Wandering in Alzheimer's disease may be particularly associated with parietal involvement" (de Leon et al., 1984). Each patient was tested on the Kahn-Goldfarb Mental Status Questionnaire and several parietal test which included matchstick construction, left-right orientation, finger writing (graphesthesia test), finger agnosia, tactile object identification, two point discrimination test and clock reading. Significant differences in the cumulative parietal test score were found between wanderers and non-wanderers. Since the Mental Status Questionnaires scores were not significantly different, it was concluded that wandering may be significantly associated with parietal lobe signs.

Although the sample size in this study was small, it contributes toward the need for greater understanding of the etiology of wandering behavior. In this study, the use of parietal test were for diagnostic purposes. However, some of these tests also had potential for the systematic assessment under discussion were those of left-right orientation, finger writing and tactile object discrimination.

In evaluating left-right orientation a patient is asked to identify the right and left hand, to touch the left ear and right eye with the right and left hand respectively, to touch the examiner's left and right hand, and to imitate the various positions of the examiner's hands and arms. The abilities elicited from the preceding include, (i) differentiation of left from right at simple self and other, and complex self levels; (i.e., to respond to directions using left or right, then left and right in combination and finally the left or right of an other person); (ii) comprehension of one and two-verbal instructions and of specific verbal cues such as the words right and left; (iii) attending and relating to another person and (iv) imitation skills. How can the identification of abilities such as these influence clinical practice? The presentation of the clinical relevance is at this stage experiential and speculative since it reflects an evolving approach to developing specific nursing approaches based on specific findings. They do require testing and evaluation in practice. Based on the study findings, the absence of these abilities suggests that some judgement can be made regarding the potential for wandering. However, the presence of left-right discrimination may indicate that cues for wandering such as turn right, turn left, can be used to guide the patient who wanders. The use of such verbal cues can also facilitate performance in activities of daily living. I recently found that a patient with a diagnosis of multi-infarct dementia was able to execute activities of daily living with much greater ease when cued with left-right verbal guidance. Comprehension can be facilitated through demonstration when imitation skills are present. Finally the ability to attend to another person may mean that contact with other on an individual or group basis is an approach which can be used to prevent the excess disability of withdrawal or social isolation. These suggestions are only a beginning in examining the clinical relevance of the abilities under discussion. However, I find that these suggestions are adding meaning in my clinical practice and in the practice of nurses with whom I work.

When left-right orientation skills are broken down into simple, complex and other for the twenty patients whose abilities I've assessed (see Table 1) greater difficulty is seen in combining left and right directions within a single instruction than with the single use of left or right instructions. The ability to attend to the left and right of another person at a single level is greater that combining left and right together. The more complex ability of combining is retained by fewer of the twenty patients. However, half of these patients can combine left and right and for them, excess disability can only be prevented by appealing to this level of ability. On the other hand, expectations of performance at this level for the remaining patients might reinforce feelings of loss and incompetency leading to withdrawal and agitation. Thus, individual assessment is necessary for the selection of caregiving approaches.

The graphesthesia test or finger writing was assessed in the following manner. With dull pencils, numbers were drawn on the index fingers of each hand and the patient was asked to close his eyes and identify the number. Again this was a test of parietal functioning and also assessed for fine tactile discrimination. This assessment method could again provide some basis for judging the potential of wandering. As well, it could provide some measure of the patient's ability to discern by touch and to manage fine motor activities. However, because of the aging process per se, the majority of patients were unable to demonstrate sufficient ability on this test to continue its use. Therefore, this component of the assessment has been omitted in further revisions of the assessment.

The third test which was incorporated into assessment of patients with intellectual psychopathology was that of tactile object discrimination. Rather than numbers, patients closed their eyes and identified small objects such as a key and elastic band through touch. Two coins are put into the hands and the patient identifies which hand holds the larger coin. In addition to assessing parietal functioning, this provides another method of assessing tactile ability and the extent to which touch can be used to facilitate activities of daily living. In other words, the use of objects such as a washcloth may provide tactile stimulation and evoke a life-long skill such as washing one's face. When these abilities are present, the patient may be able to engage in self care with greater ease when tactile cues are combined with verbal or object cues. The selection of appropriate cues for their specific use in ability enhancement can be based on some objective method of assessment.

Table 1.  Right-Left Orientation - Percent Ability

|         | Total Group (20) | Wanderers (9) | Non-Wanderers (11) |
|---------|------------------|---------------|---------------------|
| Simple  | 80               | 78            | 82                  |
| Complex | 50               | 56            | 45                  |
| Other   | 65               | 61.5          | 68.5                |

The response to these assessment methods by twenty patients with Intellectual psychopathology suggests that for some, these abilities are present (see Table 2). The ability to differentiate right from left, especially at a simple level is retained by the majority of these twenty patients. Imitation skills and the potential for demonstration also apply to a majority of these patients. Tactile object discrimination poses greater difficulty and will facilitate for fewer patients. The differential response of the patients who wander with those who do not wander is unexpected since it is inconsistent with findings of the study cited earlier. The patients who wander performed as effectively, or better, as those considered to be non-wanderers. Since these twenty patients are referred population and not a randomized or in any way controlled sample, it is inappropriate to draw conclusions. However, the level of ability retention of these patients on these measures is sufficient to support their continued evaluation in guiding nursing practice.

The second study entitled "The Challenge of Time: Clock Drawing and Cognitive Function in the Elderly", forms the basis of another component of the abilities assessment for patients with intellectual psychopathology. The investigators proposed the clock drawing may have clinical value as a sensitive indication of cerebral-organic dysfunction (Shulman et al., 1985). The subjects included seventy-five persons sixty-five years and older who were in-patients and outpatients at Sunnybrook Medical Centre. The patients were categorized according to the diagnoses of Organic Mental Disorders or Major Affective Disorders, and compared with a group considered to be "normal". The standardized clock test employed was simply asking the patient to draw a clock face which would indicate three o'clock on a pre-drawn circle. Other measures included the Mini-Mental State Exam (MMSE) (Folstein et al., 1975), the short Mental Status Questionnaire (SMSQ) (Robertson et al., 1982), and the Geriatric Depression Rating Scale (GDR) (Yesavage et al., 1983). It was found that five levels of clock drawing error scores correlated significantly with scores on the Mini-Mental State Exam and the shore Mental Status Questionnaire. However, no significant correlation between the Geriatric Depression Scale and scores on the Mental Status Questionnaire or the Clock drawing test emerged. The investigators concluded that clock drawing was useful as an adjunctive screening instrument for cognitive dysfunction which is free of cultural and educational bias.

This study is of interest in light of the frequently recommended practice of relating information such as time to help orient patients with intellectual psychopathology. If such information exceeds the ability level of the patient, then it can be incompetency reinforcing and overburdening to the patient. Therefore, consideration must be given to each individual patient's ability to relate to time. In the ability assessment, patients are asked to read time and also to draw a clock face on a circle. This provides a basis to determine the extent to which the patient is able to relate to time. The ability of the patient to write and sequence numbers is also examined and the spacial distribution of numbers may suggest areas where compensation by caregivers is required. Assessment of the ability to relate to time is useful in clinical practice to determine the extent to which time and numbers can facilitate competency and orientation. If time telling ability persists, time frames can be used to provide a structure for the patient's day. However, if such an ability is not present more general time markers such as morning, afternoon or mealtimes may be of value. This information will also indicate whether numbers can be useful in orienting someone to place or whether an alternative, such as symbols, would be more appropriate. One patient, who has not been able to find his room for a number of years, was assisted to locate his room by placing a red circle as a symbol outside the door of his room. He was able to learn the association between the red circle and the location of his room when symbols were used

Table 2. Percent Abilities of 20 Patients with
Cognitive Psychopathology in Parietal
Test Performance

|  | Total Group (20) | Wanderers (9) | Non-Wanderers (11) |
|---|---|---|---|
| Right-Left orientation | 64 | 65 | 63 |
| Imitation skills | 69 | 80 | 60 |
| Tactile Object Discrimination | 47 | 46 | 27 |
| Total Parietal | 58 | 64 | 52 |

rather than numbers. If the spacial distribution of numbers is to one side there may be neglect or interruption of the visual field. In such a case attention to the arrangement of the environment to enhance the patient's abilities is proving to be useful. Finally the occasional patient who demonstrates spacial orientation through the arrangement of numbers on the clock face has been able to spend diversional time attempting to do jigsaw puzzles. These suggestions for care continue to speculative and based on limited experience. However, the discernment of the abilities suggested by examining the use of time by patients enables nurses to select interventions more specifically. May interventions are suggested in the literature but rationale to support the selection of caregiving approaches tends to be general rather than based on specific assessment findings.

To what extent would time information assist the twenty patients? As shown in Table 3, the ability to tell time is retained by less than half of this group. Clock reading was one of the measures of parietal functioning used in the first study and as with the previous parietal tests, the patients who wander retain a greater level of ability than those who do not wander. Because time telling ability is retained by some and not by others in this group of patients, the use of time for orientation and structure in the context of clinical practice would vary depending on the assessment findings of each patient.

The third study which has influenced the development of the abilities assessment is part of a larger study examining the differential diagnosis of Alzheimers disease. This is a three year prospective, longitudinal study which is being conducted at Sunnybrook Medical Centre (Tierney et al., 1983). The three-hundred and sixty subjects in the study are in-patients, out-patients and older volunteers living in the community. The purpose of this study is validate current approaches in the differential diagnosis of Alzheimer's disease and to follow the progress of the disease for a period of three years. Subjects in this study have been classified into the following diagnostic categories which are: 1) demented non-Alzheimer, 2) combined dementia, 3) non-demented, 4) Alzheimer (pure) and 5) neurologically normal. This multi-disciplinary study employs a wide battery of measures. This discussion will focus on one component of the study which related to the findings regarding primitive reflexes. In Table 4, differences are shown in the incidence of the primitive reflexes between the diagnostic categories and in particular, the incidence of the suck and grasp reflexes between those with Alzheimers disease and dementia and those without such diagnoses. Consequently a further ability for assessment is

Table 3. Percent of Patients Able to Read Time

| Total Group (20) | Wanderers (9) | Non-Wanderers (11) |
|---|---|---|
| 40% | 55.5% | 27% |

that of active and passive extension of the fingers. Passive extension of the fingers is comprised when the grasp reflex is present. The grasp reflex is considered positive when having instructed the patient to relax, stimulation of the palmar surface of the patient's pronated hand causes fingers flexion and grasping of the examiner's finger (Robertson et al.,1981). The purpose of assessment then is to determine if palmer stimulation produces flexion. When the grasp reflex is present, staff may interpret a patient's tendency to grasp and hold on to objects as resistance or aggression when in fact it is simply a neurological response. Therefore, in recognizing its presence, measures can be taken to avoid stimulating it during care. For example, hands can be washed at the end of the bath rather than at the beginning of the bath. It can also be stimulated to help the patient initiate feeding activities.

A positive suck reflex is not an ability, but if it is present, it can have implications for nursing care. The suck reflex is elicited by stroking the lips with the curved tip of a tongue blade or a flexed joint of the index finger (Tweedy et al., 1982). If the lips close around the object, the reflex is present. This is to determine the response of the patient to light pressure along the lips. If it is present and eliciting the cooperation of the patient with fluid intake of fluid, a straw will stimulate this response and facilitate the intake of fluid. Recently we were able to reduce the incidence of shouting in a noisy patient by stimulating the suck reflex and providing lady fingers. However, the effect of the intervention lasted only as long as the lady finger and we had to balance the prospect of considerable weight gain with noisiness. We have also found that some patients who become agitated with the stimulation of the bath will remain calm if given a biscuit or cookie to suck during this period. When a positive suck reflex is seen, one also realizes that objects which could be brought to the mouth by the patient need to be edible and safe.

A third neurological response which has relevance for caregiving is that of the Gegenhalten response. In the study cited, the incidence of a positive Gegenhalten response is significantly greater with those who have Alzheimer's disease and dementia as compared with those who do not. It is positive when resistance is felt to attempts to extend the arm and so the ability of passive extension of the arms is compromised. It is assessed by simply extending the arm to see if flexion is stimulated (Pryse and Murray, 1978). If it is present, one can avoid stimulating it during care. The extremities can be bathed after the trunk. Articles of clothing are more easily put on the patient when the patient is standing and the arms are in extension.

The incidence of positive neurological responses is fairly low in the population of twenty patients which have been assessed with the abilities assessment (see Table 5). However, for caregiving purposes the fact that they exist at all requires their inclusion in an assessment of patients suffering from Alzheimer's disease and dementia. We have found that by adjusting caregiving approaches when these responses are present, that it is facilitative for both the patient and the care caregiver.

Table 4.  Diagnosis and primitive Reflexes (Chi Square)

| | Normal | Alzheimer | Combined Dementia | Dementia | Non-Demented |
|---|---|---|---|---|---|
| Palmomental 24.23 | 10 | 31 | 31 | 39 | 17*** |
| Suck 2.84 | 0 | 4 | 7 | 5 | 0* |
| (R)(L) Grasp 7.99 | 0 | 14 | 16 | 16 | 0*** |
| Pout 49.48 | 21 | 69 | 72 | 69 | 32*** |
| Glabellar | 6 | 44 | 66 | 55 | 20*** |

*    p = 0.05                              (Tierney et al., 1986)
***  p = 0.0001

The three studies under discussion have had relevance for nursing decision making and caregiving.  The purpose of each study is different than the purpose for which they have been used in practice.  For the most part it has been the methods rather than the findings which have had the greater relevance to the assessment.  However, the findings have provided the rationale for inclusion in the assessment.  It has only been recently that I have been searching the literature with this intent and am finding greater clarification and direction in my clinical practice.

The preceding has served to illustrate how research can influence practice.  However, clinical practice guides research.  The example which will be discussed today is the phenomena of wandering which is often observed in patients with diagnoses such as Alzheimer's disease and dementia.  Patients demonstrating wandering behaviours pose caregiving, ethical and legal dilemmas for caregivers and health professional.  As was stated earlier, excess disability can result from over protection as well as from under protection of such patients.  Until recently the subject of wandering has had limited attention in the literature.  We conducted a study in the attempt to gain understanding of the phenomena of wandering behaviour (Dawson and Reid, 1986).  Previous studies had differentiated character- istics of wanderers and non-wanderers but the variables or characteristics within these studies have been pre-determined.  We questioned that these behaviours or variables represented the totality of behaviours which might be related to the phenomena of wandering.  Therefore, we undertook a descriptive study to look at the characteristics which described what we consider to be a vulnerable population of patients at Sunnybrook Medical Centre.  It is a practice at Sunnybrook Medical Centre to photograph patients who may be at risk for harm due to frailty, wandering or unpredict- able behavior.  This was the population defined as vulnerable.  From this population we hoped to assess if there were characteristics that were more specific in describing or identifying the patient who wanders.

The purposes of the study were: 1) to identify specific features nursing staff found to be characteristic of patients at "risk for harm", 2) to analyze data to identify the basic factors to describe the above population, and 3) to test the ability of these factors to differentiate wanderers and non-wanderers.  One hundred patients in the Department of Extended Care had photographs on their chart at that time.  A short list of potential descriptors was developed and the head nurses on eight units and primary nurses on one unit were interviewed about each patient.  The interview began by asking whether or not these descriptors applied to the patient under discussion and then further descriptors, specific to each patient, were sought from the interviewee.  The interviews were repeated with the nurses on all patients until each patient had been rated on all descriptors. We ultimately found fifty-seven descriptors which had been used in relation to these patients.

Each patient was classified as a wanderer, wanderer-improve, (wandering had declined or was less or a problem ), and non-wanderers. Wandering was defined as frequent and/or unpredictable pacing with no discerning or achievable goals.

When all the information was collected on all the patients, a two-stage statistical analysis was done to determine: 1) the characteristics of the overall population and 2) the ability of these characteristics to differentiate wanderers and non-wanderers. Descriptors identifying less than 15% of the population were dropped and twenty-five behaviours were analyzed. From the factor analysis, three factors or clusters of behaviours emerged to identify the populations of one hundred patients. These were cognitive deficits, agitation/aggression and hyperactivity. The descriptors within each factor were as follows: 1) cognitive deficits - constant disorientation; 2) agitation/aggression - sleep disturbances, agitation, aggression, strong, shouts, angry; 3) hyperactivity - not withdrawn, hearing normal, a good gait, perpetual motion, and socially skilled. The factor sub-scores were compared between wanderers and non-wanderers. Wanderers who had improved and wanderers were analyzed together since initial analysis showed no differences between these two groups. Differences were found between wanderers and non-wanderers on the two factors of cognitive deficits and hyperactivity. Correlations were found between these factors and risk items on which each patient had been rated during the interviews.

From this study a profile of wanderers was developed. Wanderers were described as having difficulties with speech, reading and incontinence. They had constant rather than transitory disorientation and an inability to discern when they were lost. On the other hand they were more socially skilled, had better hearing, were less withdrawn and were more mobile in that they had a good gait and were perpetually active. It seemed that patients who wandered had cognitive impairment sufficient to become lost, but appear socially skilled.

The use of these findings in practice could only be speculative at this point. However, the descriptors and factors which identified wanderers who were at high risk for harm could form the basis for an assessment instrument and assist in management decisions. For example shirts and sweaters which are specially marked are provided to those patients in our population judged to be at risk of harm from wandering. From this data one could speculate on interventions which may be effective if directed at the behaviours associated with wandering. For example, the factor of cognitive deficits could provide a basis on which to develop some group work to divert the interest and attention of the wanderer at the level of their capability. The descriptors also could be used to form a basis for intervention,. For example, there has been no determination made of the influence of incontinence as a stimulus to wandering. Perhaps attention to incontinence care may influence the incidence of wandering.

Shortly we will be undertaking further study which evolves from the findings presented here and in this study prospective longitudinal research will be done to test the predictive validity of the descriptors and to further refine the instrument. For instance, we believe there would be value in developing another factor based on the findings of the Monsour and Robb (1982) study which assessed the influence of past behaviours and coping styles on the phenomenon of wandering. The relationship between wandering behaviour and environmental factors will also be undertaken in this study.

256

Table 5.  Percent Incidence of Neurological Responses
in 20 Patients with Cognitive Psychopathology

| | Total Group (20) | Wanderers (9) | Non-Wanderers (11) |
|---|---|---|---|
| Grasp Reflex | 15 | 11 | 18 |
| Suck Reflex | 20 | 11 | 27 |
| Gegenhalten | 22.5 | 22 | 23 |

It is our hope that the findings of this next study will further enable caregivers to formulate approached to the phenomena of wandering which ultimately will result in avoidance of the excess disability from either the extreme of over protection or under protection of this vulnerable group of patients.

Although the influence of research on practice and practice on research as reflected in my practice is only at an initial phase, it is providing a process and frame work upon which ongoing work will proceed.  The caregiving implications relative to the phenomenon of wandering continues to be elusive.  Research based practice is providing more information about caregiving for patients with Alzheimer's disease and dementia rather than for patients who wander.  Perhaps through a dual approach of systematic practice and research, further hypotheses relevant to the caregiving of patients who wander can be developed and evaluated.  At its current stage, this approach is demonstrating for me a persistence of ability retention in spite of intellectual psychopathology and the potential of ability assessment in guiding nursing practice intended to prevent excess disability.  Through this inter-relationship of research and practice, I believe nursing can acquire and then teach knowledge and skill to caregivers so that the intent of care for patients with Alzheimer's disease and dementia is therapeutic.

REFERENCES

Brody, E.M., Kleban, M.H., Lawton, M.P., and Silverman, H.A., 1971, Excess disability of mentally impaired aged:  Impact of individualized treatment, The Gerontologist, 2:124.
Brody, E.M., Kleban, M.H., Lawton, M.P., and Moss, M., 1974, A longitudual look at excess disabilities in the mentally impaired aged, Journal of Gerontology, 29:79-84.
Dawson, P. and Reid, D.W., 1986, Behavioural dimensions of patients at risk of wandering, The Gerontologist, (in press).
deLeon, M.J., Potegal, M., Gurland, B, 1984, Wandering and parietal signs in senile dementia of alzheimers type, Neuropsychobiology, 11:155-157.
Folstein, M.F., Folstein, S.E., and McHugh, P.R., 1975, Mini-mental state:  A practice guide for grading the cognitive state of patients of the clinician, Journal of Psychiatric Research, 12:189-198.
Kahn, R.L., 1966, Mental impairment in the aged, in:  "Philadelphia Geriatric Centre," M.P. Lawton and F.G. Lawton, eds., Philadelphia.
Monsour, and Robb S.S., 1982, Wandering behaviour in old age:  A psycho-social study," Social Work, 3:411-416.
Pryse, P.W., and Murray, T.J., 1978, "Essential Neurology," Medical Examination Publishing Co. Inc., Garden City, N.Y.
Robertson, D., Rockwood, D., and Christ, L., 1981, Abnormal reflexes in dementia, in:  "XII International Congress of Gerontology," Hamburg, Germany.

Robertson, D., Rockwood, K., and Stolee, P., 1982, A short mental status questionnaire, Canadian Journal on Aging, 1:16-20.

Shulman, K.I., Shedletsky, R., and Silver, J.L., 1985, The Challenge of time: Clock drawing as a cognitive screen in the elderly, in: XIIIth International Congress of Gerontology," New York, N.Y.

Tierney, M.C., 1983, The differential diagnoses of Alzheimer's disease: Clinical features and their assessment, in: "Alzheimer's Disease: Psychologist's contribution to research and treatment," Canadian Psychological Association, Winnipeg, Manitoba.

Tweedy, J., Reding, M., Garcia, C., Shulman, P., Deutch, G.L., and Antin, S. 1982, Significance of cortical disinhibition signs, Neurology, 32:169-73.

Yesavage, J.A., Bink, T.L., Rose, T.L., Lum, O., Huang, V., Adey, M., and Leiner, V.O., 1982, Development and validation of a geriatric depression screening scale: A Preliminary report, Clinical Gerontologist, 1:37-49.

SLEEP AND DEMENTIA: NURSING CARE CONSIDERATIONS

Judith A. Floyd

Wayne State University
Detroit, Michigan

The sleep-wake process is a basic component of human experience.
When a person's life is altered by social or emotional upheaval or by
physical illness, the quality and quantity of both sleep and waking
undergo change. We know that sleep-wake patterns also undergo change
as the individual grows older. When growing older coincides with an
illness such as Alzheimer's Disease the changes in sleep-wake patterns
become more exaggerated.

Our current understanding of sleep-wake patterns was greatly
enhanced when the electroencephalographic techniques developed by
Berger (1929) were applied to the study of sleep. Early researchers
were able to classify five types of electrical activity which they
labeled A through E. Using this classification system, sleep of any
night could be categorized and the rhythmicity of sleep could be
described in terms of the frequency and duration of each stage.

A major breakthrough occurred in the early 1950's when Aserinsky
and Kleitman discovered rapid eye movement sleep. This discovery led
to the numerical classification of stages of sleep: In stages 1, 2, 3,
and 4, there were no eye movements or only very slow ones. These were
referred to collectively as Non-Rapid Eye Movement, or NREM sleep. A
fifth stage was called Rapid Eye Movement, or REM, sleep (Dement &
Kleitman, 1957).

In the 1960's research in sleep laboratories began in earnest with
the describing of sleep stages and the regularity of changes throughout
a typical night. It is now known that as an average adult person falls
asleep, the brain waves go through certain characteristic changes. The
waking electroencephalogram (EEG) is characterized by alpha waves (8-12
cycles-per-second) and low voltage activity of mixed frequency. As the
person falls asleep, there is a disappearance of alpha activity. Stage
1, the lightest stage of sleep, is characterized by low-voltage,
desynchronized activity and sometimes by low-voltage, regular, 4-6
cycle-per-second activity as well. After a few minutes, or sometimes
only seconds, this gives way to Stage 2, a pattern showing frequent,
13-15 cycle-per-second spindle-shaped tracings known as sleep spindles,
and by some high-voltage spikes known as K-complexes. In a few more
minutes delta waves, high voltage activity at 0.5 to 2-cycles-per
second, occur (Stage 3). Eventually these large slow waves occupy the
major part of the encephalograph and the sleep is termed Stage 4.

Sleep is cyclical throughout the night with four or five periods of emergence from Stages 2, 3, and 4 to the REM stage. The first REM period occurs about 90 to 100 minutes after the onset of sleep. The lengths of the REM periods increase during the typical night. The first REM period tends to be the shortest, often lasting only five or six minutes. The later REM periods may last 20 to 40 minutes. Most REM time occurs in the last third of the night, while most Stages 3 and 4 sleep, also called delta sleep, occur in the first third. The total time taken up by REM periods during a typical night is about 20 percent of the total sleep time (Cartwright, 1978).

NREM sleep can be organized according to depth: Stage 1 is the lightest and Stage 4 the deepest stage. Depth is manifest by arousal threshold measures, as well as by appearance of the EEG. However, REM sleep does not fit into this continuum. During REM sleep the arousal threshold is higher than in NREM sleep, and the resting muscle potential is lower. Thus, REM sleep is neither light sleep nor deep sleep but a different kind of sleep (Hartmann, 1979).

SLEEP AND AGING

In recent years the focus of sleep research has been influenced by an increased national interest on research in aging. Studies of the sleep-wake patterns in the elderly have revealed a number of changes that occur with aging. The elderly spend an increased amount of time in bed at night, awaken more frequently during the night, and have a shorter total sleep time at night than younger persons. Of equal importance, the elderly nap more often during the day (Roehrs, Zorick & Roth, 1984).

Changes in sleep associated with the aging process have been documented by continuous recording of various physiological parameters throughout the night. These parameters include the electromyogram (EMG) from the submental muscle, and the electrooculogram (EOG) as well as the electroencephalogram (EEG). The characteristics of these recordings are used to score each 30 seconds of time as either awake, or one of the four NREM stages of sleep, or as REM sleep (Hauri, 1982).

One of the pervasive signs of aging is decrease in delta EEG activity, which defines Stages 3 and 4, or deep sleep. In addition, Stage 1, or light sleep, tends to increase in the elderly. Absolute amounts of REM sleep decrease slightly, but relative to total sleep amounts the percentage of REM remains constant for the healthy elderly. Also, more and longer episodes of waking occur during the night. Thus, the nighttime sleep of the elderly is shorter, lighter, and more disrupted than that of younger people (Roehrs et al, 1984).

Other research has shown that the quality and quantity of night-time sleep are directly related to one's ability to maintain alertness when awake. People usually want to be alert with a low tendency to fall asleep throughout the day. Using sleep-laboratory techniques, it is possible to precisely measure the daytime tendency to fall asleep. The Multiple Sleep Latency Test (MSLT) involves recording the time it takes to fall asleep repeatedly throughout the day. The test is given for 20 minutes every two hours. Prepubescent adolescents, who typically sleep more than 9 hours at night, remain awake for each 20-minute nap opportunity throughout the day. Normal adults sleeping seven to eight hours at night fall asleep during the day on the average between 12 and 15 minutes, with a small increase in sleepiness at midafternoon.

It has been found that sleepiness increases when the normal adult's nighttime sleep length is held constant but the sleep is interrupted by brief arousals (Carskadon & Dement, 1981).

The elderly person who is reasonably healthy has been found to be more sleepy during the day than normal younger adults and adolescents. Often the elderly person is not aware of this and does not complain about it. This increased daytime sleepiness is believed to be directly related to the naturally occurring fragmentation of their nighttime sleep. It appears the fragmentation of sleep in the elderly results from the increase in light sleep. It is influenced by internal events such as arthritic pain or the urge to urinate, and external events such as noise or a cold room (Roehrs et al, 1984).

SLEEP AND ALZHEIMER'S DISEASE

Research on Alzheimer's Disease indicates that patients' sleep deteriorate as they loose cognitive abilities (Prinz, Perskind, & Vitaliano, 1982). Although it is now fairly clear that Alzheimer's Disease is not an acceleration of normal brain aging, many of the changes found in sleep of Alzheimer's patients can be viewed as exaggerations of the normal aging of sleep (Wagner, 1984). For instance, the Alzheimer's patient's sleep shows reduction of Stages 3 and 4 sleep early in the course of the disease. Late in Alzheimer's Disease, Stages 3 and 4 sleep disappear completely. As happens in normal aging, the sleep spindles of Stage 2 sleep diminish in Alzheimer's Disease. Unlike healthy elderly, however, the sleep spindles eventually disappear entirely as Alzheimer's Disease progresses. Also, there is a marked increase in sleep interruptions and stage changes in Alzheimer's Disease patients. Finally, REM sleep, which normally continues to occupy 20% of the night in reasonably healthy elderly, gradually decreases during the course of Alzheimer's Disease although it does not disappear completely (Lowenstein, Weingartner & Gillin, 1982; Prinz et al, 1982).

As might be expected from the research on the relationship between fragmented nighttime sleep and daytime sleepiness, Alzheimer's Disease patients frequently begin dozing during daytime hours. This daytime napping often accompanies increased waking with attendant wandering, confusion, and agitation in the evening and at night. Thus, as nighttime sleep deteriorates progressively in Alzheimer's Disease, so does the ability to maintain wakefulness (Wagner, 1984).

Data from a case study of an 86 year old man with Alzheimer's Disease reported by Wagner (1984) serves as an example of changes in the sleep-wake pattern of the Alzheimer's Disease patient. The patient was studied in a sleep laboratory that had been designed to eliminate the usual environmental cues to time of day. The subject's sleep consisted only of Stages 1 and REM, and was extremely fragmented. The longest period of uninterrupted sleep lasted just one-half hour. Numerous 10 to 60 minute episodes of dozing occurred, and the sleep was scattered across the 24 hour day. Slightly more sleep was present during the 12 hours between noon and midnight than the other 12 hours of the 24 hour period. Because of the frequent dozing and awakening the overall result was a sleep-wake pattern with numerous sleep-wake cycles per 24-hour period. Despite these numerous cycles there were two 3-hour periods each day during which the subject never chose to begin sleep. A similar phenomenon has been noted in healthy adults (Strogatz & Kronauer, 1985).

THE RHYTHM PERSPECTIVE

Paralleling the development of sleep research has been research on human rhythms. The variety of rhythmic phenomena studied in humans includes very short rhythms such as brain waves or heart rhythms, as well as very long rhythms such as the life-span cycle. Between these two extremes are rhythms of varying lengths such as the daily rhythms of body temperature, urinary output, and sleep, the monthly menstrual cycle, and the childbearing year.

A rhythm is sometimes described as wholly dependent upon some external periodicity such as an environmental cue or a habit. When a rhythm is thought to be dependent upon an external periodicity, it is described as exogenous. If, on the other hand, the oscillation continues in the absence of external rhythms, it is considered to originate within the living system and is referred to as endogenous. If an environmental rhythm is thought to influence or entrain the rhythms of living systems, it is called a "zeitgeber," a German term which means time-giver. When a zeitgeber is suspended, an endogenous rhythm may continue but show some alteration in frequency. The rhythm is then said to be free-running.

Most of the literature on human sleep-wake patterns describe sleeping and waking as an endogenous rhythm for which the 24-hour rhythm of terrestrial rotation serves as a zeitgeber. This view is supported by empirical evidence of the sleep-wake rhythm becoming free-running in the absence of environmental cues regarding the time of day (Control & Mills, 1970).

A central focus in the study of rhythmic phenomena in humans has been the question of their origin. Is the observed behavioral rhythm generated by the organism itself and then synchronized with the environmental periodicity at a particular phase, or is it the external rhythm which causes the periodicity in the organism directly? There is still considerable debate about these alternatives with some theorists continuing to seek support for each of the positions (Floyd, 1982).

Within nursing the theorist who has discussed rhythmic phenomena most directly is Rogers (1970, 1980). According to Rogers, rhythmicity is a concomitant of life and its environment. Rhythmic phenomena are viewed as expressions of the complementary relationship between human beings and their environment. Rogers conceptual system postulates that rhythmic patterning develops in the direction of increasing complexity and diversity of rhythmic patterns and toward rhythms with increasing frequency. Furthermore, changes in human beings rhythmic patterning are postulated to occur more rapidly in response to disruptions. According to Rogers, the increasing frequency of cycles may become so rapid that the rhythm appears continuous.

A number of specific predictions influenced by Rogers conceptual system regarding the evolution of sleep-wake rhythms have been identified (Floyd, 1983). Essentially, the predictions describe ways in which rhythmic patterns such as the sleep-wake pattern could manifest the increasing complexity and diversity described by Rogers (1970). A prediction that appears to be supported by the changes observed in the sleep-wake pattern of older people including those with Alzheimer's Disease is the increase in the number of sleep-wake cycles per unit of time. In the case of the Alzheimer's patient, the frequency of the sleep-wake cycles may increase to the point where the rhythm appears continuous.

## IMPLICATIONS OF INTERVENTION

The rhythm perspective may have implications for working with Alzheimer's patients and their families. It has been reported by Sanford (1975) that primary caregivers of the cognitively disabled find that night wandering and agitation are among the least tolerated of the symptoms that such caregivers must handle. The use of major tranquilizers is the usual treatment. Prinz and Raskind (1970) found that these medications appear to work well initially in the majority of patients. However, this approach is not effective with all Alzheimer's patients and even when beneficial, the use of these medications involves a number of adverse side effects including: over sedation, increased confusion, paradoxical agitation, ataxia, and parkinsonian-type stiffness.

Temporal pattering is another approach to the management of nighttime agitation and confusion. It is suggested by the rhythm perspective. If nighttime agitation and confusion are manifestations of abnormal sleep-wake cycling in Alzheimer's Disease, it may be possible to intervene by temporal pattering, e.g., by planned enhancement of the synchronizing power of the zeitgebers in the patient's environment. Such an approach would involve an individualized but consistent scheduling of nighttime sleep hours, daytime naps, daytime (or if necessary, nighttime) activity periods, and mealtimes.

To attempt temporal pattering in the home, it is recommended that baseline data be collected to determine the 24 hour patters of the individual. Attempts can then be made to reinforce the temporal structure if it is a workable pattern or to influence it if changes are needed. Zeitgebers that have been found to influence sleep-wake patterns including environmental rhythms such as the light-dark cycle, the food-intake cycle, and the rest-activity cycle. Therefore, these are the zeitgebers in the physical environment which may be influential. It is important to identify psycho-social cues that also may serve to structure time. Since even healthy individuals differ in terms of how they organize their sleep-wake pattern with respect to environmental cues, a highly individualized approach will be necessary in clinical practice.

For each Alzheimer's patient there may be periods of time when the initiation of sleep is highly unlikely. If the timing of these periods can be identified it may be easier for caregivers to cope with them although the hope is that the timing and nature of these periods can be influenced by manipulation of environmental cues.

Wagner (1984) reported that one nursing home has used a consistent scheduling approach and has found that many patients can do with little or no medication. No reports of the effect of counselling families to try temporal pattering in the home has been published. Thus, nothing specific is known about the realities of instituting such an approach. However, the difficulties encountered in carrying out such an program in the home may be preferable to the agonizing decision to institutionalize a loved on who is disrupting the family's sleep.

Much has been learned in the past few decades about the rhythmicity of sleep and how it develops with aging. This knowledge is basic to understanding the sleep disturbance experienced by the Alzheimer's patient. It also may be basic to discovering interventions that assist the Alzheimer's patient and his caregivers.

REFERENCES

Berger, H., 1929, Uber des elekrenkephalogramm des menschen, Archives of Psychiatry, 87: 527-570.
Carskadon, M., and Dement, W.C., 1981, Respiration and sleep in the aged human, Sleep, 2: 527-570.
Cartwright, R.D. 1978, "Primer on Sleep and Sleeping," Addison-Wesley, Reading, Massachusetts.
Conroy, R.T., and Mills, J.N., 1970, "Human circadian rhythms," J and A Churchill, London.
Dement, W.C. and Kleitman, N., 1957, Cyclic variations in EEG during sleep and their relation to eye movements, bodily motility, and external stimuli to dream content, Electroencephalography and Clinical Neurophysiology, 9: 673-690.
Floyd, J.A., 1982, Rhythm theory: Relationship to nursing conceptual models, in: "Nursing models and their psychiatric mental health applications," Fitzpatrick, ed., Robert J. Brady Co., Bowie, MD.
Floyd, M.A., 1983, Research using Rogers' conceptual system: Development of a testable theorem, Advances in Nursing Science, 5: 37-48.
Hartmann, E.L., 1979, What we know about sleep, Medical Times, 107: 1d-19d.
Hauri, P.O., 1982, "The Sleep Disorders," Upjohn Company, Kalamazoo, MI.
Lowenstein, R.J., Weingartner, H., and Gillin, D.C., 1982. Disturbances in sleep and cognitive functioning in patients with dementia. Neurobiology and of Aging, 3: 371-377.
Prinz, P.N., and Raskind, M., 1978, Aging and sleep disorders, in: "Sleep disorders-diagnosis and treatment," L. Williams and I. Karacan, eds., John Wiley and Sons, New York.
Prinz, P.N., Perskind, E.R., and Vitalinao, P.O., 1982, Changes in the sleep and waking EEG's of nondemented and demented elderly subjects, Journal of the American Geriatric Society, 30: 86-93.
Roehrs, T., Zorick, F., and Roth, T., 1984, Sleep disorders in the elderly, Geriatric Medicine Today, 3: 76-86.
Rogers, M.E., 1970, "An introduction to the theoretical basis of nursing," F.A. Davis, Philadelphia.
Rogers, M.E., 1980, Nursing: A science of unitary man, in: "Conceptual models for nursing practice," J. Riehl and C. Roy, eds., Appleton-Century Crofts, New York.
Strogatz, S.H., and Kronauer, R.E., 1985, Circadian Wake-maintenance zones and insomnia in man, Sleep Research, 14: 219-229.
Wagner, D.R., 1984, Sleep, Generations, 9: 31-37.

NURSING CARE OF THE HUMAN WITH COGNITIVE LOSS

Mary Opal Wolanin

Associate Professor, Emeritus, University of Arizona
Tucson, Arizona    85721

I have always believed that what we call something determines our
attitude toward it.  Perhaps a rose by any other name would smell as sweet,
but when we refer to something as rose-like we add the softness of velvety
petals and dewy fragrance of early morning and an illusion of beauty.  For
this reason I have deplored our use of the word patient in referring to the
human being who must adapt to a new life with diminished cognitive
resources.  I believe that by emphasizing his humanity we stress the
positive aspects in him, and think in terms of assets rather than
liabilities.  When we speak of dementia we are forgetting the person and
emphasizing the pathology.  When I hear someone refer to the Alzheimer's
patient I cringe, for I realize that for the speaker, the humanity no longer
exists, only the disease.  This is the reason for the title being distorted.
It is my own concept of how as nurses we should view the problem we face.

For the caregiver this is doubly important.  Most of us have been
disease- or system-oriented in our educational backgrounds, and in practice
in our huge institutions, we tend to depersonalize.  If ever a person needs
to maintain his personhood, it is the human being whose cognitive function
is diminishing, leaving him bewildered and frightened in a world he can no
longer understand or deal with.  Depersonalization is found everywhere--if
you do not have your correct number--matriculation, registration, license,
social security, telephone or bank account--you may not exist.  I find
myself replaced by little plastic cards which have a number on them that is
now assuming the role of my identity, leaving me wondering who and what I
am.  For the older person with cognitive loss and problems in processing
information, there is a constant need to relate to a better and earlier
life--his history as a person.

I am making a big point of all this because I want to bring out how
hard the care of the human with cognitive changes is to face, as one human
being facing and interacting with another.  As human beings, and nurses,
(but apply this to any service provider) we have a need for our own stable
world.  We have lived in a culture that arouses certain expectations in
relationships.  Even one as transitory as the one with a parking lot
attendant has certain rules and expectancies about it.  He will indicate
where we should park--give information, and a ticket at the least.  And he
will likely thank us for our patronage, and we will thank him for his
courtesy.  Then we will smile and nothing more is expected unless we pay

at that time.  A parking attendant in Kalamazoo, Michigan, or one in Seattle will probably react much the same as one here.  We base our dependable world upon every one having learned and remembered the rules and expectations and following them.  When someone forgets, it surprises us, and if we cannot account for it, we are troubled by the event.  We pass on to other things but the memory of the unexpected haunts us.

When we care for the person with cognitive loss, we are frequently faced with a human being who does not remember his proper responses to our half of the interaction.  We are bewildered.  We are uncertain, and as human beings we do not handle uncertainty well.  It is easy to pretend the encounter does not exist and to treat the human being with his ambiguous reaction as a non-human, for the person who cannot remember what we expect and need him to remember becomes an ambiguous human being.  We cannot tolerate ambiguity.  Preston in his book The Dilemmas of Care (1979) points out that the disabled, the deformed and the aged all represent ambiguity to us-- deviations for our expected normal.  For most people with cognitive loss, there may be a fourth cause of ambiguity--the person who does not respond as we expect.  For some of us older people this means that we will represent ambiguity on four levels, disability, disfigurement (many of us aren't our beautiful youthful selves), aging and inability to process information.  This is to explain why we have the tendency to avoid the human with cognitive loss--he interferes with our dependable world.

Theoretically, explaining something makes all our attitudes change--I am not sure this is the case.  It does make it easier to care for the older person whose memory is decreasing, and whose ability to function is being lost as a result, if we know why we react as we do.  This is a truism I want to leave at this point--it was best said by Cassius in Shakespeare's Julius Ceasar, "The fault, dear Brutus, is not in our stars, but in ourselves, that we are underlings."  We too, are human beings, and unfortunately we bring to our work the meanings of our culture.  The word dementia and the Alzheimer's are burdened with a freight of unpleasant meanings for us--frightening even; so much so, that we have forgotten the quintessential human being and focused on the ambiguity.  Finally, I have tried to show that it is our own reaction that sets up the barriers--that puts distance between ourselves and this ambiguous person in order to protect ourselves from encounter.  Until we face the facts, we, as personnel who are the service-givers, cannot take information and use it.  We have to climb our own barriers and recognize this person for what he is--an older person who is suffering cognitive loss, who cannot process the information that our world is so full of.

I prefer cognitive loss.  The word cognition is not so freely used as many others we use in describing the forgetfulness of the person with dementia.  It isn't a household word, so I would like to share meaning with you that I have been able to use in planning this paper.  If the cognitive processes were a system such as the gastro-intestinal tract which gives forth hunger pangs when the stomach is empty, which cramps when the gut is in distress, that locks up with constipation, or pours forth diarrhea when abused--or which talks to us in terms of nausea, or vomiting, or indigestion or gas--we would know a lot more about it, and probably have little home remedies.  If it were a bone--the size of a femur, which showed a fracture on X-ray, and pain on movement, we would be concerned, and not only that, but we would insure freedom from movement by splinting, relief from weight bearing, etc.  But memory seems to be composed of far subtler chemicals than calcium and phosphorus, and the fracture is not visible by simple tests such as X-ray.  So the ambiguity.  Do me the favor of thinking of the processes underlying memory or cognition as a bone and the person with cognitive loss as one whose bone integrity has been compromised.  Now, we need an emergency room, a radiologist, an orthopedic surgeon, pins, casts--the whole bit.

Do we have such treatment for the human being whose memory is not functioning? I know we have no magic bullets, no memory transplants, no Jarvik 7 to
implant. What do we have? I contend that at this time, we have human
beings functioning in the helping role as caregivers. They include us. But
not if we are afraid of these "non-humans," or if we cannot face their
ambiguity. This point has been well belabored.

So we start with a constant--a human being--who has the same basic
needs from birth to death--oxygen, fluid, nutrition, communication,
activity, safety or freedom from pain, elimination, and the need to see oneself reflected as a loving person worth loving, in another person's eyes.
For the last one might substitute a dog--they seem to be very successful in
loving and taking love. Remember I said this was a constant--the human
being with cognitive loss is never any less a human being. And as an older
person, he has one more characteristic--he is subject to all the problems
that his age mates are subject to. Having cognitive loss does not immunize
one from fractured hips or myocardial infarctions. However, the inability
to process information as well, or finally, perhaps not at all, makes this
human being more vulnerable to the world and its vagaries. If you the caregiver cannot stand uncertainty with your intact mental processes, and great
support system, you may find it easier to understand the need of the person
with cognitive loss. We need to deal with a stable world--a world with few
surprises, one which has reduced stress. The need for stability is shown
best in this equation:

$$\frac{Change}{Support\ Systems} = \text{Likelihood of stress related problems in the elderly such as depression and or confusional states.}$$

This is a guideline that can be used as a planning principle. For each
change that is introduced there must be a support system that neutralizes
the consequences. Whenever the older person with a cognitive problem comes
into the health system he is facing change--we are part of it. I challenge
us to look hard at our settings and our systems to see where we can reduce
the stress of change. Fortunately, we can also function as support systems.
But not if we are uncertain of ourselves and refuse to face our uncertainty.

The most important single action that we perform in any encounter is an
estimate of the situation--using our cognitive qualities to the fullest. An
assessment of this individual--not just of his ability to remember recent
events such as who the last president was, and what day it is today---must
spell out how this person is functioning as a human being in meeting his
needs with a broken memory. There are 7 parts to this assessment. The
first factor is, naturally, the extent of memory loss. Instead of measuring
this on a Short Portable or an MSQ or Folstein, I am putting it in less
quantifiable terms. I am suspicious of nonqualifiable items that give a
score that can be used to separate the moderately from the severely
demented, etc. I express this as a stage of memory loss. Any memory loss
is severe to the person who has it. (See Table 1).

The next factor to be considered is the setting (Table 1). On a grid
that has setting and extent of memory loss one can see that the greater the
support, the more memory loss can be tolerated before the situation becomes
critical. Again, the general health of the individual is important.
Maintenance of health status and prevention of illness require planning and
problem solving for the elderly, and are as dependent upon an intact and
well functioning memory as on physical factors. The quality of the support
system is a factor which makes a difference as change and discontinuities
force the diminishing cognitive functions to cope with what become the new
reality. Since change and discontinuities are part of the older person's
life, to what extent is the lifestyle threatened?

Table 1.  Factors which must be assessed and used to titrate the amount and quality of nursing care needed by the human with memory loss

A. Extent of memory loss
   1. First stage or insidious (Human can cope with support and this stage is often recognized only in retrospect).
   2. Advanced or second stage (Human functions independently with good support) Needed help organizing or with calculations.
   3. Far advanced or third stage. Orientation problems, distinct memory loss. Totally dependent upon supports.
   4. Fourth or terminal stage. Totally dependent upon supports for all care—unable to perform any self care. No memory.

B. Setting
   1. Long familiar such as home, loving support by familiar persons. (A continuation of life setting style and history).
   2. Home setting with lesser degree of human support.
   3. Home without family but with good community support.
   4. Home without family or community support.
   5. New setting: Institution with staff supportive of memory loss.
   6. New setting: Institution with staff not supportive of memory loss (hospital, nursing home, etc.)

C. General health of the person who has memory loss
   1. Good health, fully mobile; good sensori-perceptual ability; no dental problems other than maintenance.
   2. Good health, impaired sensori-perceptual abilities and/or activity level.
   3. Impaired health with no problems of chronicity, sensori-perceptual deficits, dental and/or foot problems.
   4. Acute illness, or need for surgery.

D. Quality of support system (family or secondary supports)
   1. Large family in which relationships have been strong and loving.
   2. Very small family, but excellent relationships in past.
   3. Spouse or significant other only. Good relationship.
   4. Spouse only—poor relationship/poor health/aged.
   5. No primary support. Good secondary support.
   6. Poor secondary supports.

E. Previous lifestyle
   1. Motoric or active. Athletic.
   2. Sedentary.
   3. Many educational advantages.
   4. Good source of self-esteem.
   5. Loner.
   6. Recent change due to illness or disability.
   7. Recent change due to memory loss.

F. Ability of the human with memory loss to perform self-care.
   1. Needs no assistance with self-care activities.
   2. Performs most activities of self-care but needs some prompting.
   3. Performs activities of self-care if helped with organization and some reminding.
   4. Unable to plan ahead or organize activities, remember dental or root care, or to perform self-care without close supervision.
   5. Unable to take responsibility for self-care including toileting, feeding and grooming.

G. Ability to communicate
   1. Articulate, may need help to remind of recent events.

2. Unable to recall nouns and proper names, but recognizes them. Can express himself. Needs help remembering recent events, routine affairs, and appointments.
3. Unable to organize coherent sentences, but recognizes communication of others. Uses nonverbal communication.
4. Initiates little conversation. Depends more on nonverbal communication. Gives up easily. Problem understanding. Remembers no previous verbal interchange. Recognizes feeling or affect of others.
5. Rarely uses words to communicate. Recognizes affect of others.
6. Unable to communicate verbally—diminished ability to communicate non-verbally.

---

and finally, to what extent can the older person with memory loss still perform the personal and valued self-care. It is at this point that self-esteem becomes endangered. Now included in Table I is ability to communicate. We all know that there is a continuum from the usual abilities or optimum sharing of meaning by the person, to the sad state when we all search for meaning in wordless noises and frustrated motions.

The above seven categories of change should give an estimate of the extent to which a human being has suffered human functional losses from memory, and the extent to which supports help to buffer the losses from memory. With an analysis of the assessment we can place this human being into a fair estimate which cargivers need to base their plan of care. The focus is not on the memory—but the human being with a memory loss which is subject to changes—and is never stable unless we provide the stability. We may not be able to change the cognitive status. I am not sure that we can restore lost memory, even with all the interesting approaches that we experiment with. I am certainly not against experimentation though, for I should be happy to be found wrong. The memory crutches such as reality orientation, etc, probably don't work in the long term. But one thing does work. That is human interaction on a feeling level. When words no longer seem to have meaning---approval and kindness communicate well. The person with cognitive loss is still a human, and just as the infant knows when he is held by a frightened new parent and screams and panics, so too, the human being with memory loss senses feeling. They do not remember what happened a few minutes before, but they remember if the caregiver was patient or not. Communication takes place on the feeling level—two way communication. Per Sanderson of Sweden studied the ability of patients with the diagnosis of Alzheimer's disease to participate in their own morning care. He found that personnel who were non-critical and accepting were able to achieve much higher levels of performance from the person with cognitive loss. The answer is on the feeling level which brings us back to my opening statements—that we must look at ourselves and how we interact with the ambiguous person. Are we taking on a job that demands more maturity than we have?

I have watched staff members trying to follow protocols that have been set out for them by therapists who have a different orientation. Some recognize the embarrassment that memory drills cause the human being who simply cannot remember—the sense of frustration and futility. Other's follow the routines in a wooden manner which does not let the unique human being come through. Keeping the human being and his needs as a human centermost helps to place his loss in perspective even if we cannot see a fractured bone or atrophied brain substance.

Our institutional needs of safety pervade all of our planning. What if this person loses himself, wanders away or harms another person, gets angry, has a catastrophic reaction? This last worry may take precedence over the need to meet his human needs--our human needs or institutional needs come first.  Prevention is the key.  What causes frustration in this human being with memory loss?  His needs to express anger do not differ from yours or mine, yet his provoke fear in us and in our attempts to insure our own peace of mind, we may overlook the triggering mechanisms that arouse his anger. Usually increased activity and tension become apparent to the keen observer early on.  Is the environment full of distraction--sound, movement, surprises, instability, lack of privacy, impersonal staff, lack of touch? Closing one's eyes and listening to what is heard--background noise, music, or clatter, can sound like pandemonium if not understood.  Constant movement requires information processing that never catches up.  Slow the world down. But first keep it slow and stable.  Except for these catastrophic episodes, the human being with memory loss is like the rest of us.  For that matter, we all blow at regular intervals, too.

Remember what Shakespeare said when he wrote the wonderful passage in the Merchant of Venice where Shylock defends his humanity.  I will paraphrase using human being with memory loss instead of Jew.

> I am a human being with memory loss.  Hath not such a human
> being eyes?  Hath not a human being hands, organs, dimensions,
> senses, affections, passions fed by the same food, hurt
> by the same weapons, subject to the same diseases, healed by
> the same means, warmed and cooled by the same winter and
> summer as you are?  If you prick us do we not bleed?  If
> you tickle us do we not laugh?  And if you wrong us shall we
> not revenge?  If they are like us in all the rest, they resemble
> you in that.
> (Merchant of Benice, Act III, Scene 1, lines 60-71)

REFERENCES

Preston, R.P., 1979, "The Dilemmas of Care, Social and Nursing adaptations to deformed, the disabled and the aged," Elsevier North Holland, New York.

PATIENT BEHAVIOR, CARE NEEDS, PERSONALIZED COMMUNITY RESOURCES OF BOTH

INSTITUTIONALIZED AND NON-INSTITUTIONALIZED ALZHEIMER'S PATIENTS

Christine Gmeiner

Lafayette Clinic
Detroit, MI 48207

Nursing homes are a phenomenon of the past two decades. Approximately 5% of the over sixty-five population are being cared for in a nursing home at any one time. Twenty percent of those over sixty-five will have spent sometime in a nursing home before they die. The cost of this nursing home care in 1979 was approximately 18 billion dollars (Crystal, 1982). The demented are estimated to occupy 50-70% of nursing home beds (Reisberg, 1981). Alzheimer's type dementia accounts for at least 50% of all dementia's. The incidence of Alzheimer's disease is 15% of persons in their sixties and seventies and 50% of the persons over eighty (Bartol, 1979). Both the over 65 population and the over 80 population are expected to continue increasing into the early 2000's (Department of Health, Education and Welfare, 1977). Therefore, if percentages of afflicted and nursing home placement remain proportional, the numbers and cost of nursing home placement due to Alzheimer's disease will be astronomical.

Some factors are known to correlate with institutionalization in general. Brody and Spark (1966) reported that one fourth of persons within nursing homes were placed after the death or illness of a spouse and another fourth after the death or illness of an adult child or child-in-law. Findings cited by Crystal (1982) calculated from the 1976 Survey of Institutionalized Persons from the Bureau of the Census support the hypothesis that married persons and persons with living children were the least likely to be institutionalized.

Assuming that the demented population has a similar proportion of spouses and children as the cognitively intact population, what accounts for the higher percentage of institutionalized demented persons? One hypothesis might be that affection of families for their demented relative is less then affection for non-afflicted members. However, studies cited by Robinson and Thuruber (1979) refute the hypothesis of decreased caring on the part of relatives. Butler and Lewis (1977) also found children caring for demented parents to be motivated by genuine affection. The research by Murray, Hrielskoltter and O'Driscoll (1980) reported similar findings for spouses.

Research reported on the decision to institutionalize an older person is minimal. Grauer and Birnbom (1975) present data supporting the hypothesis that institutionalization occurs when a person's physical and/or mental disabilities outweigh his/her functional abilities and the support available from relatives and community resources. Sanford (1975) states that relatives of geriatric patients hospitalize patients primarily due to the patient's problem behaviors, the families' limitations in caring for the patient and environmental and social conditions. Wheeler (1981) compared female caretakers who had institutionalized their demented relatives with those who had not. The significant finding was a perceived lack of community services by females who had placed their demented relative.

RESEARCH PROBLEM

The reseach problem addressed in this descriptive study was to compare patient's behaviors, care needs and use by spouses of personal and community resources to determine if there was a difference between institutionalized and non-institutionalized patients with Alzheimer's. This research problem was considered not only in light of previously reported findings, but also, because of it's possible relevance to nursing practice.

Nursing personnel are often in the unique and crucial position of providing services to the Alzheimer's patient and family while the patient is being cared for in the home. The scope of nursing practice includes intervening in patient's behaviors, providing for patient's care needs, teaching family caregivers, and promoting use of personal resources and community services. If findings indicate that institutionalized patients exhibited problematic behaviors and required different care then non-institutionalized Alzheimer's patients, nurses could design interventions for changing or coping with the problematic behaviors and specialized care. Some interventions might be directly provided by nursing personnel. Other interventions could be taught to family caregivers and community agencies.

INSTRUMENT

The instrument was a questionnaire used in a structured face-to-face interview with the non-afflicted spouse. Sixty-one behaviors thought to be symptomatic of Alzheimer's disease such as restlessness, wandering, inability to remember dates, to read and fix meals were listed. If the behavior did not occur it was scored as a "0". If the behavior occurred, questions about the degree (minimal, moderate, or severe) to which the caretaker found the behavior a problem was included.

A list of 25 care needs was developed. These items were thought to be care required by the patient as a result of the symptom's of Alzheimer's disease. Care needs included making major decisions for the patient, preparing food, helping bathe, reminding to go to the bathroom, and providing constant supervision. Again, questions about the degree of problem that providing the care posed were asked (minimal, moderate, or severe).

This questionnaire was developed by the researcher prior to the publication of Reisberg, Ferris and Crook (1982). However, most of these behaviors and care needs were also reported in Reisberg's research on the stages of symptomology of Alzheimer's disease.

Personal resources included family, friends, neighbors and the use of prayer, exercise and hobbies. Questions were asked about the number of hours of care per week provided by family, friends and neighbors. Also, questions were asked rating the perceived helpfulness (not helpful, a little helpful, moderately helpful, very helpful) of any personal resources utilized.

Community resources included either free or paid services that assisted with housekeeping, patient care, or support of the caregiver. Examples of community resources were physicians, religious affiliations, Alzheimer's Disease and Related Disorders Association, registered nurses and day care programs.

Spouses who had institutionalized their patient were asked to answer the questions retrospectively, that is, to report the behaviors and care needs of the patients and the resources utilized at the time when spouse made the decision to institutionalize the patient. Spouses who were caring for the patient at home were to report their current situation.

DATA ANALYSIS

A chi square 2 X 2 analysis with one degree of freedom was used to compare the two groups on prevalence of behaviors, care needs, and resources utilized. The Kruskal-Wallis was applied to questions of the degree to which something was problematic or helpful. Although the Kruskal-Wallis is a less well known statistic then a "t" test to compare ranking, the computer was programed for the Kruskal-Wallis.

SAMPLE

A convenience sample of 60 spouses (whose Alzheimer's spouses were alive) who spoke English, had no psychiatric history, and were living in Michigan were interviewed. Thirty of the spouses were caring for the patient at home and thirty had institutionalized the patient within these years of the interview. Volunteers were obtained through contacts with persons at a research facility and community organizations providing information and support to Alzheimer's families.

The respondent spouses were white. Ages ranged from 48 years old to 81 years old (mean age = 65, SD = 6.47). Forty-three were female and 17 were males. Fifty-nine had at least a high school education and 50 had a college education. Mean reported income was $21,000.00 (range $7,000.00 to over $70,000.00 gross annual income—1983 dollars). The majority owned their own homes (62%) and had worked as professionals, managers, business owners, office or sales personnel before retirement (60%). The sample was representative of the socio-economic class persons belonging to the volunteer organization, but not of the general population. When comparing the two groups, the only demographic variable significant to the $p < 0.01$ level was the age of the spouses respondent. The mean age of the caregiver spouse in the institutionalized sample was 66.7, SD = 6.26 compared to 63.3 mean age, SD = 5.77 spouses caring for the patients at home.

Comparison of patients age, education, income, home ownership and previous occupation revealed no statistically significant difference (alpha =0.05) between the home and the institutionalized groups.

FINDINGS

Four behaviors occurred more frequently in the patients that were subsequently institutionalized. Frequent night wakening ($X2 = 6.94$) was significant to the p<0.01 level. Night wandering (X2 = 5.71), inability to drive safely (X2 = 4.63) were significant to the p<0.05 level. Seven patient behaviors were rated as more problematic by those who then institutionalized their spouses.

RATING OF BEHAVIORS

## TABLE I

### PROBLEMATIC RATING OF PATIENT BEHAVIORS

| Behavior | Group With Higher Mean | H |
|---|---|---|
| Inability to Find Bathroom | 1 | 14.280**** |
| Occasional Night Waking | I | 8.218*** |
| Night Wandering | I | 5.109* |
| Inability to Recognize Spouse | 1 | 4.327* |
| Inability to write | 1 | 4.076* |
| Inability to Drive | 1 | 4.028* |
| Patient's Depression | 1 | 3.905* |

NOTE:   I = Institutionalized Group
        * = p < .05
      ** = p < .01
    *** = p < .005
  **** = p < .001

Six care needs depicted in TABLE II: Prevalence of Care Needs were required more frequently by the patients who were subsequently institutionalized. The home and institutionalized group differed on only two variables rating the degree of difficulty providing for the Alzheimer's patient care needs. The home group reported preparing of patients food was more problematic (H = 3.85, p<0.05). Spouse deciding to institutionalize rated keeping the patient occupied (H = 4.63, p<0.05) more difficult.

## TABLE II

### PREVALENCE OF CARE NEEDS

| Behavior | Group With Higher Mean | X2 |
|---|---|---|
| Help Bathe | I | 9.820*** |
| Take to Bathroom | I | 5.406* |
| Be Accompanied At All Times | 1 | 4.800* |
| Lay Out Clothes | 1 | 4.705* |
| Help Dress | 1 | 4.565* |
| Help Brush | 1 | 4.344* |

NOTE:    I = Institutionalized Group
        * = p < .05
    *** = p < .005

Utilization of the personal or community resource variables was not significantly different (p<0.05) between the two groups. However, the institutionalized group more frequently declared a need for additional respite care.

In order to further explore the differences between the two groups, six predictor variables, identified by multiple regression analysis, were used in a Discriminate Function Analysis. The six predictor variables were the perceived rate of patient's decline, patient's inability to talk, patient's restlessness, patient's need to have food prepared, age of the caretaker, and spouse and fatigue of the caretaker spouse.

The more rapid the perceived rate of patients decline, the less verbal and more restless the patient, the older the caretaker and the greater the fatigue reported by caretaker the more apt the patient was to be institutionalized. The converse of these along with reporting food preparation to be quite problematic, predicted the probability of the patient being cared for at home. Using these variables, group membership of fifty of the sixty patients (83%) was accurately predicted. Four institutionalized were predicted to be cared for at home. Two of these four had scores close to the cut-off between the groups. Six of the home group were predicted as belonging to the institutionalized group. Of these six, four were placed within a year of the interview.

NURSING IMPLICATIONS

Since Alzheimer's disease is progressive and of approximately a five to 25 year duration, the stress on the spouse-caregiver is phenomenal. The behaviors and care needs occurring more frequently in the group at the time of institutionalization are those described by Reisberg, Ferris, and Crook (1982) as presenting in the fifth and sixth stage of the seven stage progression. The caregiver is usually very fatigued by the burdens assumed during the earlier stages of illness. Night-waking and wandering then disrupts the sleep of the caregiver, often pushing fatigue to the exhaustion point. Nurses can provide information to the spouse. Keeping the patient active during the day may aid the patient to sleep. If not, medication may be helpful. Providing a safe confined area within which the patient can wander or securing respite care would allow the caretaker time for rest. Caregiver fatigue was a predictor of institutionalization. Decreasing caregiver fatigue may increase the time that the caretaker may be able to cope with the patient at home.

The spouses reported of distress over lack of recognition by the patient. Every human being needs recognition. Nurses can acknowledge the tremendous job the spouse is doing in caring for the patient, as well as encourage respite care so the spouse's psychological and social needs can be met by persons other then the incapable patient (Grossman, London and Barry, 1981)

The patient's inability to drive presented more hardship to the spouses of the institutionalized group. These spouses also tended to be older females. Older women are less apt to drive than younger women (Treas, 1979). Nurses should familiarize themselves with both the variety of transportation services available for their clientele and the types that the spouse and patient are capable and willing to use.

Incontinence was an undesirable behavior in this study as in Stanford's study (1975). Diapering, condom catheters (for men); regular toileting schedule, sufficient fluids, high fiber diet and use of rectal suppositories aid in urine and feces regulation. Easy to wash clothing such as sweat suits and protection of furniture with plastic facilitate easier cleaning after incontinent episodes.

The care needs of bathing, toileting, dressing, mouth care and supervision of the patient at the time of institutionalization require considerable skill to elicit the demented person's cooperation. One technique nurses can teach the spouse is to break down large tasks, such as dressing, into smaller tasks that the patient can manage. For example, the spouse can lay out the patient's clothes in the order which the patient would put them on. Then the patient is not faced with the complexity of decision-making and organization.

In summary, institutionalization tends to occur in the late stages of Alzheimer's disease when the patient becomes restless, incontinent; requires constant supervision and loses his ability to care for basic needs. The care required by the Alzheimer's patient is primarily nursing. Nurses working with Alzheimer's patients can play important teaching, caregiving and emotionally supportive roles with patients and spouses. Through these roles the nurse may prevent the institutionalization of the Alzheimer's patient.

REFERENCES

Bartol, M.A., 1979, Nonverbal communication in patients with Alzheimer's disease, Journal of Gerontological Nursing, 5:21-36.

Brody, E.M., and Spark, G.M., 1966, Institutionalization of the aged: A family crisis, Family Process, 5:76-90.

Crossman, L., London, C., and Barry, C., 1980, Older women caring for disabled spouses: A model for Supportive Services, The Gerontologist, 21:464-70.

Crystal, S., 1982, "America's Old Age Crisis: Public Policy and the Two Worlds of Aging," Basic Books Inc., New York.

Department of Health and Welfare, 1977, "Our Future Selves: A Research Plan Toward Understanding Aging of the Population," (HEW Publication No. 77-1096), U.S. Government Printing Office, Washington, D.C.

Graurer, H., Birnbom, F., 1975, A geriatric functional rating scale to determine the need for institutional care, Journal of the American Geriatrics Society, 33:472-76.

Murray, R., Hrielskoltter, M., O'Driscoll, D., 1980, "The Nursing Process in Later Maturity," Prentice Hall, Englewood Cliffs.

Reisberg, B., Ferris, S., and Crook, T., 1982, Signs, symptoms and course of age-associated cognitive decline, in: "Aging in the 1980's: Alzheimer's Disease: A Report Progress in Research," S. Corkin, K. Davis, J. Growdon, E. Usdin, R. Wortman, eds., Raven Press, New York.

Reisberg, B., 1981, "Brain Failure: An Introduction to Current Concepts of Senility". The Free Press, New York.

Robinson, B., Thuruber, M., 1979, Taking care of aged parents: A family cycle transition, The Gerontologist, 19:586-93.

Sanford, J., 1975, Tolerance of ability in elderly dependents by supporters at home: Its significance for hospital practice, *British Medical Journal*, 3:471-73.

Treas, J., 1977, Family support systems for the aged: Some social and demographic considerations, *Gerontologist*, 17(6):486-91.

Wheeler, J.C., 1981, A comparison of stressors and supports reported by females in caring for age relatives with senile dementia, Unpublished Master's Thesis. Wayne State University, Detroit.

CREATING TIES AND MAINTAINING SUPPORT:   NETWORKING AND SELF HELP

Lambert Maguire

School of Social Work
University of Pittsburgh
2331 Cathedral of Learning
Pittsburgh, PA   15260

Alzheimer's disease strikes families, not just individuals.  It is a degenerative disorder which has no known medical cure.  Neither the affected individuals nor their families are allowed much hope and without hope we frequently find despair.  This despair on the part of the Alzheimer's patient and his or her family members can occasionally lead to depression which in turn leads to isolation and to a subsequent cutting off of family and social ties.  In other instances, this dismal prognosis spurs people on to strengthen their ties with family, friends, and similarly afflicted people.  The former response is generally considered maladaptive and frequently exacerbates the depression and isolation on the part of both the patient and the concerned family members.  The latter response tends to help enable people to deal better psychologically with the very real and genuine pain of losing a loved one.

Creating Ties and Maintaining Support: Cultural, Interpersonal, and Cognitive Factors

There is no single way to help the families cope better with their own feelings, but there are rather specific factors which health and mental health professionals can consider in designing a supportive and even therapeutic intervention with them.

Primary among those is the rather consistent research finding that a positive support system or network of family and friends serves as a buffer against stress (Lin, et al, 1979).  Families dealing with the tremendous stress caused by the effects of a member with Alzheimer's will either succeed or fail in their coping capacity based upon their ability to find and use their social networks.  Whether we are referring to the enhanced ability of families of unemployed workers (Gore, 1978), the families of pregnant women (Nuckolls, et al, 1972), or the families and networks of schizophrenics (Pattison, et al, 1975; Tollsdorf, 1976), the research is unambiguous.  The families which are strongly linked together and strongly associated with other family members, friends, neighbors, professionals, and others in an interactive social network seem to cope better and are more healthy and supportive of themselves and their afflicted family member than socially isolated families or individuals.

Before trying to develop healthy family networks, professionals must first recognize that there is a very wide range of "appropriate" responses on the part of family members which are related to fairly idiosyncratic cultural, interpersonal, and cognitive factors. Culturally, families differ both in the way and the extent to which they want other family members and friends to be involved or even informed. Within some cultures, the immediate family takes care of its own and to go outside of the family is considered an insult and could undermine further family support. This attitude can be easily perceived by many professionals as maladaptive, but in many cases, it is not. In fact, these small, dense family networks can be very emotionally supportive. Although they may be limited in their capacity to efficiently find and utilize diverse health, mental health, and community resources, they do serve a socially supportive function quite well (Walker, et al, 1977).

Interpersonally, some families are more emotive and verbally more interactive than others. Families which have long standing traditions of discussions at the dinner table or elsewhere will no doubt continue to be more comfortable with those exchanges than less verbal families. Professionals need to assess the capacity of the family realistically and not make demands upon them which will only add to, rather than diminish, the degree of perceived stress.

Cognitively, families use and interpret data and facts differently. Some families can handle a great many facts about Alzheimer's, its causes, its effects, and their own medical and psychosocial options extremely well. These families can and should be given as much information and in as detailed a form as they are able to digest. Other families may use combinations of denial and defenses to misinterpret even small amounts of information, or will perceive the giving of such information as being either cruel, overly pessimistic, or defeatest in its intent. Still other families and individual members may be poorly helped when we give them more information than they can intellectually comprehend, with the outcome being increased confusion rather than a greater understanding.

The research on Alzheimer's and working with family members certainly supports supplying families with cognitive guidelines or information (Wasow, 1986). This is as it should be since families need to know what the disease is, its prognosis, and its etiology, at least to the extent that it is known by any of us. However, many of the caregivers come from an era and tradition where is was not considered helpful to dwell on one's problems and where family and friends would try to protect each other from certain hard facts rather than consciously and deliberately attack those problems or issues. We have probably all had the experience where spouses or other family caregivers and friends seemed personally hurt or offended by the fact of our giving either too much information or information which allows relatively little hope. When that attitude, on the part of family members, is combined with our own self protective distancing which we often affect for our personal sakes, it can be perceived as not only cold but cruel.

These three areas and the general caveats within each are mentioned only because traditional mainstream mental health work with families may not be the best approach with the families of those with Alzheimer's. For instance, the psychodynamic approaches which value disclosure, introspection, and the gradual breaking down of defense mechanisms may be appropriate for family therapy, but not for all families who may need to be more self protective (Riesberg, 1981). The family members of one with Alzheimer's may need a tremendous amount of psychic reserve or resources for a long period of time. To "open up" too quickly to one's own most primitive fears of loss too early could prove to be counterproductive in

the long run.  What is needed instead is a careful and sensitive assessment
on the part of the social worker, nurse, or physician concerning the family
members ongoing capacity to help themselves as well as the member with
Alzheimer's (Steinberg, 1983).

Culturally, the mental health professions have only rather recently
recognized that there are variations within families based to a limited
extent on ethnic and racial traditions.  We are not all middle class
Viennese from circa 1890.  Cultural traditions of some families allow for
the inclusion of wide networks of professionals, community leaders, neighbors, work colleagues, and others.  However, some traditions prefer to
include only the immediate family and appropriate professionals when necessary.  This cannot be labeled as deviant or maladaptive.  If families or
individual caregivers isolate themselves to the exclusion of others who
could and would be genuinely and perhaps unobtrusively helpful to them,
then they may need help to see this.  However, families cannot be forced
against their heritage and tradition to turn over the care of a loved one
to "strangers" and institutions until they have at least been allowed to
use their own resources appropriately.

In summary, it seems that the current thinking regarding working with
the families of Alzheimer's patients support the belief that families should
be given as much clear information as possible and provided with help in
networking with familial and community resources.  Professionals must,
however, be cautious in recognizing that families have differing cultural,
interpersonal, and cognitive coping and adaptive strategies.  For some
families, a great deal of caution and sensitivity must be used by professionals in their networking endeavors, or else those efforts will be
seen as an insult to the family and can actually undermine their efforts.
Furthermore, the manner in which the needed information is given may have
to vary from one family to another, as well as the amount of data which
they are willing or able to digest.  It may be necessary to slow down the
process of providing information and the process of developing networks
for certain families with more traditional coping strategies.

## Networking and Self Help

Networking with the families where a member has Alzheimer's involves
linking concerned caregivers with potentially supportive family members,
professionals, neighbors, and friends.  The purpose is to provide resources,
information, a protection against stress and a psychological support system
for both family caregivers and the member with Alzheimer's.  Furthermore,
it enhances the self help capacity of the family at a time when it needs
a great deal of help.

The process itself involves three stages: assessment, mapping, and
linking (Maguire, 1983).  In the first stage, the social worker, nurse,
or physician needs to interview the family to establish their potential
as a supportive network.  This stage is also used as a way to develop
rapport and a relationship with the family members and the patient.  It
should take the tone of a low key, casual but caring and concerned discussion.  For the purposes of potential networking, certain information
must be gathered which is more relevant to social supports than the typical
background histories.  In this initial phase or assessment stage, the
worker must begin evaluating the strength or capacity of the family and
the individual's social networks.

Variations of the following questions are therefore indicated:  Could
you tell me about your friends?  Are there family members with whom you
feel comfortable in discussing problems?  Are there neighbors or friends
who have had a relationship in the past with your husband (or wife or

whomever the patient may be). Are you or your family members active now or in the past with any church, union, social group, or ethnically oriented organization? The data you gather in this stage must be gathered in such a way that the cultural, interpersonal, and cognitive histories and capacities of the family and the patient with Alzheimer's are all considered. This general discussion is a precursor of the second stage which involves a more in-depth analysis of the social network.

The social network analysis goes beyond just gathering more information. It is the means by which the professional can help the patient and the family members begin to think in depth about their own existent and potential social supports. Whereas stage one is a more general discussion used partially to get people to begin to think in terms of social networks, stage two is a more rigorous and detailed analysis. A network diagram (Maguire, 1983) is often used at this stage to graphically examine the network. This diagram entails four concentric circles with the middle circle labeled with the name of the family member. The circles are divided into three pie shaped wedges which are labeled family, friends, and others. The worker then asks the family member to begin with the family section, and put the names of their closest family members in the inner circle, closest to their own names. The definition of "closest" varies with the individual, but generally it refers to the family members whom they rely upon, confide in, or love the most. This discussion itself further sensitizes people to the nature of their relationships with family members. The next concentric circle as one goes farther away from the individual is for family members who are a bit more psychologically distant. Typically, married people put their spouses, children, and occasionally their parents into the closest circle. The next circle may include brothers and sisters, close cousins, and concerned aunts or uncles. Finally, the outer circle may have relatives who are uninvolved or even antagonistic in their relationship. The same pattern is used for the "friends" wedge, and finally the "other". For others, one may include professional caregivers such as doctors, lawyers, pharmacists, nurses, social workers, police and neighbors or work colleagues who do not qualify as friends. It also may involve individual members of various self help or support groups for the family members or the patient with Alzheimer's.

Once the social network diagram has been completed, there is a series of questions which one needs to ask pertaining to each person designated on the diagram. These questions include: what is their relationship to you (e.g. neighbor, cousin, doctor)? How often do you see them? Who initiates this contact? Do you feel that you get more or give more in this relationship? How long have you known them? What do you get from them (e.g. personal support, financial aid, information, etc.)? The last question entails more than just a brief response. At this point, you need to discuss the nature of the relationship with that designated person and the issue of whether they might be both willing and able to provide support. The support can take many forms such as watching the family member with Alzheimer's, going out to dinner with the primary caregiver, or just being available for discussions on the phone when the family member needs someone to emotionally help them deal with problems. This information becomes the basis for the self help and networking strategy of phase three.

Phase three is the linking stage where the real networking takes place. At this point, the professional knows who each of the family members and the Alzheimer's patient's actual and potential support contacts are and how they might help. The intervention at this phase is directed toward developing and maintaining supportive ties with as many helpful network members as possible. This linking process flows from the needs and capacities of each family member with a focus upon the primary caregiver and the patient himself or herself.

As a case example, the professional may work with a working class Italian Catholic family.  In the worker's initial assessment, he finds that the Alzheimer's patient, a 68-year-old male, has been retired for three years and has had some symptoms for the past year.  He has two daughters and a son who are all married as well as a brother and a sister who are also married and who all live in the same general vicinity.  The wife is the primary caregiver and is 66 and has arthritis, but is otherwise in good health.  She has one sister who lives out of town.  She has a very close relationship with one of her daughters but refuses to speak to her other daughter since she married a man three years ago whom the family disliked.  Her only sources of social support consist of the one daughter and her family with some limited visiting with the son, along with frequent phone calls to her sister and occasional involvement with friends at the parish church.  She does not trust that professionals would be willing or able to provide her husband with the affection and support which his own close knit family has provided for so many years.

To help this woman and her husband, the worker will have to develop the linkages with a small but already cohesive family unit.  A couple of family sessions which would include the entire social network (Attneave, 1976; Rueveni, 1979) might even be considered.  These family network sessions have been known to pull together as many as 80 people who are all directed and coordinated through five stages of development, culminating in a detailed plan for the provision of social support.  An open and frank discussion of the wife's need for social support from family members should be discussed.  Furthermore, she might be encouraged to visit her sister for occasional brief vacations while the "closer" daughter moves in to watch her father.  The son can be encouraged to come over at least weekly to take his father out for a dinner and walk.  The parish priest should also be asked to join in on the social network to provide help and support to the wife and the husband and also to engage his help in leading the wife to further interaction with other women from the parish.  There are invariably groups of women within every parish who volunteer to help with a variety of activities.  These women may be of a similar age and background to the primary caregiver and with permission from the priest and support from the family, she can allow herself to get out of the home occasionally.  She needs to share her concerns with other women who may have similar concerns themselves.  The homogeneity of some of these church groups contributes to their being relatively cohesive and supportive systems.

In a more typical example, the worker may be presented with a family which has a 58-year-old woman as the patient.  She and her 60-year-old husband have no strong ethnic or religious identification.  He is an engineer with mid-level administrative responsibilities with a locally based corporation.  They have three children, two of whom are married with children, and only the 23-year-old unmarried son remains at home.  The son has been increasingly staying away from home, leaving the father to care for his wife.  On his occasional business trips out of town, he has hired a nurse to watch her, but finds that his wife intensely dislikes that arrangement, and he can no longer afford it.

In this instance, a less familial and more professional social network might be considered.  The husband, who has become increasingly depressed and has begun drinking to excess, should be referred to an individual therapist for supportive counseling which will also occasionally include the son.  The daughter from out of town should be contacted and encouraged to agree to at least watch their mother when the father goes away on business.  The husband should also be referred to a support group for the family members of those with Alzheimer's.  The names and meeting times and places for these groups can generally be found by calling the local community mental health/mental retardation center, any hospital which has a geriatric program, the John Hopkins Dementia Research Clinic (301-955-6792) or a local self help clearinghouse such as New Jersey's (201-525-9565) or Pittsburgh's (412-521-9822), which will provide information about local Alzheimer's support groups.

The supportive and therapeutic effects of support groups are tremendous (Schmidt and Keyes, 1985; Barnes et al., 1981). The common bond is based upon the high level of stress and feeling of isolation and loss by its support and understanding but also information and resource sharing. Occasionally, members exchange times when they will watch or be with each other's afflicted family members. In instances where there is no strong family network, such groups are essential for the primary caregiver and often for any other family member who is very closely affected.

In summary, the networking process itself involves three stages of assessing, mapping the network, and linking supportive family, professionals, friends, and neighbors together. It is a process which must be sensitive to cultural, interpersonal, and cognitive needs and capacities. Furthermore, it should focus first upon strengthening and supporting the immediate family supports, but recognize that the family, and particularly the primary caregiver, may need outside help as well. That help may involve counseling on an individual basis, but in most instances a support group for fellow caregivers for Alzheimer's patients will prove to be particularly beneficial.

REFERENCES

Attneave, C., 1976, Social networks as the unit of intervention, in: "Family Therapy" P. Guerin, ed., Gardner Press, New York.
Barnes, R.F., 1981, Problems of families caring for Alzheimer's patients: Use of a support group, Journal of the American Geriatrics Society, 29: 84-85.
Gore, S., 1978, The effects of social support in moderating the health consequences of unemployment, Journal of Health and Social Behavior, 19: 157-165.
Lin, N., Ensel, W.M., Simeone, R.S., and Kuo, W., 1979, Social support stressful life events, and illness: A model and an empirical test, Journal of Health and Social Behavior, 20: 108-119.
Maguire, Lambert, 1983, "Understanding Social Networks," Stage Publications, Beverly Hills, CA.
Pattison, E.M., Francisco, D., Wood, Frazier, H., and Crowder, J.A., 1975, Psychosocial kinship model of family therapy, American Journal of Psychiatry, 132: 1246-1251.
Riesberg, B., 1981, "A Guide to Alzheimer's Disease: For Families, Spouses and Friends," Free Press, New York.
Rueveni, U., 1979, "Networking Families in Crises," Human Science Press, New York.
Schmidt, G.L. and Keyes, B., 1985, Group psychotherapy with family care givers of demented patients, Gerontologist, 25: 347-350.
Steinberg, G., 1983, Long-term continuous support for family members of Alzheimer's patients, in: "Alzheimer's Diseases: The Standard Reference," B. Riesberg, ed., Free Press, New York.
Toffsdorf, C.C., 1976, Social networks, support and coping: An exploratory study, Family process, 15: 407-417.
Walker, K.N., MacBride, A., and Vachon, 1977, Social support networks and the crises of bereavement, Social Science and Medicine, 11: 35-41.
Wasow, M., 1986, Support groups for family caregivers of patients with Alzheimer's disease, Social Work, 31: 93-98.

THE FAMILY CAREGIVING ROLE:  STRESSES AND EFFECTIVE COPING

Beverly A. Baldwin

University of Maryland
School of Nursing
Graduate Program
Baltimore, Maryland

Conservative estimates suggest at least 5 million people in the U.S. are involved in parent care at any given time (Brody, 1985).  Another 4-5 million assume some type of family responsibility for elders, whether on a consistent or transitional basis.  The components of family caregiving have shifted significantly over the past 10 years.  Where once family members offered support and kinship ties, they are now responsible for the management of chronic physical and psychological/emotional disorders which increase in complexity and intensity as a person ages.  The fact that families of today are committed to and responsible for their elder members is indeed interesting, given the nostalgic myth that families do not care for their elders today as they did in years past.  Ninety-five percent of America's elderly reside in homes with their spouses, other family or friends, or live alone.  Shanas (1979) found that over twice as many frail and ill elderly are cared for by spouses or children than live in institutions such as nursing homes.  Families of today provide over 80 percent of the home care needed by elders (Springer and Brubaker, 1984; Horowitz, 1985).

The members of the family who are consistently identified as principal caregivers are adult daughters, representing approximately 40 percent of family caregivers.  Spouses, specifically wives, constitute the largest group of family caregivers, approximately 50 percent (Shanas, 1979; Poulshock and Deimling, 1984).  Eighteen percent of all elders (approximately 5 million) live with an adult child.

The responsibilities of family caregiving carry with them stress, strain, and, for some, a sense of burden.  As the dependency of older adults increases, conflict may arise, placing stress on individuals and the family system as a whole.  Emotional, physical, and financial strain may be accompanied by unresolved family issues or conflicts or historical events which influence the roles of various family members.  Adult children, particularly, may feel reluctant or resentful in assuming a "parent role" in the care of the elder.  The increasing dependency of frail and ill older adults raises many concerns related to the role reversal between parent and adult child, and becomes especially difficult for middle-aged women who care for an aging parent (or parents) in addition to their own spouse, children, and sometimes grandchildren.  Francis (1984), in a kinship comparison study of American and English older adults, found contrasting patterns of adjustment to retirement and old age in these groups with similar ethnic and religious backgrounds. One difference of significance here was the degree to which elders relied on family support and maintenance of socialization, particularly in the American community. The difficulty in making new friends and social support networks was evident as elders relied more on the family to meet both kinship and friendship needs. Given present knowledge of family caregivers of elders, there is little doubt that the role has inherent strain with an increasing need for coping strategies. To date, little empirical attention has been given to the possibility that caregiving has emotional and physical costs as well as rewards for the caregiver, and that long-term caregiving may indeed alter the quality of life of the family member assuming primary responsibility for an aging parent.

A series of pilot studies was conducted by this author and others in 1984-85 to identify some of the stresses and coping strategies of family members caring for an older adult in their home. Caregivers were contacted through adult day care centers used for socialization and rehabilitation of the elder and respite for the families. Twenty family members were contacted and agreed to participate in a comparative study of two types of groups for stress management: educative/didactic and psychotherapeutic/ supportive.

Although the length of the participation was less than a month, the family members (10 daughters, 2 sons, 7 spouses, and 1 cousin) were actively verbal in both groups, and there appeared to be no hesitancy to become involved in the interaction and affective exchange. Caregiver roles, trials, joys, and burden were shared, in addition to attempts at problem solving and decision making surrounding anticipated or real crisis events. The impact on the individuals was readily explored and included depression, stress-related physical symptoms (heart palpitations, shortness of breath, gastrointestinal distress) and altered self-esteem. Family impact was expressed in terms of conflict and marital (spousal) strain, "acting-out" by teenage children, altered lifestyle, and role reversals. Most of the participants had read (and brought to the group sessions) The 36-Hour Day (Mace and Rabins, 1981), a book specially written for families regarding the day-to-day issues, concerns, and problems confronted by caregivers. Questions arose as to the application of many of the suggestions in the books, as a way of validating and verifying the information their own particular situation.

Examples of physiological and psychobiological symptoms of stress experienced by these family members included changes in sleeping patterns, especially if the older parent/spouse was a restless or "unpredictable" sleeper, altered eating habits or patterns, most often noted in crisis events or when the family as a whole appeared stressed, increased blood pressure, and, with some, the onset of hypertension, gastrointestinal changes or upsets, including gastroenteritis, bouts of diarrhea, vomiting or abdominal pain, bouts of depression (often experienced somatically, as in G.I. symptoms, insomnia, wakefulness) and loss of motivation at work, headaches, either persistent or intermittent, extreme mood swings and, in all cases, fatigue. Varying in combination and degree, the onset of these symptoms was specifically identified since the period of time the caregiving responsibilities began.

Many psychosocial stressors were identified by the families in the group sessions. These included feelings of alienation from friends and from other family members not involved in direct caregiving (some participants expressed feelings of being abandoned by other family members or the lack of desire of other family members to assist in the care-giving responsibilities); feelings of being "trapped" in a situation in which there was little outlet or relief; feelings of isolation or aloneness in the situation (no one to turn to for help or for understanding) a marked decrease in socialization or participation in social activities once taken for granted or treasured (eating out with friends, visiting neighbors, travel, having friends into their home for social events); decreased work enjoyment and productivity, especially where caregiving duties were heavy in the evening or on weekends and particularly among participants who viewed career and their job as a high priority in their lives; feelings of resentment, anger, and frustration over their responsibilities, over promises made earlier in life without knowledge of the consequences, or over their perceived lack of ability to cope well with the caregiving role; and guilt, a feeling shared in common in both groups--guilt of omission and commission in actions and thoughts provided a consistent theme--wrestling with this overpowering and often all-consuming feeling required much energy and investment of self.

More positive consequences of caregiving expressed by the family members included being forced into getting their lives more organized and planned, involving other family members who otherwise might not have had the opportunity to get to know the elder well (particularly if, before the caregiving began, the elder did not reside in the same geographic area), and an opportunity to repay the dependent elder for caregiving or support they received at an earlier age or time.

Regardless of the type of consequence identified by the family members, it was clear from the group discussions that the stressors were not linked to the strain of caregiving. The lack of awareness of the result of caregiving on physical and emotional health status was profound. Denial of burden permeated the discussion on the one hand, yet the consequences for the individuals and their families of caregiving dominated the interactions. Recognizing and labeling stressors appeared to be a new experience, easily and validated in the group settings.

Coping strategies initiated by the family members demonstrated ingenuity, creativity, and a commitment to their caregiving responsibil- ities. The frequent and deliberate use of humor was evident throughout the group sessions. Problem solving, using solutions cited in professional or lay literature provided a sense of control over the situation and enhanced self-confidence. Getting away from the responsibility on a consistent basis (i.e., which the adult day care center provided for many) offered coping and "refueling" opportunities, particularly if the guilt or anxiety over leaving the elder had been adequately resolved. Changing family expectations and goals often precipitated more involvement of other family members in the day-to-day caregiving activities. Some participants expressed attempts at getting professional counseling or psychiatric support when they realized their ability to cope with a particular situation or the long-term perspective was limited. Those utilizing special community support groups (stroke, Alzheimer's, day care, etc.) found them helpful in that sharing and validating common experiences allowed the family caregiver an opportunity to look at his/her situation from another perspective. The use of support groups varied widely among the participants.

Suggestions of other coping strategies by group leaders and other members were readily accepted by the participants. Some homework trials of new alternatives to handling "problem" behaviors (i.e., wandering, agitation, incontinence) were initiated and reported back to the group. Little resistance was observed in these family members to new options for their own methods of handling caregiving. On the contrary, they eagerly sought the assistance of the group members in more clearly delineating problem situations and potential solutions.

Preliminary data from these pilot studies are currently being used in a long-term, large-scale study of 80 adult daughters in the Baltimore-Washington metropolitan areas. The commitment of these families to providing care to their elder family member is clear, reinforcing Brody's (1981) contention that families of today do not abandon the elderly. The thought of institutionalization of the elder parent or spouse was consistently expressed by the 20 family members, along with the agony of the decision and the resistance to such a measure except as a last resort.

The impact of caregiving on families will continue to be felt in the increased longevity and the potential for a longer, more active older age. The consequences of four-generation families living in the same household are being realized for the first time in our society. Many middle-aged women and older female spouses will not experience the "empty next syndrome" once anticipated as children grow up, leave home, and start their own families. Many younger adults, after short leave from parents' homes, are returning for employment or economical reasons. On the same wake of this unexpected return is the need to become caregiver for a frail and growingly dependent older parent.

Data from these preliminary studies indicate that family caregiving is a stressful experience for many. Long-term effects of this stress remain to be realized. Effective coping strategies can be introduced during the caregiving experience which, when measured long-term, may significantly alter the negative stressors inherent in family caregiving.

REFERENCES

Bohn, L.C., and Rodin, J., 1985, Aging and the family, in: "Health, Illness and Families," D.C. Turk and R.D. Kerns, eds., John Wiley and Sons, New York.
Brody, E., 1981, Women in the middle and family help to older people, Geront., 21:471-480.
Brody, E., 1985, Parent care as a normative experience, Geront., 25:19-29.
Brody, E., et al., 1983, Women's changing roles and help to elderly parents: Attitudes to three generations of women, J. Geront.,597-607.
Clark, N.M., and Rakowski, W., 1983, Family caregivers of older adults: Improving helpers' skills, Geront., 23:637-642.
Francis, D., 1984, "Will You Still Need Me, Will You Still Feed Me, When I'm 84?" Indiana Univ. Press, Bloomington.
Horowitz, A., 1985, The role of the family in providing long-term care to the frail and chronically ill elderly living in the community, Geront., 612-617.
Johnson, C.L., and Catalano, D.J., 1983, A longitudinal study of family supports to impaired elderly, Geront., 23:612-618.
Mace, N.L., and Rabins, P.V., 1981, "The 36-Hour Day," Johns Hopkins Press, Baltimore.
Maples, L., 1985, Patient-family responses to the DRG system, Ger. Nurs., 6:271-272.
"The Maturing society in the Maturing Health Care System" (Report of the Second Ross Health Administration Forum), 1983, Ross Laboratories, Columbus.
Poulshock, S.W. and Deimling, G.T., 1984, Families caring for elders in residence: Issues in the measurement of burden, J. Geront., 39:230-239.
Rabins, P.V., et al., 1982, The impact of dementia on the family, JAMA, 248:333-335.
Shanas, E., 1979, The family as a support system in old age, Geront., 19:169-174.

Springer, D., and Brubaker, T.H., 1984, "Family Caregivers and Dependent Elderly:  Minimizing Stress and Maximizing Independence," Sage Publications, Beverly Hills.
Springer, D., and Brubaker, T.H., 1984, "Family Caregivers and Dependent Elderly:  Minimizing Stress and Maximizing Independence," Sage Publications, Beverly Hills.
Who's taking care of our parents?  1985, 6 May, <u>Newsweek</u>:  60-70.

PATTERNS OF FUNCTIONING AND COPING IN BLACK FAMILIES:  CARING FOR

PHYSICALLY DISABLED ELDERS

Gaynell Walker-Burt

Michigan Department of Mental
Health
Lewis Cass Building, 6th Floor
Lansing, Michigan 48926

Betty M. Morrison

School of Education
The University of Michigan
Ann Arbor, Michigan 48109

INTRODUCTION

This paper examines patterns of functioning and coping among black family members who assume caregiver functions for their physically disabled elderly relatives.  There are few studies which focus on the experiences of black family members who provide care for their older relatives.  Previous studies indicate that black older persons requiring personal care look within their household or immediate community for assistance (Jackson, 1980; Archbold, 1980; Shanas, 1979).  Shanas (1979), for example, found that for both whites and blacks the provider of physical health care services is often a spouse if the older person is married, a child, or other relative living in or outside the household.  Paid helpers or social/public services were rarely reported as providing these necessary services to the sick older person.  In the black family, it is the women (wife or daughter) who usually provides these services.  The elderly wives who assume primary caregiver roles are often faced with chronic disabilities themselves.  Brody (1978), reported that the middle-aged daughter of aging parents often carries the burden of both older and younger generations.  Many black women who act as primary caregivers for their disabled elderly parent experience social as well as economic problems which make parental caregiving difficult.

CARE OF PHYSICALLY DISABLED BLACK ELDERS IN THE HOME

There is evidence that disabled black elders are cared for in the community rather than in nursing homes.  A survey of the nursing home population revealed a disproportionately white (96%), female (70%) and widowed (64%) population.  Only 4% of nursing home residents in the U.S. are members of a minority group (Harris, 1978).  The disabled elderly black make up about 1% of the population who are institutionalized.  Explanations regarding this situation include: 1) the lack of facilities willing to accept black clients; 2) the lack of financial resources; and 3) the fact that elderly blacks tend to rely on the supportive services of their families, often because blacks have had limited access to outside supportive services.  In addition, family cohesion has traditionally been a strength of the black family with an elderly person being the focal point of that cohesion (Hill, 1972).  Kinship ties are frequently sustained through religious values as well as of economic necessity.

Health status among the elderly is considered to be disabling or poor when the elderly person is not able to function with reasonable independence (Hoffman and Thomas, 1970). In examining the impact of federal health care policy on the health status of the black elders, Taylor (1980) found that black elders tended to be lower on social indicators (i.e., income, education, and housing) related to health status than white elderly. Black elderly tended to have lower health status than white elderly, evidenced by a number of indicators (i.e., bed disability days, restricted activity days and shortened life expectancy). When the black disabled elderly person is in a dependent role she may experience feelings of being a burden to the family, fears of receiving inadequate care, and generalized depression.

The extensive health problems of black elders and the provision of care by their family members increase the probability that the elderly as well as the caregiver will use coping behaviors as adaptive strategies to handle the health problems encountered. These health problems often occur as a result of changes in life situations generated by physical illness, mental illness, or the normal process of aging. Lazarus and Olbrich (1981) point out that how a person copes with any stressful encounter determines the emotional response. This occurs in two ways: by changing the troubled person-environment relationship; or by changing, through realistic or defensive reappraisal, the way an encounter is construed.

Little is known about the black family's capacity to function and cope with different types of impairments and disabilities of their elderly relatives. Several issues must be considered when a family member assumes a caregiver role. The caregiver role can be viewed as both satisfying and stressful. Whatever the experience, the family member involved as primary caregiver will at some point experience psychological stress or strain. Troll (1979), for example, points out that many of the stresses and distresses experienced by the middle-aged women, as caretaker, occur because she is caught between concern for her own immediate family and her job. Family caregivers in general have many responses to the caregiver role including feeling burden, fears of inadequacy in carrying out prescribed medical regime, depression due to social isolation, and frustration in their efforts to find enough money to survive.

A HOME CARE STUDY OF BLACK FAMILIES

This study investigated the impact of the relationship between physically disabled black elders and their family members who provide care in the home environment. A total of 30 physically disabled black elders and their primary caregivers were interviewed in the home. The sample of disabled black elders was obtained from active cases of a Visiting Nurses Association. These clients had been active cases for no more than 6 months. Five of the disabled elders and four of the caregivers were not included in the data analysis. None of these five disabled elders could respond to the interview and two of these had Alzheimer's Disease. Disabled black elders (N=24) with physical health problems and their primary caregivers (N=24) were included in the present data analyses. The age range of the disabled elders was 61-96 years. Most disabled black elders had achieved less than a 10th grade education and had an income over $5,000 but less than $10,000. These data are consistent with data reported by Swanson (1971) and Dancy (1977). Most primary caregivers were either the spouse (N=12) or daughter (N=9). The age range of the caregivers was 26-88. Family caregivers had a range of 7 months to 2 years of experience in the caregiver role. Although most caregivers reported educational levels at high school and below, there was a higher incidence of post high school education than among the disabled black elders. These data also revealed that two and three generations were a part of the same household.

All caregivers and their disabled relatives were interviewed in the home for approximately 1 1/2 hours. Each of them was interviewed separately and in a private area of the home. The data collection instrument was developed to measure levels of functioning in physical health and mental health. The number of caregivers problems and ways of coping with them was also determined. Interviews were conducted by two research faculty and two black graduate students in nursing.

Correllograms were constructed for each scale to determine internal consistency among items. The small sample size did not permit more sophisticated techniques for data reduction. After examining these correllograms, indices were developed for each construct. Measures of physical health functioning were determined by using a list of common illnesses. Disabled black elders were asked to report illnesses that a doctor, nurse or someone else had told them that they had. Overall health status was determined by responses to two questions: "In general, how would you rate your health?" and "How do you think your health is compared to other people your age?" While there is some disagreement regarding the utility of self-reported health status, there is evidence to suggest that self-reported health status correlates highly with physicians' ratings.

Measures of mental health functioning were determined by using Duke University's (1978) OARS Mental Health Screening Test. A mean score on this 15 item yes-no scale was derived to obtain a rating of overall mental health. A high score was judged to be indicative of good mental health functioning.

A measurement of caregiver problems and how they managed these problems was also obtained. A low mean score on these items indicated having problems with caregivers.

Measures of coping were determined for both the caregiver and the disabled elder by using Lazarus' concept of coping. Ten items were designed to determine the way caregivers coped with problems encountered in the caregiver's role. Two ways of coping were measured in this present study - "seeks emotional support" and "reducing or minimizing threat". A high score on these scales indicates use of these ways of coping strategies.

A measure of black elders' morale was determined using a modified version of the Philadelphia Morale Scale. "Morale is viewed as consisting of a series of interrelated parts that can be measured by self report items (Lawton, 1975). This 17 item scale measures three factors: "agitation", which characterizes the anxiety experienced by the older person; "attitude toward own aging", which relates to the older person's attitude toward the aging process they experience and captures the individual's perception of the changes taking place in his or her life; and "acceptance of life situations", which represents the older person's acceptance or dissatisfaction with the amount of social interaction they are presently experiencing and with their life situation in general. This factor measures the individual's reaction to the social relationships he or she maintains. A sum of these factors was obtained and a high score indicates high morale.

Mean scores and standard deviations on characteristics of the black families are found in Table 1. The mean score on caregiver's mental health functioning was 1.70. This finding indicates that caregivers reported relatively good mental health functioning. Caregivers reported feeling happy, useful and full of life. Given the length of caregivers experience, in this study one wonders how long the caregivers could maintain their mental health if they continued in the caregiver role for long periods of time. Table 2 shows the percentage responses on mental health items.

TABLE 1:   Mean Scores and Standard Deviations on Characteristics
of the Home Care Sample of Black Families

| Variables | Family Caregivers (N = 24) | | Black Elders (N = 24) | |
|---|---|---|---|---|
| | Mean | Std. Dev. | Mean | Std. Dev. |
| Mental Health | 1.70 | .21 | -- | -- |
| Caregiver Problems | 4.46 | 3.08 | -- | -- |
| Coping: | | | | |
| Emotional Support | 1.49 | .34 | -- | -- |
| Reduce Threat | 1.75 | .18 | -- | -- |
| Morale: | | | | |
| Agitation | -- | -- | 4.13 | 1.42 |
| Attitude Toward Own Aging | -- | -- | 2.04 | .99 |
| Acceptance | -- | -- | 4.79 | 1.02 |
| Physical Health | 2.38 | .65 | 3.08 | .65 |
| Health Compared | 1.88 | .61 | 1.88 | .80 |

TABLE 2:   Percentage Responses on Caregiver Mental Health
(N = 24)

| Mental Health Items[a] | % Yes | % No |
|---|---|---|
| Do you feel useless? | 8 | 92 |
| Are you being plotted against? | 15 | 85 |
| Even when you are with people, do you feel lonely most of the time? | 19 | 81 |
| Are you happy? | 81 | 19 |
| Does it seem that no one understands you? | 23 | 77 |
| Do you wake up fresh and rested in the mornings? | 77 | 24 |
| Have you had difficulty in keeping your balance in walking? | 27 | 73 |
| Are you bothered by heart pounding and shortness of breath? | 27 | 73 |
| Are you troubled by headaches? | 35 | 65 |
| Is your sleep fitful and disturbed? | 39 | 61 |
| Feeling like leaving home? | 42 | 58 |
| Have you, at times, wanted to leave home? | 46 | 54 |
| Do you often worry about things? | 56 | 44 |
| Is your daily life full of things that keep you interested? | 46 | 54 |

[a]In order of the most positive mental health responses.

A mean score of 4.46 was obtained on measures of caregiver problems.
This finding indicates that caregivers experience a moderate number of problems in providing home care to black elders.  Caregivers reported having
problems with "carrying out treatments", "having to keep close watch on
elder", "time for vacation", and "time to do housekeeping".  (Table 3 illustrates the percentages of caregiving problems identified by caregivers.)

TABLE 3: Percentage Responses on Caregiver Problems
(N = 24)

| Problems | % | Ability to Manage Problem | | |
| --- | --- | --- | --- | --- |
| | | Manageable % | With Help % | Unmanage-able % |
| Carrying out treatments | 80.0 | 25.0 | 75.0 | -- |
| Having to keep close watch on elderly | 73.1 | 5.3 | 68.4 | 26.3 |
| Time for vacation | 57.7 | 26.7 | 60.0 | 13.3 |
| Time to do housekeeping | 53.8 | 25.0 | 75.0 | -- |
| Time for getting out with friends | 42.3 | 50.0 | 50.0 | -- |
| Transportation | 38.5 | 30.0 | 60.0 | 10.0 |
| Caring for personal needs | 30.8 | 50.0 | 50.0 | -- |
| Shopping | 26.9 | 14.3 | 85.7 | -- |
| Knowing how to care for elderly | 19.2 | 20.0 | 80.0 | -- |
| Your own health | 19.2 | -- | 100.0 | -- |
| Preparing proper food | 19.2 | 50.0 | 50.0 | -- |

After caregivers had identified caregiving problems they encountered in providing care for their elderly relative, they were asked to identify the one problem which caused them the most worry and concern. For this one problem, they were asked to respond to ways they handled their concerns about this problem. Caregivers reported a relatively high use of emotional support (mean = 1.45) as a way to handle problems. For example, they used "prayer", "asked the advice of a friend", and "consulted persons who experienced the same problem". Caregivers used strategies to reduce anxiety (mean = 1.56) such as "telling self things could be worse", and "keeping busy". Table 4 shows the percentage responses on caregiver ways of coping.

TABLE 4: Percentage Responses on Caregiver Ways of Coping
(N = 24)

| Ways of Coping | Caregiver % |
| --- | --- |
| Emotional Support | |
| Do you pray or get someone to pray for you? | 96.0 |
| Do you ask the advice of a friend or neighbor? | 52.0 |
| Do you try to find people who have experienced the same thing to see how they dealt with it? | 52.0 |
| Do you ask the advice of relatives? | 48.0 |
| Have you read any books to help you? | 32.0 |
| Reduce Threat | |
| Do you remind yourself that things could be worse? | 88.0 |
| Do you do things to keep busy like watching TV, knitting, etc? | 71.4 |
| Do you try to ignore difficulties by looking only at good things? | 68.0 |
| Do you eat too much or too little? | 40.8 |
| Do you drink alcoholic beverages (beer, wine, etc.)? | 16.0 |

The mean score for disabled elders' perceived physical health status was 3.08 indicating that they tended to perceive their health status to be "not too good". When comparing their health to other persons their age, disabled elders obtained a mean score of 1.88, suggesting that disabled elders thought that their health was about average. To further assess physical health functioning, disabled elders were asked to indicate from a list of common health problems, if a doctor, nurse or someone else had told them that they had the illness. Most physically disabled elderly persons reported health problems in the following areas" "hypertension" (83%), "circulation problems" (79%), "arthritis" (71%), "problems with sight" (63%), "heart problems" (50%), and "foot problems" (50%). Most disabled elders reported two or more health problems. It is not surprising that multiple health problems were found. Dancy (1977) pointed out that factors contributing to the overall poor health reported by black elderly include lack of money, poor transportation, and the unavailability of suitable health care in the black community.

Scores on measures of morale of disabled black elders ranged from low to medium. Disabled elders obtained a mean score of 4.13 on agitation suggesting that they experienced a medium amount of anxiety. On measures of "attitude toward their own aging" disabled elders obtained a mean score of 2.04. This score suggests that disabled elders experience a lower morale, when considering the changes that are taking place in their life. A mean score of 4.79 was obtained on measures of "acceptance of life situation", indicating that disabled have moderately high levels of acceptance with the amount of social interactions they are presently experiencing. Table 5 shows the percentage responses on black elders' morale.

In this study we also attempted to predict the mental health status, coping behavior and the perceived problems of the caretaker from the morale and physical health of the black elderly. Zero-order correlations were obtained for all variables and are reported in Table 6. Relationships[1] were found between the positive mental health of the caregiver and the following caregiver variables: low number of caregiving problems and (high emotional support). High caregiver mental health was also associated with the following characteristic of the disabled black elder: acceptance of present life situations; (low agitation; positive attitudes toward own aging; better physical health; and better physical health in comparison with others). These findings suggest that the caregiver's mental health is influenced by the morale and (perceived health status) of disabled black elderly.

When the number of caregiving problems was considered, a correlation was found with (low emotional support). In terms of the elderly, when the caregiver perceived a large number of problems, the elderly reported less positive attitudes toward own aging, greater dissatisfaction with their present life situation, (high agitation, and poorer physical health in comparison with peers). When the caregiver reported high emotional support the elderly accepted their present life situation, reported better physical health, and perceived themselves in better physical health in comparison with peers. These findings suggest that caregiver problems increase when there is low emotional support. Since emotional support includes "advice from friends", and "contact with someone who experienced similar feelings", these findings suggest the need for support for caregivers who report increased numbers of caregiver problems. Zarit, et al. (1980) found, in his study of caregiver burden, that subjects receiving more visits from family other than the caregiver reported less caregiver burden.

---

[1] Since the sample size is so small, relationships that were not significant at .05 are reported to suggest possibilities for future research. These are presented in parentheses.

TABLE 5: Percentage on Responses of Disabled Black Elders High Morale
(N = 24)

| Morale Categories | High Morale Response | N | % |
|---|---|---|---|
| **CATEGORY 1 - Agitation** | | | |
| Do little things bother you more this year? | No | 23 | 38 |
| Do you sometimes worry so much that you can't sleep? | No | 24 | 63 |
| Are you afraid of a lot of things? | No | 24 | 79 |
| Do you get mad more than you used to? | No | 24 | 79 |
| Do you take things hard? | No | 24 | 75 |
| Do you get upset easily? | No | 24 | 67 |
| **CATEGORY 2 - Attitude Toward Own Aging** | | | |
| Do things keep getting worse as you get older? | No | 24 | 63 |
| Do you have as much pep as you had last year? | Yes | 24 | 42 |
| As you get older, are things worse, the same or better than you thought? | Better | 24 | 44 |
| Are you as happy now as you were when you were younger? | Yes | 24 | 33 |
| **CATEGORY 3 - Acceptance** | | | |
| How much do you feel lonely? | Not Much | 23 | 87 |
| Do you see enough of your friends and relatives? | Yes | 24 | 62 |
| Do you sometimes feel that life isn't worth living? | No | 24 | 79 |
| Do you have a lot to be sad about? | No | 24 | 83 |
| Is life hard much of the time? | No | 24 | 83 |
| How satisfied are you with your life today? | Satisfied | 24 | 87 |

TABLE 6: Correlations Between Major Characteristics of
the Home Care Sample of Black Families
(N = 24 pairs)

| Variables | Caregiver Mental Health | Caregiver Problems | Caregiver Coping-Support | Reduce Threat | Elder's Agitation | Elder's Attitude | Elder's Acceptance | Elder's Physical Health |
|---|---|---|---|---|---|---|---|---|
| Caregiver problems | -.43* | -- | | | | | | |
| Caregiver coping support | .22 | -.24 | -- | | | | | |
| Reduce threat | -.10 | -.31 | .09 | -- | | | | |
| Elder's agitation | .24 | -.28 | -.04 | .16 | -- | | | |
| Elder's attitude | .16 | -.47* | -.02 | -.15 | .21 | -- | | |
| Elder's acceptance | .50** | -.45* | .43* | -.19 | .32 | .18 | -- | |
| Elder's physical health | -.30 | .29 | -.39 | .20 | -.39 | -.34 | -.56** | -- |
| Elder's health comparison | -.32 | .27 | -.41* | .01 | -.22 | -.32 | -.19 | .44* |

\* p < .05
\*\* p < .01

It is also important to note the relationship between the elderly persons' morale and their perceived physical health status. The elderly were more accepting of their life situations, (less agitated and had a more positive attitude) when they were in better physical health. These findings indicate black elders' perception of their physical health status will influence the ability to successfully cope with their social environment through acceptance and tolerance of their everyday life. Edwards and Klemmock (1973) found that the best predictors of life satisfaction were socio-economic status, perceived health status and informal participation with non-relatives. When considering formal participation they found that involvement in church activities was directly related to life satisfaction.

Stepwise, forward, multiple regressions were used to predict characteristics of the caregivers from attributes of the black elderly. The small sample size (N=24 pairs) limited the number of variables that could be entered in the equations. Indeed, even these results should be interpreted with care.

Three morale measures of the elderly were used to predict the mental health, care giving problems, and coping behavior of the caregiver. This decision was made because: 1) morale was a variable that could be more readily changed by intervention than physical health; and 2) there was a high correlation between physical health scores and measures of morale.

The results of the Multiple Regressions are reported in Table 7.

TABLE 7: Stepwise Multiple Regression of Disabled Black
Elders Morale on Caregiver Characteristics
(N = 24 out of 24)

### MENTAL HEALTH

| SOURCE | DF | SUM OF SQRS. | MEAN SQUARE | F-STAT | SIGNIF |
|---|---|---|---|---|---|
| REGRESSION | 1 | .24360 | .24360 | 7.1649 | .0138 |
| ERROR | 22 | .74798 | .33999 −1 | | |
| TOTAL | 23 | .99158 | | | |

MULTIPLE R = .43565     R-SQR = .24567     SE = .18439

| VARIABLE | PARTIAL | COEFFICIENT | STD ERROR | T-STAT | SIGNIF |
|---|---|---|---|---|---|
| CONSTANT | 1.2160 | .18439 | 6.5948 | .0000 | |
| ACCEPTANCE | .49565 | .10083 | .37671 −1 | 2.6767 | .0138 |

| REMAINING | PARTIAL | SIGNIF |
|---|---|---|
| AGITATION | .10379 | .6374 |
| ATTITUDE | .08499 | .6998 |

### PROBLEMS OF CAREGIVING

| SOURCE | DF | SUM OF SQRS. | MEAN SQUARE | F-STAT | SIGNIF |
|---|---|---|---|---|---|
| REGRESSION | 2 | 83.316 | 41.658 | 5.8854 | .0093 |
| ERROR | 21 | 148.64 | 7.0782 | | |
| TOTAL | 23 | 231.96 | | | |

MULTIPLE R = .59932     R-SQR = .35919     SE = 2.6605

| VARIABLE | PARTIAL | COEFFICIENT | STD ERROR | T-STAT | SIGNIF |
|---|---|---|---|---|---|
| CONSTANT | | 23.750 | 2.7453 | 8.6509 | <.0001 |
| ATTITUDE | −.44671 | −1.2914 | .56441 | −2.2880 | .0326 |
| ACCEPTANCE | −.41733 | −1.1627 | .55251 | −2.1044 | .0476 |

| REMAINING | PARTIAL | SIGNIF |
|---|---|---|
| AGITATION | −.09495 | .6743 |

When considering the caregiver mental health, the elders' acceptance of present life situations accounted for approximately 25 per cent of the variance and was significant at the .01 level. That is, knowing how well the elderly person accepted her/his social interactions predicted, to some extent, the mental health of the caregiver. For example, when disabled black elders had high level of acceptance of their life situation, did not feel lonely, and saw enough of their friends, the caregiver had more positive mental health. (The level of agitation and attitude toward own aging reported by the disabled elders did not improve the prediction.)

The second regression analysis attempts to explain the number of problems the caregiver perceives. When elders' attitude toward own aging was entered into the equation as a single independent variable, 22 per cent of the variance in the number of problems that the caretaker perceived was explained (p <.02). However, when acceptance of present social interactions was added to the equation, 36 per cent of the variance was explained (p = .009). Thus, when a knowledge of the elders' acceptance of present life situation was introduced, 15 per cent more variance was explained. Therefore, one can predict the number of problems that the caretaker perceives from a combination of the elder's attitude toward aging and acceptance of the present life situation scores. When disabled elders reported a poor attitude toward aging (felt that they did not have as much pep as last year, felt less useful and felt things were worse as they got older) caregivers had more problems with providing care for their disabled relatives. Agitation had no predictive power.

Disabled black elders acceptance of present life situations, agitation and attitude score accounts for 22 per cent of the variance when the caregivers use of emotional support was considered. This was not significant at the .05 level.

DISCUSSION AND RECOMMENDATIONS

In recent years more attention has been given to the factors associated with home care of the elderly. There is a paucity of research which addresses the needs of black families who act as primary caregivers for disabled elders. Although the physically disabled elders in this study were intact cognitively, some of the problems faced by caregivers are consistent with findings regarding persons who care for relatives with Alzheimer's Disease as well as other disorders associated with cognitive impairment. One of the problems with doing research with elderly who have cognitive impairment is their difficulty or inability in responding to the interview instrument (Kolata, 1982). Though several problems experienced by a relative who provides care to an elderly person with Alzheimer's are unique to this disorder, the relationship between variables associated with caregivers and those variables associated with disabled elders appear similar. Mental health and psychosocial problems such as feelings of isolation, lack of support by other family members, feelings of not being able to handle the needs of the disabled person are some common problems associated with the role of caregiver whatever the level of functioning of the elderly person. Caregivers seem to have more positive mental health and experience less problems with providing care when disabled elders are more acceptive of their present life situation and have a more positive attitude toward their own aging.

Because providing care to dependent relatives impacts caregivers' mental health, attention must be given to the caregiver's psychosocial supports, such as support groups, education and counseling. An untapped resource which should be considered by health professionals who provide service to black families is the church. The use of the church as a means to provide educational information regarding physical and/or mental health problems as well as to conduct support groups is a viable alternative to traditional health delivery approaches.

The findings of this study have implications for professional and community agencies who provide services to black families. Strategies to facilitate caregivers should include physical assistance such as respite care and homemaker assistance; and financial assistance such as tax credits, family subsidy and vouchers. Financial assistance for the family in providing care for its elderly is becoming a promising possibility. According to Callahan et al. (1980), awarding cash payment and/or tax credits to families who assume responsibility for the elderly may be more cost effective than long term care provided in institutional settings.

Although institutional care may be more costly, some black families may need assistance in choosing this type of care as an option. For many black families, institutional care is not usually considered for disabled black elders because symptoms associated with physical or mental illnesses are often accepted as part of "just getting old". The need to support black families in whatever setting they choose to provide care for their disabled black elders is clear.

REFERENCES

Archbold, P.G., 1980, Impact of parent caring on middle-age offspring, Journal of Gerontological Nursing, 6:79-85.
Brody, S.J.S., Poulchock, W., and Masciocchi, C.F., 1978, "The family caring unit: A major consideration in the long-term care support system, Gerontologist, 18:6.
Callahan, J.J., Diamond, L.D., Giele, J.Z., and Morris, R., 1980, "Responsibility of families for their severely disabled elders", Health Care Financing Review, 3:29-48.
Dancy, J., 1977, "The Black Elderly--A guide for Practitioners", University of Michigan-Wayne State University, The Institute of Gerontology.
Duke University Center for the Study of Aging & Human Development, 1978, "Multidimensional Functional Assessment: The OARS Methodology", Duke University, Durham, N.C.
Edwards, J., and Klemmock, D., 1973, Correlates of life satisfaction: A re-examination, Journal of Gerontology, 28:497-502.
Hill, R., 1972, "The Strength of Black Families", Emerson-Hall, New York.
Jackson, J.J., 1980, "Minorities and Aging", Undsworth Publishing Co., Belmont, CA.
Kolata, G., 1982, Alzheimer research poses dilemma, Science, 215:47-48.
Lawton, M.P., 1975, The Philadelphia Geriatric Center Morale Scale: A Revision, Journal of Gerontology, 15:85-89.
Lazarus, R., and Olbrich, E., 1983, Problems of stress and coping in old age, in: "Aging in the Eighties and Beyond", M. Bergener, U. Lehr, E. Lang, R. Schmitz-Scheszer, eds., Springer Publishing Co., New York.
Swanson, et al., 1971, How do elderly blacks cope in New Orleans? Aging and Human Development, 2:210-216.
Taylor, R.J., 1980, The impact of federal health care policy on the elderly poor: The special care of the black elderly, The Gerontologist, 20:211.
Zarit, S., Reeves, K., Back-Peterson, J., 1980, Relatives of the impaired elderly: Correlates of feeling of burden, The Gerontologist, 20:649-655.

DESIGNING SERVICES FOR THE MINORITY AGED

Harold R. Johnson

Dean
School of Social Work
The University of Michigan
Ann Arbor, Michigan

Let me begin by saying that research on the utilization of services by minorities and minority elderly is a relatively underdeveloped area of scholarship. Some case studies have been published, and they present illustrative profiles of particular client groups in specific locales; but it is exceedingly dangerous to generalize from the findings of such small-scale, descriptive studies.

Only a few large quantitative studies have been conducted that shed some light on this topic and can be used for designing services for the minority aged (e.g., Mindel and Wright, 1982). With regard to the Black community, the National Survey of Black Americans, conducted by The University of Michigan's Institute for Social Research, has pioneered in providing initial data on service utilization based on the first nationally representative sample of American Blacks. Interviews for this study were conducted in 1979-80 on a sample of about 2,000 Blacks, ranging in age from 18 to 101.

Findings from this and other studies have highlighted several trends in the Black community. One is the strong relationship of family income to the use of social services; low income Blacks were over twice as likely (as high income Blacks) to use social services, even when the effects of education, gender, and age were taken into account (Neighbors and Taylor, 1985:13). A second is that informal family support was more important for Black elderly than White elderly, and a third is that family aid was found to be supplementary rather than an alternative support system (Mindel & Wright, Jr., 1982:107). Finally, Blacks in distress who seek some kind of professional assistance are more likely to turn to traditional health care providers (doctors, hospitals) and ministers than specific mental health caregivers (community mental health centers, psychiatrists or psychologists)(Neighbors, 1985).

Findings such as these are helpful in beginning to understand the utilization of both informal and familial supports as well as professional and community resources by Black elderly. And, I hope that further systematic studies will be launched to further aid us in design of such services. But, the overall paucity of such utilization behavior research has led me to decide to share with you this afternoon a number of impressions and concerns I have developed about what I perceive as the underutilization of social services by minorities in general, and the Black elderly in particular.  Hopefully they will provide some ideas that we can discuss in the latter part of this session.

Social services have never been adequate in the United States.  And, in recent years, the lack of many services has become increasingly serious as a result of underfunding.  Many of the programs designed for special populations such as the elderly and minorities were the first to be cut back or terminated.  Although I am appalled and angered by such actions, I do not believe we can afford to spend our time and talents simply bemoaning program reductions.  We must redouble our efforts to use our very scarce resources more efficiently and more effectively.  Therefore, I would like to identify a number of critical factors to be considered in the design, organization, and delivery of social services for minorities, in general, and the minority aged, in particular.

At this point, let me note that the single most common characteristic of all minorities -- including Blacks of all ages -- is their individuality.  Each person is an unique individual, shaped by a particular combination of cultural, geographic, social, and economic circumstances.  And, as we process and label minorities as "old," "Brown," "Black," "Red," "Spanish speaking," "Asian American," and so on, we increase the likelihood that their individuality will be ignored by those persons planning and delivering community services.  To state my proposition somewhat differently, our perception of "homogenized" special populations increases the barriers to social services for all people, but particularly for minorities.

Yet, as different as people and their circumstances may be in different regions of the country, the need for the development of more effective services for Blacks is general and dramatic.  Population mobility, unemployment, and changes in our social values have modified the supportive role of the Black family.  Segregation, crime, and a lack of public transportation have served to increase the social isolation of Blacks in many areas of the country.  This isolation is particularly true for the Black elderly, the majority of whom, coincidentally, are women (Jackson, 1980:31).  As a result of the abovementioned factors, we see in our central cities not only a substantially larger minority population but one with many more aged persons who have fewer resources and more extensive needs than heretofore identified and served.

As a society we tend to <u>prescribe</u> policies that establish priorities and dictate the development of specific programs in our communities:  urban renewal, delinquency prevention and control, war on poverty, war against crime, cancer crusade, adolescent pregnancies, and so on.  We have prescribed overlapping and competitive structures to carry out programs: anti-poverty agencies, model cities agencies, area agencies on aging, regional transportation authorities, regional criminal justice programs, regional health planning groups -- the list is endless.  We have prescribed the clients for most of our programs -- by age, income, gender, religion, place of residence, disease, and so forth.  We have prescribed agencies' hours of operation, the number and kinds of their board members, and the fees for consumers and service providers.  We have prescribed patterns of fiscal and program evaluation, and formats of reports that are rarely read or used.  In other words, we are an <u>overly-prescribed</u> society.  And these prescriptions change at a glacial rate, thus, remaining out of balance with the problems they are intended to correct.

Please do not misconstrue my comments as a criticism of program standards -- <u>they are essential</u>.  And, in most instances, should be developed at the national and state levels.  Rather, my comments reflect my concerns about the emphasis and specificity we place on process to the detriment of the responsiveness and quality of service programs for minorities.

On the one hand, local community leaders are wondering what they can do to prevent and control community problems. On the other hand, they feel increasingly distant from major institutions with prescribed programs that do not appear to address local problems. It appears that in too many instances we are designing programs to prevent abuses by the providers, rather than to provide appropriate services. The federal and state governments must provide local communities with more resources and more authority so they can plan and implement social services to meet the needs of their residents.

We need to become more concerned about outcomes. We need to find a way to assist each local community to mobilize its distinctive resources, in combination with state and federal resources, as imaginatively as possible. I often wonder what would happen if we insisted that every symphony orchestra must have a specific number of strings, brass, woodwinds, and so on. Should every conductor be a pianist? Can you imagine what would happen to the creativity of artists if we were to prescribe their structures and behaviors as we do in the human services?

If the senior levels of government wish to play a more responsive role -- and do it with imagination -- let them prescribe outcomes instead of procedures. As an example, the federal and/or state government may require local communities to have a prescribed set of services (health, housing, transportation, counselling, education, etc.) available to qualify for federal and state funds; but, they need not prescribe the size, shape, or color of the service package. Compliance would be determined by outcome-centered evaluation -- not by the process employed.

We then come to the question: if local communities are given more resources and more flexibility, how can they improve services for minorities? When I think about increasing the effectiveness of services, I become very pragmatic. I want to know why particular groups have been unable to utilize services. What are the barriers? How can we eliminate or circumvent them? Let me mention some of the barriers that I believe are significant and put them in a conceptual framework that may be helpful in our later discussions.

These barriers fall in five rather discrete categories: personal and social, economic, geographic, organizational, and suppositional. In each of the five, permit me to offer a few examples of specific barriers to the utilization of social services:

A. Personal and social barriers

1. Many minorities have insufficient information about their problems and appropriate resources to aid them. And, they are often of the opinion that service providers are not interested in them. Therefore, they often do not seek assistance.

2. Ageism, racism, and sexism are reflected in negative attitudes toward minorities on the part of service providers.

3. In this era of specialization, it is nearly impossible for individuals to receive services focused on their total well-being rather than on discrete problems. This fragmentation of services is a particular problem for aged persons.

B. Economic barriers

1. Minorities suffer disproportionately from low incomes. Again, this is particularly true of the minority aged. In 1983, the poverty rate among Black elderly (36.3%) was triple the poverty rate among the White elderly (12.1%), and poverty rates were highest among minority women living alone; nearly two out of every three (63.4%) elderly Black women not living with family had an income below the poverty level (U.S. Senate Special Committee on Aging, 1985:39-40). The lack of discretionary income prohibits the purchase of "non-essential" services and products.

2. Medicare requires that the elderly individual pay a significant portion of the costs of health care services. This is a particular burden for Black families attempting to care for their elders.

3. Medicare is acute-care oriented and often forces chronic-care patients into underfunded institutions.

4. In many parts of the country, Medicaid is crafted to be primitive and degrading and is used only as a last resort. In the states populated by the poorest minorities, the benefits are the most inadequate. In my judgment this is not accidental.

5. Highly mobile and intrusive community services for special populations are viewed as being too expensive.

6. State and local units of government do not have the resources to support adequate services. The federal government must assume greater -- not less -- financial responsibility for health and social service programs.

C. Geographic barriers

1. Lack of adequate public transportation, and the high cost of private transportation, makes many services remote for minorities. And, because the minority aged tend to be concentrated in poor neighborhoods with the fewest transportation resources, services are most remote for them.

2. Poor health status and reduced physical mobility of the Black elderly compounds the difficulties related to public and personal transportation, accessibility of buildings, and the utilization of specialized services.

D. Organizational barriers

1. Bureaucratic policies and procedures prohibit or stultify the development of creative solutions at regional or local levels.

2. Interagency conflict is generated where similar responsibilities are assigned to multiple agencies.

3. We lack agencies with the primary goal of service innovation -- thus, innovation becomes secondary to the maintenance of ongoing programs. Note that I do not particularly blame the providers -- they are too busy coping with crises to be able to figure out better ways of doing things.

E. Suppositional barriers

1. The way in which we generalize about minorities throws us off the

track. If, for instance, service designs for Blacks are based on middle class images, the underclass -- who need the services -- probably will not use them.

2. The way in which we conceptualize the roles of professionals decreases the effectiveness of services. Should physicians be the focal point in community based health care programs? Their time is expensive, and they are not trained to utilize community resources. Moreover, they tend to have a narrowly-focused, exclusively medical, view of the needs of minorities. And, often they find it more convenient to institutionalize the aged than tailor a set of services to maintain them in an independent living arrangement. And yet, we know from the research of one of my University of Michigan colleagues, Dr. Rose Gibson, that older Black women who use formal services for mental distress most often look to medical personnel for assistance and advice rather than mental health practitioners (Gibson, 1981).

The major challenge facing us at the present time is: how can we begin to forge the scores of social service programs into an adequate and flexible system of services? The pluralistic nature of our society and the unique "partnership" of federal, state, and local units of government with the voluntary sector makes this goal much more elusive for us than for many other countries in the world.

Paranthetically, it should be noted the problem is further complicated by the active intervention of the courts into the field of human services. The courts have said that neither the lack of funds nor current service models can be accepted as excuses for the public dereliction of duty. To date, these court rulings have been focused on institutional programs, but a current case in New York City is intended to improve services for the chronically mentally ill who are coincidentally homeless.

We cannot hope to resolve our dilemma easily or quickly. I believe the best chance for a solution rests on our willingness to create an economic policy and program environment that will permit local officials to develop imaginative human service programs which are in keeping with local problems and support the integration of local resources. I should emphasize that as we encourage local initiatives and more responsive programs, we cannot permit local prejudices to interfere with the availability of service to minorities. We must build in appropriate standards and safeguards, but in a less repressive manner.

It seems to me the first step that must be taken to achieve comprehensive, integrated human service programs is agreement in principle that local units of government will be given the resources, responsibility, and freedom to organize services at the local level. The current administration's style of federalism provides the freedom, but not the resources. State politicians are behaving similarly, and, in my judgment, this is socially irresponsible behavior.

In response to the current situation, a number of local units of government have attempted to cope with the shortage of resources by experimenting with a variety of intervention strategies and tactics. They include the following approaches:

1. In some places, local or regional units of government have established umbrella agencies to plan and integrate human services. Federal policies impede, and in come cases prohibit, the comprehensiveness and the flexibility desired in such an organization. As an example, workers employed in certain categorical programs cannot be freely used to carry out related or diverse assignments. Conceivably workers engaged in such organizations could become the instrumentality to unify otherwise

fragmented services in keeping with the needs of their clients.

2. Many localities have experimented with single-entry or one-step human service agencies. This approach has proved useful to consumers who are spared the time, expense, and travail of being referred around town. Also, it serves to encourage the coordination of services. However, a number of studies reveal that the scale of programs in such centers and a lack of good transportation may well limit their appeal and accessibility to minorities.

3. Large numbers of communities have experimented with the involvement of consumers in policy making and planning as a mechanism to improve the organization and quality of services. This experiment is rooted in the last century, but was given new impetus over the past 30 years. The idea has great merit. At the present time, however, we have multiple federal and state programs that require various degrees and kinds of consumer participation in single programs. Seemingly, this has contributed to the increased fragmentation and complexity of services, rather than infusing consumer policy and program perspectives into the development of a local network of services. In many instances, minorities have tended to be excluded from -- or minimally represented -- in these kinds of positions. Frequently social class related behavior prompts counter-productive "solutions." I can recall scores of instances where upper middle class Blacks were the least understanding participants on committees planning social service programs for lower class Blacks.

4. Many human service programs have been vastly improved at the local level through the development and utilization of good management techniques. As an example, the collection and analysis of systematic data have assisted many communities to better identify problems, predict needs, and evaluate programs. By contracting-out, or purchasing services, the quality of care has often been improved. The development of sound employment practices, training programs, promotional policies, etc., will serve to improve the quality of service programs. Such techniques are not frills -- they are essential.

The above approaches, singly or collectively, will not resolve all of the problems mentioned earlier. However, if the federal and state governments were to adopt policies and develop programs to encourage -- rather than discourage -- such approaches, we would finally be moving in the right direction -- toward an era of more creative intergovernmental and public/voluntary sector relationships.

Next, let me mention five points at the operational level that are of particular importance for the minorities:

1. Services must be sensitive to and affirmative to special populations. This suggests training all personnel in human service organizations to reduce the deleterious effects of prejudice and discrimination based on age, race, sex, ethnicity, etc.

2. Services must be known to and viewed positively by prospective clients. We should make better use of the media, threshold agencies (police, visiting nurses, mailmen, homemakers), organizations of the aged, block clubs, churches, housing managers, etc. The complex of services is so vast in our major urban centers that "advocates" may be required to assist consumers through the maze.

3. Services should be organized and delivered to maintain people in

independent living situations.  This suggests more home services, decentralized settings, supportive transportation, and so on.  This would eliminate or reduce geographic barriers.

4.  We must place more emphasis on prevention and rehabilitation, particularly for the aged.  We must better inform minorities about health matters, including the appropriate use and interactions of medications.

5.  Services should be designed to make greater use of the intelligence, experience, and other resources of consumers and especially elderly people -- they should be viewed as a service resource instead of as a group of pathological consumers.

Finally, let me offer two more general suggestions that could countervail against some of the organizational and suppositional barriers listed earlier.  First, as a matter of public policy, we must cease and desist from prescribing the form of service programs aimed at minorities. We can guarantee standards and still be able to facilitate the development and utilization of social services at the local level.  Local service designs will permit the creative mobilization and combination of local/state/federal resources to meet local problems.  Second, we should develop a number of innovation-oriented organizations, free from the pressures of ongoing service programs and interorganizational competition, to test new programs.  This could be done in selected program areas and for particular populations.

The kinds of problems and service improvements that I have touched on are not meant to be exhaustive.  Rather, they are intended to provoke discussion and generate ideas.  We must rise above our organizational allegiances to create an environment more conducive to experimentation -- an environment characterized by improved personnel and improved services for all Americans, irrespective of race, age or gender.

REFERENCES

Gibson, R., 1981, Stressful life events:  Use of the formal and informal networks, in:  "Aging and Aged Black Women:  Factors Impacting Well-Being," final report to Administration on Aging, grant 90-AR-2183-01, U.S. Government Printing Office, Washington, D.C.
Jackson, J. J., 1980, "Minorities and Aging," Wadsworth Publishing Co., Belmont, CA.
Mindel, C. H. and Wright, Jr., R., 1982, The use of social services by black and white elderly:  The role of social support systems, Journal of Gerontological Social Work, 4:107-125.
Neighbors, H. W. and Taylor, R. J., 1985, Seeking professional help for personal problems:  Black Americans' use of health and mental health services, Community Mental Health Journal, 21:156-166.
Neighbors, H. W. and Taylor, R. J., 1985, The use of social service agencies among black americans, Social Service Review, 59:259-263.
U.S. Senate, Special Committee on Aging, 1985, "America in Transition:  An Aging Society," Serial No. 99-B, U.S. Government Printing Office, Washington, D.C.

ENVIRONMENTAL DESIGN AND MENTALLY IMPAIRED OLDER PEOPLE

Lorraine G. Hiatt

Consultant in Environmental Psychology/Gerontology
200 West 79th St.
New York City, NY 10024

INTRODUCTION

Not so long ago, it was assumed that only fully alert older people
could respond to their physical surroundings. "She's too 'far gone' to
care what the room looks like," was voiced by those I encountered on study
tours of several hundred U.S. institutions.

On more recent site visits I have met administrators and caregivers
who are curious about how the environment may interact with the behavior
of mentally impaired older people and how physical premises might be
coordinated with programs of care.

The purpose of this chapter is 1) to outline some issues in care of
older adults who are mentally impaired, particularly by Alzheimer's
disease (Alzheimer, 1981; Miller & Cohen, 1981; Katzman, Terry & Bick,
1978) and 2) to relate research on the capacities as well as the needs of
people with cognitive impairments to facility and interior design.

WHAT ARE "ENVIRONMENTAL CONSIDERATIONS?"

A first step in using environments effectively is to understand the
many elements which define the term and which influence human responses.

Environmental psychology, a branch of social science, focuses upon
the interactions between people and their surroundings (Ittelson, Rivlin,
Proshansky & Winkel,1974; Stokols, 1978; Sommer, 1969). One contribution
of environmental psychology has been to help health professionals
recognize that there are elements outside of the individual's diagnosis or
disease which may contribute to one's feelings, well-being (Lawton, 1982)
and ability to remember (Fozard, 1981). Behavioral scientists and
caregivers used to think that difficulties in recall were primarily the
result of organic changes. More recently, researchers have suggested that
while organic changes may indeed exist, features of the physical and
social environment itself may contribute to diminishing attention span or
to apparent problems in recall (Cohen & Wu, 1980; Siegler, 1980).

What is the physical environment? The physical environment may include a variety of resources. Sights such as outlines, contours or shapes, colors, contrasts or movement and light (brightness, dimness, directness or natural and mechanical); sounds; textures ranging from roughness/smoothness and moistness to weight; temperature; and smells. Elements of the physical environment include qualities of air (breeziness, stillness, freshness, or pollen count). The physical environment usually refers to many characteristics of space itself: length and width of floor areas, volume or ceiling height, relative openness or fenestration and objects ranging from furnishings to clothing and possessions. All of these elements are resources in environmental design.

Caregivers of memory impaired persons may be more familiar with another aspect of settings, the social environment. The social environment may be thought of as the numbers of people who occupy a space, their characteristics and activities, their positional relationships to each other, and their effects upon each other.

Beyond the social and physical aspects of environments, individuals harbor many psychological responses to settings (Howell, 1980a, 1980b). These are a function of cultural, social, geographic and economic factors which subtly influence likes, feelings and preferences. Typically, caregivers have little control over these aspects of an older person's (or any person's) environmental responses. Knowledge of the individual's preferences and environmental history may, however, be useful in understanding patterns of behavior.

Environments are also characterized by norms or expectations and policies (Parr, 1980). Caregivers, or perhaps managers, have a great deal of influence over norms. Examples of environmental norms influencing mentally impaired older people include 1) the distance or area a person is allowed to roam; 2) possessions permitted and whether they can be placed on walls; 3) practices regarding use/non-use of restraint; and 4) what is expected of or taught to mentally impaired persons.

How an individual older person experiences the environment may require a special understanding of the person: knowledge of the physical and social aspects of a place, a person's preferences and the setting's norms will not sufficiently predict personal reactions to surroundings. The responses of older people to settings is likely to be affected by interacting physical and mental capabilities (Fozard & Popkin, 1979). Perceptual abilities of older people in terms of vision, hearing, olfactory sensitivity, touch and kinesthesis, locomotion and balance may all be influential. Individual differences in physical and perceptual skills may alter the effects of space, light, sounds and people on behavior (Fozard, 1980, 1981). Like personal responses, knowledge of 1) how older people normatively respond to environmental stimuli and 2) how a particular person responds may both be useful in developing care plans and in design.

While defining environments and qualifying environmental responses on so many levels may at first seem overwhelming, differentiating physical, social, psychological issues from environmental norms may reveal clues to behavior (Parr, 1980). Researchers working in retirement facilities suggest that even the very confused individual typically responds to selected attributes of the physical and social environment (Rosenfield, 1978; Lawton, 1981) though mentally impaired older people may not attribute their reactions to design.

ENVIRONMENTS AND THE BEHAVIOR OF MENTALLY IMPAIRED OLDER PEOPLE

Environments may...

1) help elicit appropriate behaviors by conveying expectations;
2) minimize agitation or belligerence by providing exercise and energy outlets; (Sawyer & Mendlovitz, 1982; 1984).
3) provide comfort and security through features, textures, spatial configuration and orchestration of stimuli;
4) evoke cognitive development (as manipulation of textures and utensils contribute to language development in children); (Vygotsky, 1978);
5) cue or prompt recollections such as wayfinding, or externalizing memory so one need not rely solely on mental recall;
6) assist one in locating self in time (as using photo collections or museum tours or halls as a "memory lane");
7) arouse or stimulate awareness and pique curiosity by providing variety and the freedom to explore action, changes, surfaces and details;
8) connect one with other people, living things (animals and plants), places, times and personal experiences (through use of icons, actual stimuli and personal possessions); and, perhaps most important:
9) structure attention span and
10) shift emotional states (i.e., discharge anger and sadness) when speaking or other conventional means are untenable.

Mental impairment is probably not caused by environmental design, however, some of the confused behavior that is problematic for caregivers and for the individual may be exacerbated by inappropriately detailed physical and social environments.

Consider the case of the wanderer. By understanding his/her life history we may find that personal expression through movement was a common lifestyle attribute of the person (Monsour & Robb, 1980; Hiatt, 1985). However, institutional life and even home care may define pacing and puttering, fidgeting and fingering as atypical and problematic. In observing perhaps a hundred wanderers in the past fifteen years, I have come to respect some as problem solvers. The motion serves as a coping mechanism. What makes wandering difficult is the risk of a person out of control. The environment could be restructured to facilitate expression, support the individual's need for movement, stimulation and exercise, and provide the safety and security required. I am equally concerned about the 89% of the average nursing homes who do not move more than 4% of their wakeful hours (Snyder, et al., 1978) as the 11% who wander. (Runaways are another issue, Hiatt, 1985.)

Before caregivers exploit the potential of environments, they need to think functionally about older people-- that is, to begin to enumerate what older people with cognitive deficits can do (Morscheck, 1984; Mace, 1984). The point is that the physical and social environment is more than a backdrop in mental function. Sometimes environments act upon the individual's mood states. Other times, the setting serves as a prop, connecting a person to present circumstances.

WHY HAVE ENVIRONMENTS BEEN OVERLOOKED?

Sometimes environments are overlooked out of sheer ignorance. Well trained professionals of one discipline may have had no introduction to environmental issues. Only recently have nursing texts in gerontology, for example, begun to address environmental design (Burnside, 1980).

Few measures of mental functioning include specific questions about previous environments (Monsour & Robb, 1980; Hiatt, 1985). As a consequence, much of the science of health, psychology, gerontology and even social work has overlooked the interactions between older people and their settings (Howell, 1980a,b; Fozard & Popkin, 1979).

A DESIGN AGENDA FOR THOSE PROVIDING CARE TO MEMORY IMPAIRED PEOPLE

What are the issues in environmental design for mentally impaired older people?

1. Expand the potential of the sensory environment (Marsh, 1980; Fozard & Popkin, 1979).
     a. Minimize noxious stimuli such as background noise, glare, shadow and dimness;
     b. Increase lighting on tasks that require concentration: eating, dressing, focused conversation;
     c. Rely on textural variety and touchable surfaces within reach of the individual(s) for stimulation that younger people may be able to obtain from people or visual design features such as color.

2. Provide opportunities for energy outlet and for exercise.
     a. Fresh air, a walk or changes in scenery may allow one to vent emotions when speaking or other conventional means of communication are difficult;
     b. Physical exercise, whether in formal groups (using objects like balls, parachutes or balloons) or motor release through safely selected rocking, swiveling or bouncing chairs may all help people deal with agitation.
     c. Walking can be very therapeutic. Where can it occur for memory impaired people and how can assistance be provided to minimize the risks to those who are unsteady?

3. Stimulate the sense of touch and need to clutch (Hiatt, 1980c).
     a. Surfaces of walls (fire rated carpeting, for example), materials for pillows or chairs, and finger foods may all satisfy the needs of touching, manipulating and holding. Therapeutic gardening, bathing, grooming the scalp, massaging back or feet, and applying hand lotions are other sources of textural stimulation.
     b. Human and animal contact are also viable sources of stimulation and are central to the emotional comfort of some individuals.
     c. Some tactile-motor experiences need to be developed to allow for violent, aggressive, exuberant non-verbal expression of frustration. What can be tugged, dug, torn, socked, smashed, struck, thwarted or squeezed? Demented individuals need acceptable means of venting anger.

4. Develop a specific program for orientation to place and to build up wayfinding skills (Hiatt, 1980a).
     a. Research on spatial orientation suggests that some people have never had good directional sense. Actual experience-- seeing the building from the outside, approaching from many angles-- can be helpful.
     b. Wayfinding refers to the ability to successfully get to an intended destination by using a planned and efficient method. Landmarks and practice may facilitate wayfinding and comfort those who are concerned about being lost or are proud of their independence.
     c. Places are more difficult to image or locate when they have unclear names or when names are not coordinated with signs. Name rooms and halls with familiar terms. Link names with landmarks or geography rather than obscuring them in the jargon of health care. Use the names in conversations, written materials and signs.

d. Like the barber pole to a barber shop or mail box to a post office, meaningful objects need to be coupled with significant places. Actual objects may be more helpful than abstract graphics or symbols. These landmarks need to be detectable from a distance (name plates may be useful as one gets closer to verify). Actual people (volunteers or staff in an institution) may be the best, most believable sources of information of all.

e. To minimize problem rummaging, camouflage features that should not attract the attention of the curious. This may involve use of non-distinguishable colors, hidden doors or latches. Camouflaging is not likely to be distracting unless there are at the same time appropriate, interesting places for an individual to satisfy the needs of rummaging and exploration (Hiatt, 1980b).

5. Take stock of the social environment and its effects on responses of memory impaired older people.

a. The environment as a whole might consist of a range of social options: private spaces, spaces for dyads or intimacy, spaces for family-sized groups, for classroom sized groups, and spaces for full assembly (DeLong, 1970; Snyder, 1978; Hiatt, 1983; Pastalan, 1986). Each individual typically needs some time out and some time in the company of others. An individual can often benefit from 15-45 minutes off a unit or away from a fragmented social situation-- as can caregivers.

b. Crowding or density may be problematic for some impaired older people. Too many people, especially too many similarly impaired people may contribute to heightened confusion for all. Consider ways of working with small groups, perhaps six to eight rather than 25-40 persons. This can be especially useful in dining, where the distractions of many other individuals may interrupt dining or self-feeding.

6. Use objects and possessions to cue and evoke behavior.

a. Personal objects, from familiar possessions to sounds, smells and images may all stimulate memory and encourage thinking. The environment needs to afford a safe place to hang, display or keep the objects. High shelves, tackable walls or glass cases are all possible methods of keeping items available yet safe.

b. Encourage areas where exhibits of objects may be presented and may change (this is different from using landmarks which should be stable and predictable).

c. Use objects as decorative features to extend the value of color in evoking responses and creating a "mood" (Hiatt, 1980b).

d. For particularly demanding activities of daily living, consider the use of familiar utensils or tools with a familiar way of operating. Dial clocks may work better for some than do digital ones; toilets with a conventionally placed handle are more likely to be flushed. Eating utensils of familiar weight such as cups and forks may be easier to use than styrofoam and plastic. There is a place for specially designed objects, such as those that make eating easier for one with palsy or impaired grip, but look for implements that do not challenge long-held process memories.

7. Consider the potential for rooms and places as a whole to help people shift moods or lift spirits.

a. People of many ages use a change of surroundings to stimulate fresh thinking. Develop the potential for in-house or nearby spiritual vacations, such that the environment may reach a person who is not responding to group work or other direct communications.

b. In institutions, some of the spaces that can be developed for these purposes are bedrooms (for solitude and "one-li-ness"), parlors and living rooms (for action and socialization); hallways (for exercise and perhaps manual exploration of a tactile "museum"); courtyards and secure but unusually shaped outdoor areas (for meandering and visiting); bathing rooms (which could be far less institutional and more relaxing through the use of familiar objects, textural variety, color accents and vestibular stimulation) (Snyder, 1978; Hiatt, 1980b, 1983).

8. Take advantage of natural inclinations and remembered responses.
    a. Even many confused people tend to respond to odors. The physical environment can provoke memories by providing natural odors: yeast breads, cocoa, familiar spices, popcorn, etc. Often odors are masked by body processes, by smelly pharmaceuticals and by cleaning supplies that are thought to clean better the worse they smell.
    b. Children, pets and a range of new and familiar (especially peer-group aged) faces may all be social stimulants to behavior.

9. Reinforce a positive self-image.
    a. Photographs and sounds may be useful in putting people back in touch with themselves. The environment needs to make these elements appropriately significant rather than overshadow them with excessive or distracting design features.
    b. Beauty parlors or "head shops" and physical therapy spaces could be a haven for body images which reinforce dignity of age. Other locations might become the sites of emotionally appealing images: the interactions of older people and children, humor, powerful emotions; cultural attachments (patriotism, faith, healing, former ways); and local pride. Images, sounds and textures or scenarios of these experiences may be useful as decorative details and to provide stimulus for individual expression and group work.

WHAT ABOUT SPECIAL UNITS?

Special units allow the organization to focus scarce resources on staff training, on a special group of people, and in an identifiable space. It gives the service some recognition value, and with that comes prestige. In an existing facility, one can focus special design amenities such as security features on a small area. The question of whether there is value in isolating mentally impaired people from their peers has not been well researched and continues to be controversial.

Special units presume that someone is skilled at identifying people who have Alzheimer's disease. As of this writing, diagnoses are still deductions based upon ruling out other factors (Jarvik, 1980). Policies and norms regarding special units may presume people do not change; they do. Special units may isolate staff on that unit from their peers and require special measures to overcome the feeling of extra burden that may result. Special units may become unduly enclosed and confining.

There are alternatives to special units. The Masonic Home of Wallingford, CT and Villa Maria Nursing Home, Fargo, ND have developed in-house daycare programs. People from different parts of the building come together for special services catering to their needs and strengths. Design resources were focused on one room serving some people for an hour and others for longer stretches. An "off-unit program" was developed in conjunction with a special unit by Sawyer Mendlovitz (1983).

GROUPING BY ABILITY

Special units beg the question of the value of grouping demented individuals. Grouping by ability is a choice, not a mandate. I have seen successful programs operated with people co-mingled by ability and successful programs for those grouped by similar needs. In fact, clustering by abilities is often a phase in organizational maturation. A few years after establishing special units, sponsors may find that nursing staff become attached to some residents and fail to refer them up or down the continuum.

As the population "matures" or ages and the institution becomes more skilled at and convinced of the value of services to each of its populations, the features of one unit are generalized to others and distinctions are muted. The question of grouping might better be based upon sleep cycles, sensitivity to verbalization, activity patterns, personalities, programs and staffing. Ideally, families might become adept at selecting the social and physical context most in keeping with the behavioral needs of the older person.

The extreme of integration, where people of diverse abilities dwell throughout a building, risks overlooking special needs of the mentally impaired or remanding the confused person to more time alone with no special services or attention. Institutional size may be a really significant issue here (Hiatt, 1985), because the mentally impaired person may be more easily "lost" in large and diversified organizations where smaller institutions (under 60 beds) may be more effective at dealing with the diversity.

Caution. Separation by ability does not constitute a program! The provision of unit for people of similar diagnoses, even if a few extra hours of traditional nursing assistant services are added, does not mean that there are special services. I have toured special units where motion is controlled (through the use of geriatric wheelchairs and restraints) and/or where boredom is rampant, fragmented behavior is tolerated and the normal stimuli and institutional activities are limited.


GROUP OR UNIT SIZE

One of the major long-term drawbacks of special units may be inherent in decisions regarding size. The practice of identifying a floor of perhaps 35 beds in a traditional design and making that the special unit locks one into administrative needs of finding 35 occupants.

It is my impression that:

1. Older memory impaired people need to spend significant portions of the day in smaller groups of 3-10 people. Groups larger than ten often sap attention span. There are exceptions: festivals, religious services, exercise groups (follow-along), dances, parties and music participation may all be effective for larger groups. Confining too many people of similar needs to one area without adequate small group focal points or with only the television as stimulation precludes the potential for role modeling and possibilities for interaction.

2. Larger units (35 or so) are workable when a) the majority of residents have private rooms; 2) there are at least two and perhaps three options for socializing (i.e., a dining room separate from a living room); and 3) the living and dining rooms are designed to encourage small

clusters of 6-8 people, with options for 1, 2 or 3. The space may be defined by moveable furniture such as high backed wing chairs. An example of this approach exists at Golden Acres, Dallas Jewish Home and Hospital for the Aged.

3. An alternative plan is to devise small clusters, groups of 9-12 individuals living in a circumscribed area who may take some meals in that area and have some programs and meals elsewhere. Cluster plans would also accommodate many different models of caregiving: grouping people of like needs, intermingling and focusing units on other timely issues such as stroke rehabilitation. The overall architectural design may then eliminate the hospital-like character of many nursing homes. Cluster designs have been used for years in psychiatric and rehabilitation centers. Cluster designs are being developed for the Hebrew Home and Hospital of Jersey City and Glacier Hills, Ann Arbor, MI.

Architecture, design and the issue of special units needs to follow function. 1) What types of people does the institution serve? 2) How many, on the average, of each type? 3) What types of programs does the institution have in place for its population as a whole? How might these be meaningfully extended to people with cognitive impairments? (A facility that is not doing a good job with its mainstream residents is unlikely to shine at caring for mentally impaired people merely by creating a special unit.) 4) Does the organization serve people with a range of mental impairments? Do its activities serve people all along the continuum? 5) How large is the organization and how large a proportion are the cognitively impaired people? How large should the service or unit for memory impaired people be? 6) Do people have the option of interacting with those of different abilities (or have the organization's caveats and norms made this impossible)?

A special unit should not mean that the population is confined to one set of spaces and programs offered only on the unit. Opportunities for frequent (daily) adventures off the unit and outside are essential to emotional well-being and may optimize cognitive functioning.


CAVEATS AND CAUTIONS: RECOGNIZING WHAT WE DO NOT KNOW AND CANNOT DO

We have no evidence that there are "perfect" environments. I resist a single prescription for design due to the variations in community size, former social and architectural experience and lifestyles.

Environmental design involves functioning with a series of paradoxes:

-a person may need stimulation yet be confused by too much;
-sound may be soothing at some times and cacophonous at others
-features should change enough to stimulate curiosity but total change may be unsettling;
-familiar images, motifs and design may be useful in reminiscence but should be balanced by features or programs that reflect present times and culture;
-exercise and motion can be beneficial but may also be risky;
-contact with other people may be stimulating and satisfying; too many other people, people for too long a time, or too dense a situation (people per available space) may be disturbing;
-simple building layouts may make wayfinding easier but may also facilitate the wanderer's slipping away;
-some familiar, traditional and even "historic" objects and images will be useful; contemporary implements and utensils may be easier in some respects but unacceptable in others...

316

Rather than look for one established layout, it might be better to begin creating environments which are tolerant of paradox for frail, mentally impaired older people. In the 18,000+ existing U.S. nursing homes, this might involve working at the level of objects, surfaces, furniture, utensils and decor and using technology to compensate for building inequities such as too many exits.


HOW

For institutions and for families, "how" may be as significant an issue as "what". How should changes be introduced and who should be involved? We have little research on these processes. Drawing on consultation experience, I would suggest the following:

1. Set up a systematic way of addressing environmental design: an advocate, a knowledgeable team, etc.
2. Define individuals in behavioral and functional terms, addressing topics such as socializing abilities, style of recall, sources of agitation, motor behavior, attention span, wayfinding skills, awareness of time, activity patterns, and facility with activities of daily living.
3. Take a position to limit the use of pharmaceuticals and physical restraints. Develop policies to deal with risk management so that the direct caregivers are not unduly restricting expression and motion in an effort to protect themselves.
4. Work as a team, seeking solutions involving interdisciplinary teams. Mental impairment is not just a nursing issue any more than environmental design is just a maintenance and housekeeping concern.
5. Assess what the setting does to enhance the strengths and evoke the weaknesses of the individual.
6. Plan changes; involve key caregivers of all shifts in the discussion, not just in the actions.
7. Time changes with a ceremony or formal event: rather than rearrange furniture in the night, do it in conjunction with a party. Anticipate, celebrate, report and reflect on changes to walls, rooms, objects, etc.
8. Document and evaluate. Enter into environmental design decisions with the idea that they can be evaluated and changed rather than that they are fixed for all time.
9. Be eclectic. Rely on multiple sources and upon the best quality research available.
10. Share and disseminate; look for those who are doing the same. Open up for outside evaluation. Don't expect to apply the features (or programs) of other organizations without some adaptation.

We need models that fit together people, services, programs, designs and costs, regulations, geographic variations and personal choice (Hiatt, 1986). The public and professionals alike need to be able to visit, study and viscerally understand holistic approaches to care. The idea that it is possible to do something for the individual in early to later stages of mental deterioration is still quite challenging to many caregivers and sponsors. What is innovative in design results from the increase in attention to people and to programs and a general dissatisfaction with custodial care and detached design.

REFERENCES

Alzheimer's disease, A mini-conference report of the 1981 White House Conference on Aging, Washington, DC: U.S. Government Printing Office, 1981.

Burnside, I., 1980, "Psychosocial Nursing Care of the Aged," McGraw Hill, New York.

Cohen, D., and Wu, S., 1980, Language cognition during aging, in: "Annual Review of Gerontology and Geriatrics, C. Eisdorfer, ed., Springer, New York.

DeLong, A.J., 1970, The micro-spatial behavior of the older person: Some implications of planning the social and spatioal environment, in: "Spatial Behavior of Older People," L.A. Pastalan and D.H. Carson, ed., University of Michigan, Ann Arbor.

Fozard, J.L., 1981, Person-environment relationships in adulthood: Implications for human factorsd engineering, Human Factors, 23 (1):7-27.

Hiatt, L.G., 1981, Color and care: The selection and use of colors in environments for older people, Nursing Homes, 30 (3):18-22.

Hiatt, L.G., 1980, Disorientation is more than a state of mind. Nursing Homes, 29 (4): 30-36.

Hiatt, L.G., 1983, Effective design for informal conversation, American Health Care Association Journal, 9 (2): 43-46.

Hiatt, L., 1980b, The happy wanderer, Nursing Homes, 29 (2): 27-31.

Hiatt, L., 1980c, Touchy about touching, Nursing Homes, 29 (6): 42-46.

Hiatt, L., 1985, Wandering behavior of older people, (Doctoral dissertation, Graduate Center, City University of New York), Dissertation Abstracts International, 46: 86-01, 653.

Hiatt, L., 1986, Well-being and the elderly: An holistic view, Physical and Mental Health of the Elderly, American Association of Homes for the Aging, Washington, D.C.

Howell, S., 1980a, Environments and Aging, Annual Review of Gerontology and Geriatrics, 237-260.

Howell, S., 1980b, Environments as hypotheses in human aging research, in: "Aging in the 1980's," L.W. Poon, ed., American Psychological Association, Washington D.C.

Ittelson, Rivlin, Proshanskyt and Winkel, 1974, "An Introduction to Environmental Psychology," Holt, New York.

Jarvik, L., 1980, Diagnosis of dementia in the elderly: A 1980 perspective, in: "Annual Review of Gerontology and Geriatrics," C. Eisdorfer, ed., Springer, New York.

Katzman, R., Terry, R.D., Bick, K., 1978, "Alzheimer's disease: Senile dementia and related disorders," Raven Press, New York.

Lawton, M.P., 1985, An introduction and overview to environment, Bride Institute Journal of Long-Term Home Health Care, 4:1-11.

Lawton, M.P., 1982, Competence, environmental press and the adaptation of older people, in: "Aging and the Environment," M.P. Lawton, P. Windley, and T. Byerts, eds., Springer, New York.

Lawton, M.P., 1979, Introduction: A background for the environmental study of aging, in: "Environmental Context of Aging," T.O. Byerts, S.C., Howell and L.A. Pastalan, eds., Garland, New York.

Lawton, M.P., 1981, Sensory deprivation and the effects of the environment on management of the senile dementia patient, in: "Clinical Aspects of Alzheimer's Disease and Senile Dementia," N.E. Miller and G.D. Cohen, eds., Raven Press, New York.

Mace, N., 1984, Report of a survey of day care centers, Pride Institute Journal, 3 (4): 38-43.

Marsh, G.R., 1980, Perceptual changes with age, in: "Handbook of Geriatric Psychiatry," E.W. Busse and D.G. Blazer, eds., Van Nostrand, New York.

Miller, N.E., and Cohen, G.D., 1981, "Clinical Aspects of Alzheimer's Disease and Senile Dementia," Raven Press, New York.

Monsour, N., and Robb, S., 1980, Wandering behavior in old age: A pscho-social study, Social Work, 27(5): 411-416.

Morscheck, P., 1984, Introduction: An overview of Alzheimer's disease and long term care, Pride Institute Journal, 3(4): 4-10.

Parr, J., 1980, The interaction of persons and living environments, in: "Aging in the 1980's," L. Poon, ed., American Psychological Association, Washington, D.C.

Pastalan, L., 1986, Six principles for a caring enviornment, Provider, 12 (4): 4-5.

Rosenfield, A., 1978, "New Views on Older Lives," National Institute of Mental Health, Rockville.

Sawyer, J., and Mendlovitz, A., 1984, Alzheimer's program progress report. Paper presented at the 1984 Annual Meetings, American Association of Homes for the Aging, San Antonio, TX.

Sawyer, J., and Mendlovitz, A., 1982, A management program for ambulatory institutionalized patients with Alzheimer's disease and related disorders. Paper presented at the Annual Meeting, Gerontological Society, Boston, MA.

Siegler, I.D., 1980, The psychology of adult development and aging, in: "Handbook of Geriatric Psychiatry," E. Busse and D. Blazer, eds., Van Nostrand.

Snyder, L.H., 1978, Environmental changes for socialization, Journal of Nursing Administration, 8(1): 44-50.

Synder, L.H., 1975, Living environments, geriatric wheelchairs and older persons' rehabilitation, Journal of Gerontological Nursing, 1 (5): 17-20.

Synder, L.H., Pyrek, J., and Smith, K.C., 1976, Vision and mental function of older people, Gerontologist, 16 (3): 491-495.

Synder, L.H., Rupprecht, P., Purek, J., and Smith, K.C., 1978, Wandering, Gerontologist, 18 (3): 491-495.

Sommer, R., 1969, "Personal Space," Prentice Hall, Englewood Cliffs, NJ.

Stokols, 1978, Environmental psychology, <u>Annual Review of Psychology</u>, 29: 253-295.

Vygotsky, L.S., 1978, "Mind in Society," Harvard University Press, Cambridge.

OVERCOMING PROBLEMS IN MODIFYING THE ENVIRONMENT

Dorothy H. Coons

Director, Alzheimer's Disease Projects
Institute of Gerontology
University of Michigan
Ann Arbor, Michigan

INTRODUCTION

Some biomedical scientists are predicting that it will be least fifteen more years before researchers discover the cause of, and the possible clinical treatment for, Alzheimer's disease. The fact that many nursing homes and other care settings are, at present, ill equipped to meet the needs of this special group of elderly persons compounds the situation even further. One part of a national study by the Institute of Gerontology, The University of Michigan (Coons, et al., 1983), entitled <u>Alzheimer's Disease: Subjective Experiences of Families</u> and completed in 1983, dealt with families' experiences with nursing homes. In listing problems, many felt that staff were not adequately trained to work with persons with Alzheimer's disease. We are now faced with the need to examine alternatives and explore new and innovative approaches that will provide a better quality of life for this vulnerable group and ease the distress of families who need to seek help.

For a number of years the Institute of Gerontology has been involved in the study of environmental interventions to determine ways to improve the quality of life for the long-term institutionalized elderly. In our studies, the term "environment" has been defined in the broadest sense to include all aspects of the milieu which may have impact on behaviors and on the individual's sense of well-being. With this definition, the physical environment, the staff, the opportunities to continue in normal social roles, families and friends, and the residents themselves, all are considered to have influence on the quality of the milieu.

To learn more about the type of environment that would be most therapeutic for persons with dementia, the Institute of Gerontology and the Chelsea United Methodist Retirement Home (Chelsea, Michigan) undertook a two-year project[1] which was completed in December of 1985. The investigators

---

[1]Other project staff of the Institute of Gerontology, The University of Michigan, who were involved in the development, administration, staff training, and evaluation of Wesley Hall included Anne Robinson, Director of Wesley Hall Project; Beth Spencer, Program Consultant; and Shelly F. Weaverdyck, Neuropsychology Consultant. The physician for the project was James F. Peggs, M.D., Medical Director, University of Michigan Family Practice Center and the Chelsea United Methodist Retirement Home.

designed a special living area called Wesley Hall for 9 women and 2 men diagnosed as having Alzheimer's disease or related dementias. The residents all had severe memory problems, were relatively well physically, and were ambulatory. On tests to determine their degree of impairment, they scored in the range of, or bordering on, the severely impaired.

The Wesley Hall residents had, before the establishment of the area, lived in the large retirement home where they were having serious difficulties. The wandering, incontinence, and combativeness which some displayed were resented by well residents whose reactions only increased the problems and aggravated the behaviors of the impaired persons. The residents made many changes after they moved to Wesley Hall. Incontinence, wandering, and combativeness were all reduced. There was an increase in verbal skills and an improvement in the personal appearance of most residents.

The concepts on which the project was based, staff approaches, special techniques such as task breakdown, and the designing of appropriate activities are discussed elsewhere (Coons, 1986; Coons and Weaverdyck, 1986; Misplon and Metzelaar, 1980). This paper will focus on the physical environment and on the rationale for the changes made. While much of this paper will refer to institutional settings, many of the interventions discussed are also applicable in the home situation.


THE PHYSICAL ENVIRONMENT

The alterations made in the physical environment on Wesley Hall were influenced by earlier research by the Institute of Gerontology (Coons, 1983) and by the works of others, such as Hiatt (1979, 1981, 1982), Lawton (1980), and Pastalan (1979).

The changes took into account the special needs of persons with dementia, recognizing specifically that the physical environment should:

1. provide a variety of cues to compensate for the problems of orientation;

2. accommodate sensory loss;

3. take into account the spatial problems some individuals have;

4. provide safety features and still ensure freedom to move about;

5. produce an environment that gives visual stimulation;

6. enable persons to continue in social roles that had been a part of their earlier lives;

7. offer a small, intimate home-like environment which eliminates, to the extent possible, the emphasis on illness;

8. bring about behavioral changes;

9. provide features which reestablishes individuality and a sense of ownership in his or her surroundings.

Many of the interventions described below respond to one specific need, but others served a variety of purposes.

322

## Orientation

Because orientation can be a major problem for persons with dementia whether they are at home or in institutional settings, a variety of interventions were tested. For individuals who could still read, directional signs helped them locate areas. The residents themselves were helpful in the selection of colors and lettering. Signs with different backgrounds and types of lettering were hung and several of the residents were asked to read them. There were decided differences in their abilities to comprehend words from one sign to another. Signs were finally done in a dark matte brown with white, clean, well-spaced lettering. The importance of terminology became apparent when labels were applied to kitchen drawers and cupboards. The sign "mugs" was placed on the cupboard containing coffee mugs. There was puzzlement over the word with one women pointing to her face, seeming to question if there was any connection between the label and the old fashioned slang word for face. The label was replaced with the word "cups" and the problem was solved.

Small awnings (blue for men and red for women) were placed over the bathroom doors to give residents additional help in locating them. It became obvious that some were associating the awnings with the bathrooms when one woman was overheard to say, in her efforts to help another, "Go down to that red 'light' (meaning awning)."

## Sensory Loss

Sensory loss is often a crucial problem in old age, and it may be especially so with persons with dementia. Those with hearing loss may easily be described as out of touch or disoriented; those who have difficulty seeing, especially in poorly lit areas, often must grope or move cautiously in their efforts to feel their way. This too can be interpreted as evidence of mental impairment.

Ceilings on Wesley Hall were lowered and lighting was more than doubled to assist those with sight problems. Carpeting was installed and the facility's intercom was disconnected to reduce noise. In the first several weeks before the intercom was disconnected, it became evident how disturbing the crackly noise was to residents. They would stop, become agitated, and look around frantically for the person who might be the source of the indecipherable words.

## Spatial Problems

The spatial problems some impaired persons experience are especially handicapping, sometimes affecting language as well as their ability to function. Hodge (1984) points out that "there is some controversy as to whether demented patients are truly dysphasic or have difficulty naming objects due to difficulties in recognizing them." This question has implications for designing treatment approaches for persons who have difficulty in locating items needed in activities of daily living.

Mrs. J. in the Wesley Hall study was still able to brush her teeth, but special arrangements had to be made. If the counter top contained a variety of items, her hands would move from one item to another. She seemed unable to locate her toothbrush and was uncertain about what she was expected to do. As Hodge suggests, the question was whether she was unable to see the toothbrush or whether she could no longer identify it. Staff learned quickly that a bare counter top was essential. The staff person would first place Mrs. J's hands on the lavatory edge and say, "I'll help you brush your teeth now." She would then place the tooth brush with tooth paste already applied in Mrs. J's hand and she was able to brush. She could no longer apply the tooth paste or rinse without reminding, but she seemed to take pleasure in being able to accomplish even a limited part of the task.

A number of changes were made environmentally on Wesley Hall to provide help with these spatial problems. The men's bathroom was redecorated, and the women's bathroom was totally redone. Lighting was increased, and blue fixtures, contrasting with yellow counters and matte tile walls and floors, were installed. In the dining room, white plates with dark blue borders were selected to help persons determine the perimeter of their plates. Plain placemats in the bright basic colors of blue, red or yellow were used to provide sharp contrast between plates and table.

## Safety

The essential measures to insure safety are imperative, of course. The challenge for care givers, whether at home or in treatment settings, is to protect the impaired person without stripping the individual of all freedom, of ability to function, and of dignity. Safety measures generally take a variety of forms in the current system of care, many of which may be more for the convenience of staff than protection for the person with dementia. Physical restraints and over medication are practices all too common in many nursing homes. Physical restraints, as an absolute last resort, may sometimes be essential for the protection of the individual, but it should be recognized that this is one of the most humiliating practices in institutional settings. It can cause great agitation, and it prevents the normal, healthful walking that is considered essential (Snyder et al., 1978). It also represents the power of staff and the infantilization that occurs in many settings. The story told by the daughter of a nursing home resident illustrates the attitudes that prevail in some settings. One day when she was visiting her mother, she asked a staff person why a man and women were sitting with their backs to the nursing station and tied in their chairs. Staff replied, "Charles and Mary have been a bad boy and girl, so they are getting punished." The daughter found out later that their transgressions had been a series of trips back and forth in the area's hallway. In a setting which provided no opportunities for resident involvement, this was the only activity that Charles and Mary could manage themselves.

In discussing ethical issues related to long-term care, Wetle (1985) laments that "the elderly in institutional settings are at particular risk of compromised autonomy in decision making. The very nature of the institutional setting reinforces negative feelings of dependence, encourages learned helplessness, and takes away from the individual all but the most trivial of decisions."

In the renovations of Wesley Hall, safety was carefully considered, but within the context of an unlocked area and with the expectations that residents would have access to all common space. A safety switch was installed on the stove and oven in the kitchen to prevent its being turned on without staff's knowledge. In order to reduce the focus on exit doors, they were painted to match the surrounding walls. This seemed to disguise them sufficiently that no one attempted to open them.

## Visual Stimulation

The milieu on Wesley Hall was designed also to provide visual stimulation. The traditional pastel paint was discarded in favor of figured wall paper in a number of areas. The kitchen, which was the center of much activity, was papered in white wall paper with a strawberry motif. Residents often pointed to the strawberries and made brief references to them. Wherever the basic colors of yellow, red, green, and blue could be tastefully incorporated, they were used to provide visual stimulation and better visibility for persons with poor eyesight.

Individualized door decorations and wall plaques to the left of each door with the name and an enlarged photograph of the individual added interest and also helped the individual to locate his or her room.

Slides were taken of many of the group activities and several were greatly enlarged and hung in the hallway to remind residents of their earlier involvement. They could be seen frequently together looking at the pictures and heard to comment as they were able.

A parakeet in the living room area and a fish tank in the den also were attractions. Residents fed the bird and the fishes with staff's help and the movement of the fishes and the flitting about and occasional song of the bird created a great deal of interest.

Several colorful mobiles added zest to the area and drew comments from residents from time to time. Each intervention was viewed as experimental, and any change which gave evidence of being non-therapeutic or disturbing was discarded. Visual stimulation proved to be effective and a means by which residents could still maintain contact and interact within the environment in positive ways.

Normal Social Roles

In designing therapeutic environments, Institute of Gerontology research has emphasized the need for the availability of normal social roles so that residents can continue to function and be involved in activities which had meaning to them in their earlier lives. The theory supports the idea that "roles prescribe the patterns of behavior which are socially acceptable for each position or function in a group of society. If, for example, the only available role is 'frail sick patient,' the individual will conform to the expectations embodied in that role. If, however, a number of normal nonsick social roles, such as friend, citizen, consumer, worker, or user of leisure time, are available and the individual is encouraged to choose freely among them, his or her behavior will be varied and far more therapeutic in its effects, than when it is prescribed by the sick role. These roles enable even the very frail to respond and to function in an environment which is nurturing and enabling" (Coons, 1983, 1986). With this concept in mind, the daily life on Wesley Hall was designed specifically to reinstate, to the extent possible, the roles of homemaker, family member, volunteer, and friend.

The greatest renovation was the conversion of one sleeping room to a small kitchen, with stove, refrigerator, coffee maker, popcorn popper, and a hand-crank ice cream maker. This gave a focus to their lives and enabled residents to do meaningful tasks that they had enjoyed in earlier years. The area became the center of many of the activities as residents, with the help of staff, prepared food or washed and dried dishes. Several were able to set the tables in the adjacent dining area.

Housekeeping and cleaning equipment were readily available and with the help of the housekeeper, some were able to make their beds, dust, or vacuum their rugs. Both the opportunity to be involved and the sharing of tasks with staff seemed to give them satisfaction and pleasure.

Home-Like Environment

Lawton (1981) in discussing the importance of the environment on persons with dementia states, "As individual competence decreases, the

environment assumes increasing importance in determining well-being.  One
corollary of this hypothesis is that the low-competent are increasingly
sensitive to noxious environments."  Normal social roles and a sense of well
being can hardly flourish in a setting designed after the medical model
which issues constant reminders that the individual is ill and living in an
institutional setting.  In contrast, a warm, homelike environment suggests
normalcy and deemphasizes illness.

In an effort to remove the reminders of institutional life, the decor
was altered to provide an area which was intimate, relaxing, and pleasant.
In addition to the improved lighting and wall paper, specially processed
carpeting was installed to help convert the area to a comfortable and
homelike setting.  There was no nursing station to build the clear and often
impregnable separation between residents and staff.  Staff did their
paperwork at a small desk in the kitchen or at tables in the dining area.
The telephone, bright red, was on the small white desk in the kitchen.  Two
of the residents were able to answer the phone and were taught to record
messages if staff were involved with others at the moment.  The two could
not remember the names of staff, but persons calling, who were familiar with
the area, could give a number and they were able to record it on a pad that
said, "Write down telephone numbers here."

The furniture throughout the area was selected to resemble a home.
Some of the chairs, tables, and a piano were donated by family members.
Each resident's room was individually furnished and decorated, often with
furniture, pictures, and other accessories from their own homes.  Uniform-
ity, characteristic of some settings, was considered inappropriate, non-
therapeutic, and depersonalizing.  Gradually residents began to identify the
area as their "home"; they could not recall the name of the facility or the
town they were in, but they had developed a sense of ownership in Wesley
Hall.

Behavioral Changes

A variety of interventions were tested in staff's efforts to respond to
difficult situations.  Some of the residents, for example, were particularly
resistive to bathing, and there may have been a number of reasons for this
resistance.  They may have believed, as they often said, that they had just
had a bath.  They might have been fearful of falling, or the tasks of
getting undressed and dressed might have seemed overwhelming.  Staff felt
that several of the residents were embarrassed to have someone else with
them when they were nude.  On other occasions, staff believed that they
could not comprehend what was being asked of them.

Coercion was not considered an appropriate approach on Wesley Hall, so
a variety of alternatives were considered.  A number of staff approaches
were tested, and, as with other interventions, some were effective, others
were effective part of the time, but not always, and some were never
effective.

A number of signs were tested to help residents through particularly
difficult situations.  For example, a calendar was posted in each of the
rooms of several who were consistently resistive to bathing.  After each
bath, staff marked the day the bath was taken and explained carefully that
this would help him or her to remember the date of the last bath.  When the
time for the next bath occurred, staff would point out the date of the last
one and explain it was time for the next one.  For several, this approach
reduced the anger and agitation that had occurred earlier when staff used
the direct approach of "It's time for your bath."

Several residents had periods when they searched frantically for relatives that they were sure had forsaken them even though they may have visited them a day or two before. Families were encouraged to write large legible notes to post on a relative's door. The note commented on the visit and what a good time they had had together. This proved very effective in reducing anxiety. It also gave staff a visual means of reassuring a disturbed resident.

Signs were also used to show appreciation for the help residents had given and to encourage involvement. A sign on the refrigerator said simply, "Thanks to _____, _____, and _____ for helping with the dishes today." Residents who recognized their names would often stop to look and occasionally point to it when visitors were present.

## Re-establishing Individuality

We can easily underestimate the potential of persons with dementia to feel and respond to the environment. Meacher (1972) in describing the confused elderly people in his study asserted that they could perceive their own loss of sensory powers and that of others. He found that they retained a sense of humor and could recognize ludicrousness and facetiousness. He stated further that they were disturbed by rejection and neglect and could often identify the subtle significance of social events. These conclusions parallel the findings in the Wesley Hall study.

Staff in treatment settings have the choice of providing a milieu which defines the disoriented elderly person as untreatable derelicts in our system of care, or as individuals who still have the capacity to respond and get pleasure and satisfaction from life. In the former, the individual soon becomes a non-person, learning quickly that he is sick and dependent. In the latter, with the proper interventions the older person can retain a sense of identity and self and maintain feelings of ownership in his or her environment.

Some of the changes on Wesley Hall helped residents maintain a linkage with the past. Many of the opportunities, discussed in other articles, were designed specifically to help residents continue in activities that had been important to them in earlier life. Some were able to manage tasks that had not been a part of their lives for several years. Certain features of the physical environment identified their earlier interests or types of employment. Individualized door decorations, for example, recognized that one of the women had been a life-long Detroit baseball fan. Her door sported a Tiger's pennant. The door of a former avid gardener had a basket of silk flowers, and a paper mâche loaf of bread bedecked the door of a woman who had loved to cook.

A map was hung on the wall in the hallway and flags were inserted indicating each resident's home town. This became the focus of a number of spontaneous discussions. Families were encouraged to develop photograph albums with labels of names or events, and, from time to time, staff or visitors would peruse the albums with residents. Even if they were usually unable to remember relatives or past events, they occasionally seemed to have moments of recognition.

## CONCLUSION

The emphasis in this paper is on the changes in the physical environment and their impact on the behaviors and sense of well being of residents. But these changes are not enough, because the physical environment is only one dynamic in the total milieu. On Wesley Hall, staff were carefully trained to individualize approaches and provide a supportive, relaxed environment; opportunities were introduced to enable residents to continue in normal social roles; families were helped to have pleasant and successful visits which could strengthen the feelings of kinship that may have been weakened in recent years.

It is the total environment, then, that has the potential for providing a quality of life for persons with dementia that can bring about a reduction of many of the difficult behaviors that have become a part of the stereotypical description of persons with Alzheimer's disease or other dementias. The milieu, not physical restraints and over medication, becomes the influencing factor that can reduce wandering, incontinence, and combativeness. The Wesley Hall project speaks for a need for an examination of many treatment practices that now prevail and a new look at what is possible.

REFERENCES

Coons, D.H., 1983, The therapeutic milieu, in: "Clinical Aspect of Aging," W. Reichel, ed., Wilkins, Baltimore.
Coons, D.H., Chenoweth, B., Hollenshead, C., and Spencer, B., 1983, "Final Report of Project on Alzheimer's Disease: Subjective Experiences of Families," Institute of Gerontology, The University of Michigan, Ann Arbor.
Coons, D.H., 1986, Designing a residential care unit for persons with dementia, Congressional Office of Technology Assessment, Washington, D.C., Contract #633-1950.0, (in press).
Coons, D.H., and Weaverdyck, S.E., 1986, Wesley Hall: A residential unit for persons with Alzheimer's disease and related disorders, Physical and Occupational Therapy in Geriatrics, 4:3.
Hiatt, L., 1979, Environmental considerations in understanding and designing for mentally impaired older people, in: "Mentally Impaired Aging: Bridging the Gap," H. McBride, ed., American Association of Homes for the Aging, Washington, D.C.
Hiatt, L., 1981, The color and use of color in environments of older people, Nursing Home, 30:18.
Hiatt, L., 1982, The importance of physical environments, Nursing Homes, 31:2.
Hodge, J., 1984, Toward behavioral analysis of dementia, in: "Psychological Approaches to the Care of the Elderly," I. Hanley and J. Hodge, eds., Croom Helm Australia Ltd., London and Sydney.
Lawton, M.P., 1981, Sensory deprivation and the effect of the environment on management of the patient with senile dementia, in: "Clinical Aspects of Alzheimer's Disease and Senile Dementia," N. Miller and A. Cohen, eds., Raven Press, New York.
Meacher, M., 1972, "Taken for a Ride," Longman Group Ltd., London.
Misplon, F. and Metzelaar, L., 1980, "Task Breakdown: A Teaching/Learning Technique Designed for working with the Elderly," Institute of Gerontology, The University of Michigan, Ann Arbor.
Pastalan, L., 1979, Sensory changes and environmental behaviors, in: "Environmental Context of Aging," T. Byerts, S. Howell, and L. Pastalan, eds., Garland STPM Press, New York.
Snyder, L.H., Rupprecht, P., Pyrek, J., Brekhus, S., and Moss, T., 1978, Wandering, The Gerontologist, 18:3.
Wetle, T., 1985, Ethical issues in long-term care of the aged, J.of Geriatric Psychiatry, 18:1.

WHEN TO DISCONTINUE HOME CARE:   THE CAREGIVING FAMILY'S DILEMMA

Virginia Bell

Sanders-Brown Research Center on Aging
University of Kentucky
Lexington, Kentucky 40536

The majority of persons with Alzheimer's disease (AD) live at home and receive care from a relative or friend.   There are little epidemiological data about these caregivers, but certain conclusions can be drawn from general data on the elderly population.   For example, the literature shows:

*Families care for at least as many disabled elderly as are being cared for in institutions (Brody et al., 1978).

*Families provide emotional support---the form of family help most cherished by the elderly (Shanas, 1979).

*Families provide more than 80% of needed financial and other help for community based elderly (Comptroller General, 1977).

*Families use formal support resources, such as home care aides and day care, to extend home care, thus delaying nursing home placement (Horowitz, 1985).

*Families do not dump their elderly into nursing homes.  Most often, institutional placement is preceded by prolonged, exhausting efforts to keep members in the community (Brody, 1969).

It is a myth that the family no longer cares.   The family gives more care, more difficult care, to more family members over a longer period of time than ever before.   Attitudes of the younger generation, which are clues to the future, show no weakening of the value that care of the elderly is a family responsibility (Brody, 1983).

The Family Coping With Alzheimer's Disease

Caring for an AD patient presents extraordinary difficulties as the disease progresses.  The patient not only requires assistance and supervision, but becomes increasingly impaired in language skills and social behavior.   Behaviors cited as causing serious problems are physical violence, incontinence, catastrophic reactions, belligerence, making accusations and suspiciousness (Rabins et al., 1982).   Caregiving becomes a 24 hour a day, 7 days a week marathon involving physical, emotional and financial stress.

In a study on the impact of dementia on the family, 87% of the caregivers interviewed cited being fatigued and depressed most of the time. Also, caregivers reported giving up friends and jobs and having little time for themselves. Feelings of guilt, worry, fear or illness themselves, fear of the patient and marital stress were also reported (Rabins et al., 1982).

Most caregivers are spouses. Often the spouse is old-old and very frail. AD is age related, but can appear as early as the 40's or 50's, while the spouse is still in the working force (Zarit et al., 1985).

The second most prevalent caregiver is an adult child, often a middle-aged adult, whose relief at having just finished caring for their own children is shattered by the new responsibility of caring for a demented parent. Even more traumatic is the adult child sandwiched between older children still at home and aging parents. The caregiver of a parent may also be retired; the old caring for the old-old (Zarit et al., 1985).

Other caregivers include in-laws, siblings, nieces and nephews, grandchildren and friends. A significant number of older people do not have a close family member. One in 20 (5.3%) of all people 65 and over are entirely kinless without spouse, children or siblings (National Center for Health Statistics, 1983).

Traditionally, women have been the caregivers, but many older men are now fulfilling this role. Learning how to manage a household for the first time and at the same time giving care to a demented family member can be very stressful.

## Range of Long-Term Care Facilities

Long-term care facilities range from small family care homes to large nursing homes with a full range of care, including personal, intermediate, and skilled nursing. However, most facilities are designed and operated on the basis of the medical needs of the frail dependent elderly. Throughout much of the disease process the AD patient is generally physically fit, presenting with only severe memory and cognitive deficits. The type of facility available is often not adequate or appropriate for the feeling and behaviors of an AD patient.

Few models of care especially designed for an AD patient are available for families seeking care outside the home. Preliminary studies on the dementia-specific facilities suggest that specialized management increases the quality of the patient's life and fosters "peace of mind" for the patient's family (Greene et al., 1985; Peppard, 1984). The AD patient has special needs and requires different care whether this care is given in the traditional nursing home or a dementia-specific facility.

## How Do Families Decide?

The family is complex unit. When trying to decide to discontinue home care of an AD patient it is not as simple as matching needs with facility. The decision is being made by a family with a long history. Variables unique to each family, such as size, number of available caregivers, caregiving demands, values and traditions, history of coping, socio-economic status, and community resources, all enter into a family's decision.

Each care-giving family can cope with a certain amount of stress but when pushed to the caregiving limits, the family often seeks care outside the home. However, defining and measuring this stress is very difficult for there is no clear relationship between the objective nature of caregiving, such as length or severity of problem and the degree of stress perceived by the family (Zarit et al., 1980). Caregivers differ from one another in their response to caregiving demands. Some are quickly and decisively overwhelmed and others quietly and stubbornly tackle any problem.

Functional rating scales designed to assist families and professionals in making the decision to discontinue home care must be used with caution. In a study by Hutton et al., (1985) using an informant-based functional scale, the three items most closely associated with nursing home placement were incontinence of bladder and bowel, inability to speak coherently, and inability to bathe and groom oneself.

Yet, a spouse giving 24-hour care to her non-verbal, incontinent husband in Kentucky, including bathing and dressing, literally gave up when confronted with an unlikely stressor; doctors had asked her to move a bed downstairs into her formal dining room when her husband could no longer negotiate the stairs. The thought of a hospital bed in the dining room was unacceptable. The three most likely predictors for nursing home placement were handled routinely by this spouse and an unlikely stressor pushed her beyond her caregiving limits.

Social support from family and friends is very important. Studies show that frequent visits and calls, giving "hands-on" care to provide respite to the caregiver and the existence of back-up relief, all are directly related to the family feeling less burdened (Zarit et al., 1980; Morycz, 1985). A family with strong social support is less likely to consider care outside the home.

Many families have an aversion to any institutional care. Visions of the old country poorhouse where family members were abandoned are still vivid. The traditions and values in a family may not permit the family to consider a care facility as a possibility even when it is evident that it would be best for patient and family. Families often consider care away from home only when the member is disoriented as to time and place and no longer recognizes family members.

Speaking to family members, fatigued and stressed by constant care, but unable to even consider institutional care, Dr. David Clark, Professor of Neurology at the University of Kentucky reminded them that they were already providing institutional care. Their institution has but one patient and they, as caregivers, provide all the services---nurse, counselor, telephone operator, chauffeur, financial secretary, business manager, patient monitor, cook, nutritionist aide, scrub person and case manager.

The cost of nursing home care is also a factor in a family's decision. Nursing home care is expensive. The costs may range from $17,000 to $30,000 per year (U.S. Congress, 1984). Families who can pay, may feel they need to protect the family's assets for various reasons and may not consider care in a nursing home. Families who qualify for Medicaid may decide to discontinue home care sooner than needed because they may receive more help from Medicaid in care outside the home.

Once a family makes the painful decision to discontinue home care, they are often shocked to be told that there are no available beds in the community. Long-term care facilities can be selective about filling their beds and keeping a patient once admitted (Brody et al., 1984).

At times, the family makes the decision to discontinue home care alone; other times the decision is made with the counsel of professionals or friends. Unfortunately, families most often make the decision in the worst possible way---in a crisis situation or as a last resort (Ory et al., 1985). Friends and extended family members who are not fully aware of the caregiving strain, often differ with the family's decision, causing added guilt and worry.

## Recommendations

Because the family is the primary caregiver of the AD patient today and the indications are that the family will continue to be the primary caregiver in the future, the following recommendations are suggested:

1. The whole story of each family must be known by caregiving professionals.

Each family coping with AD is unique and complex. There are many questions to ask: What is the make-up of the family size, geographic proximity, closeness in relationship, economic status, extended family network and social network? What values and traditions are woven into the fabric of the family? What has been the family's history of coping? What resources are available and how does the family feel about using these resources? It is difficult to guide a family in making major decisions without knowing the family.

2. The family must have the best information available related to their needs at each stage of care.

Given good information, most families are capable of making good decisions. Since AD affects every area of the family"s life, information and counsel from a professional team approach is suggested. Another source of conveying important information can be training sessions on all aspects of AD for the whole caregiving family network.

The danger of a family without correct information is that they may seize upon an option before it is necessary, out of fear, anger or anxiety about caring for an AD patient. Conversely, the decision may be delayed long beyond the time when the patient needs skilled care because of guilt, old problems, or a simple inability to let go (Meier, 1986).

3. More research is needed in all aspects of care and management of an AD patient. What we know about AD patients and their families has generally been based on small, nonrepresentative samples and thus should be considered suggestive, rather than definitive (Ory et al., 1985). It is often easy for both family and professionals to think in a straight line. The following are several preliminary studies on AD caregivers which suggest a departure from some formerly held assumptions:

*Caring for an AD patient does not always get worse. For many caregivers, the job gets easier over time, even though the patient's condition gets worse (Zarit, in press).

*Nursing home placement is not a cure-all for all the distress the family is experiencing. Preliminary studies show that there are no significant differences in mental health, stress symptoms and physical health between caregivers whose patients are in institutions and those caregivers whose patients live in their homes (George, 1983).

*Institutionalization is not inevitable. More caregivers than expected may be able to manage patients at home (Zarit and Zarit, 1983).

*Home care is not always better than nursing home care. It cannot be assumed that all AD patients are better off being cared for at home. Caregivers can be overwhelmed and the AD patient at home can be neglected (Brody et al., 1984).

4. The family must be supported adequately such as through formal support systems, support groups, in-home services, day care and other respite care programs, and appropriate long-term care facilities often are not available to families caring for an AD patient. A continuum of care must be available to help alleviate the pain and burden of care, often over a long period of time. The family should have good options to undergird their decisions. If the family desires home care, they should be supported with in-home services. When the family decides to discontinue home care, good care facilities must be available.

Society has a responsibility to help ease the burden of the family (the primary caregiver of the AD patient). An important role of any professional is to be an advocate for a support system which favors the family coping with AD.

The following demographic and social trends suggest that there is more need than ever for a support system for the family: increased geographic mobility; growing proportions of older people, especially among those 75 and older; decreased family size; changing sex roles, coupled with increased labor force penetration among middle-aged women; and a high rate of divorce and remarriage (Brody, 1983).

Much progress has been made in recent years in awareness of all aspects of AD. The Alzheimer's Disease and Related Disorders Association has been a strong force in this area, providing family support, research, public awareness, education and public policy. Alzheimer's Disease Research Centers have been established by the National Institute on Aging to further research in many areas of the disease. Seminars such as this one bring families and professionals together to discuss and plan for the future. Alzheimer's disease is not being ignored.

REFERENCES

Brody, E.M., Lawton, M.P. and Liebowitz, B., 1984, Senile dementia: Public policy and adequate institutional care, Am. J. Public Health, 74:1381-1383.

Brody, E.M., 1983, Testimony on the effects of Alzheimer's disease on caregiving families. Presented to the Committee on Energy and Commerce, Subcommitte on Health and the Environment, and the Select Committee on Aging, Subcommittee on Long-Term Care, August.

Brody, E.M., 1969, Follow-up study of applicants and non-applicants to a voluntary home, Gerontologist, 9:187-196.

Brody, S.J., Poulshock, S.W. and Masciocchi, C.F., 1978, The family care unit: A major consideration in the long-term care support system, Gerontologist, 18:556-651.

Comptroller General of the United States, 1977, Report to Congress: The well-being of older people in Cleveland, Ohio, Washington, D.C., General Accounting Office.

George, L.K., 1983, Caregiver well-being: Correlates and relationships with participation in community and self-help groups, Final Report submitted to the AARP Andrus Foundation, December.

Greene, J.A., Asp, J. and Crane, N., 1985, Specialized management of the Alzheimer's disease patient: Does it make a difference?, J. Tenn. Med. Assoc., 78(9):559-563.

Horowitz, A., 1985, Family caregiving to the frail elderly, in: "Annual Review of Gerontology and Geriatrics," Eisdorfer, C., Lawton, M.P., and Maddox, G.L., eds., Springer Publishing Company, New York.

Hutton, J.T., Dipple, R.L., Loewenson, R.B., Mortimer, J.A. and Christians, B.L., 1985, Predictors of nursing home placement of patients with Alzheimer's disease, Tex. Med., 104(1):98-105.

Meier, D.E., 1986, Nursing home placement and the demented patient: Case presentation and ethical analysis, Ann. Intern. Med., 104(1):98-105.

Morycz, R.K., 1985, Caregiving strain and the desire to institutionalize family members with Alzheimer's disease, Res. Aging, 7(3):329-361.

National Center for Health Statistics, Advances Report of Final Natality Statistics, 1983, Monthly Vital Statistics Report, Vol. 34, No. 6, Supp. DHHS Publication No. (PHS) 83-1120, Public Health Services, Hyattsville, MD, September 20, 1985.

Ory, M.G., Williams, T.F., Emr, M., Leobowitz, B., Rabins, P., Salloway, J., Sluss-Radbaugh, T., Wolff, E. and Zarit, S., 1985, Families, informal supports, and Alzheimer's disease, Res. Aging, 7(4):623-644.

Peppard, N.C., 1984, A special nursing home unit, Generations, 9(2):62-63.

Rabins, P.V., Mace, N.L. and Lucac, M.J., 1982, The impact of dementia on the family, J. Am. Med. Assoc., 248(3):333-335.

Shanas, E., 1979, The family as a social support system in old age, J. Gerontol., 19:169-174.

U.S. Congress, U.S. House of Representatives, Select Committee on Aging, 1984, Alzheimer's disease: A Florida Perspective, Publication No. 98-476, Washington, D.C., U.S. Government Printing Office.

Zarit, S.H., Todd, P.A. and Zarit, J.M., in press, Subjective burden of husband and wives as caregivers: A longitudinal study, Gerontologist.

Zarit, S.H., Orr, N.K. and Zarit, J.M., 1985, "The Hidden Victims of Alzheimer's Disease: Families Under Stress," New York University Press, New York, pp. 73-77.

Zarit, S.H. and Zarit, J.M., 1983, Families under stress: Interventions for caregivers of senile dementia patients, Psychotherapy, 19:461-471.

Zarit, S.H., Reeves, K. and Bach-Peterson, J., 1980, Relatives of the impaired elderly: Correlates of feelings of burden, The Gerontologist, 20(6):649-654.

DEVELOPING INSTITUTIONAL POLICIES TO OBVIATE AGONIZING

OVER COMPLEX ETHICAL DILEMMAS

Dennis A. Robbins

Director, The LeVine Institute on Aging
West Bloomfield, Michigan

On can hardly pick up a newspaper or magazine without seeing something
starting off like "one of the most complex and wrenching problems we face...
or technology has created problems which will become increasingly complex
and force difficult and agonizing decisions to be made in the future".
Ethical dilemmas cause us to scrutinize and test our own values, our moral
stances, our senses of professionalism, our sense of duty, our fear of
exposure to liability and may shape the way in which we care for our
patients in a dramatic way. When you put all these concerns together, no
wonder it appears so difficult and even mystifying to address these ethical
issues.

Most of these dilemmas or often associated with prolonged and ongoing
chronic disease or those which involve the ongoing diminishing of
competence and ability to retain lucidity so characteristic of Alzheimer's
disease. Yet, often family members are told that therapeutic modalities
must be continued despite what the patient has indicated. A distinctive
characteristic of the Alzheimer's patient is that while the prognosis may be
hopeless in terms of one suffering an ongoing deterioration with no chance
of remission, death is often not imminent. Most of the controlling case law
over the past ten years has provided guidance when both death is imminent
and the prognosis is hopeless. This, to some extent, still remains a
concern. While some states and many institutions have redressed this to
some extent through agents appointed through a durable power of attorney
(while the patient is still competent), there are still problems where
people appear to be prolonged against their earlier stated wishes or those
of their families. Rather than perceiving pneumonia as "the old man's
friend," pneumonia is now perceived as the basis for further interventions
which may often compromise the patients wishes. I in no way mean to suggest
that everyone would not want to have antibiotics or artificial feeding to
prolong his or her life, only that we assure the same self-determination
for Alzheimer's patients as we do for other citizens in this nation rather
than having them frustrate our sense of anticipating grief and their ability
to better integrate loss into life. The result would, therefore, foster the
prevention of disenfranchisement and the realization of greater autonomy and
self-determination.

A critical component in this area which is often misunderstood is the
importance and significance of patient self-determination and consent. We

frequently speak of "getting or obtaining" consents as if concent were a
piece of paper we get which we then attach to the chart, and it's over and
done with. Consent is often perceived as a legal transaction almost as if
it were a form of contract. However, since clinical care is an ongoing and
dynamic process, then consent itself must be dynamic and thus better attuned
to the ongoing process of care when the patient and family are integrated
into the decision-making process with continually renewed options for
participation.

Interestingly, most of the more troublesome issues we face are
extensions of informed consent. These often arise when one, when informed
of the consequences, may choose a course we either disagree with or one with
which we might agree but may perceive to be much more complicated than it
actually is. This may occur because of misconceptions about what we must do
and legal liability, questions and policies surrounding the removal of
respirators, whether we are required to initiate feeding supports to one who
is unable to swallow or whether we must give antibiotics to the severely
impaired Alzheimer's patient against his earlier stated wishes or his
family's currently stated wishes.

Consent allows for the performance of certain procedures in accordance
with patients' wishes. This important ingredient is often misunderstood,
particularly within the context of terminal illness or severely debilitating
and progressively degenerative diseases. This is exacerbated or complicated
when the competence of the patient is questionable or when the patient has
been determined to be incompetent. At times, patients and family members
feel their ability to make choices is jeopardized and clinicians feel
uncomfortable making decisions in this area particularly when those
decisions may involve the discontinuance of medically-supportive measures.

While making difficult decisions may be a necessary ingredient in the
clinical forum, I have found that most of the ethical dilemmas of which we
speak are indeed often avoidable when we gain appropriate understanding to
develop administrative policies to diminish the incidence and breadth of
these dilemmas through development of institutional policies so as to avert
excessive fear. By having guiding policies which integrate national
standards and guidelines with the distinctiveness of a given institution and
institutional setting, we allow clinicians to get back to the practice of
clinical medicine while better assuring the wishes of the patient and better
insulating the institution against legal liability.

While removal of respirators and other life supports have been topics
of major concern in tertiary care, historically, less attention has been
paid to addressing these topics in long-term care settings. Recent legal
decisions, however, have revived discussions surrounding removal of life
supports with dramatic implications for nursing homes. Two very recent
major court decisions in New Jersey and California have equated removal of
feeding supports with removal of respirators. These decisions indicate that
removal of feeding supports to hasten or assure death may be perceived as
"appropriate care." These new decisions require a better understanding of
surrogate decision-making and proper documentation which is now more
critical than in the past.

Over the past ten years, certain guidelines for the discontinuance of
life supports have been consistently used as precedents. Without belaboring
the legal legacy, it is important to understand some of the other
controlling considerations that are involved in removal of life supports of
incompetent patients. Besides highlighting the key elements of these
rulings, this article will discuss such vehicles for decision-making as
living wills and durable powers of attorney as well as some discussion of
proper documentations.

The right to refuse treatment as an extension of the privacy right is not new to health care. As early as 1914, Schloendorff enunciated that "every human being of adult years and sound mind has a right to determine what shall be done with his own body." Since 1976, such major cases as Quinlan (1976), Saikewicz (1977), Dinnerstein (1979), Spring (1980), Eichner v Dillon (1981), and Colyer (1983) have rendered important decisions and provided guidelines for decision-making for incompetent patients. These decisions have provided important standard and ingredients to assist caregivers in making decisions such as the significance of a prognosis of hopelessness (Quinlan, Colyer), the substituted judgment standard is an attempt to ascertain what this person would likely have decided for himself (Saikewicz), the recognition that charting DNR orders in advance is acceptable for the severely impaired Alzheimer's patient (Dinnerstein) and finally the Eichner v Dillon standard which maintained that any reasonable indication of patient intent should suffice and that there is no need to approach the courts for prior approval. These decisions have provided important standards and ingredients to assist cargivers, families and administrators in making decisions without need to routinely approach the courts for prior approval.

This issue is now on the forefront of decision-making in long-term care administration and policy. A high proportion of nursing home residents are maintained on such nutritional supports as N/G tubes and gastric tubes, only to return to the hospital on a regular basis with aspiration pneumonia. Such questions arise as to who can make the decision to remove feeding supports? "Patients' rights are not so ephemeral that a doctor or family member (or institution) can override his direction (Fowler, 1984). The President's Commission found that 36% of the public had given instructions to a friend or relative about how they would like to be treated in the case of a serious illness (Fowler, 1984).

The Supreme Court of New Jersey's decision, in the matter of Conroy (1985) (decided January 17, 1985) regarding the removal of a nasogastric tube of an 84 year old nursing home resident provides guidance in matters which, until recently, were unresolved. This is particularly interesting for us in this forum of discussion, for unlike the earlier cases noted, this involved a case where, while prognosis was hopeless, death was not imminent. This situation involved a woman who suffered from a host of maladies. Finally, her nephew approached the nursing home in which she was a resident and said he wanted her nasogastric tube removed, for it and it alone was prolonging her life and had his aunt been able to speak for herself she clearly would never have allowed it to be initiated in the first place. This is an attempt of a surrogate decision-maker acting for another to extend self-determination and patient intent. This decision argued that when the prognosis is hopeless, there is not a duty to continue even though death may not be imminent. This provided important guidance to help us in such areas for the Alzheimer's patient. It implied that feeding, administration of IV antibiotics and transfusions in the light of a prognosis of hopelessness may be contradicted. This, coupled with the Barber v Superior Court of California (October, 1983) case of a patient who suffered severe anoxic depression, had his respirator removed to allow him to die and later his IV feeding tubes removed, provides a strong basis for precedent for removing feeding supports for hopelessly ill patients when removal is consistent with patient intent. The current cases of Brophy in Massachusetts, Bovier in California and Jobes in New jersey will further clarify this domain.

Competent patients have the right to refuse treatment so long as they are clearly informed of the consequences of such refusal. When a patient specifically indicates his wishes that "extraordinary measures" or "heroics" not be employed, then the wishes of the patient, resident or as expressed by a designated agent, surrogate or family member must be honored.

Incompetent patients present different problems in terms of the writing of a DNR order. Spousal consent and designated powers of attorney can act for the patient. As already noted, a great deal of precedent exists to provide guidance in this domain dealing with such issues as "substituted judgment"; that is, what would this patient likely have decided were he able to decide for himself and other reasonable indications of patient intent, be they written or expressed by family members or designated other as well as further guidance from the President's Commission on Ethical Issues and Biomedicine and Biomedical and Behavioral Research.

A growing community of elderly persons without family where it is not clear from family members or friends what one's wishes are, complicate this domain. Some have suggested that living wills and durable powers of attorney can assist in this domain. The living will for the Alzheimer's patient is relatively useless because of the narrowness of its scope. Almost all living wills require that (1) prognosis be hopeless, (2) death be "imminent" and (3) extraordinary measures not be employed. While living wills have been notoriously ineffective in many cases, they are perhaps even worse for dealing with Alzheimer's disease. There are many situations in which one might choose in advance that his/or her suffering not be prolonged, but since death was not imminent and there is disagreement about what "extraordinary" might mean, that might undermine patient wishes. If there is ambiguity, it is very difficult for the physician who may be uneasy about making a decision to talk to a document to gain further insight. For these and related reasons, having an agent appointed by the patient while competent to represent his/or her interest through a "durable power of attorney" is much more attractive and offers much greater breadth. These are complemented by questions of whether, when, or under what circumstances one can remove life supports once they have been initiated, and finally who is the appropriate person to give consent when unresolvable conflict among family members supercedes patients' wishes at incompetence. The living will cannot help us here, while the agent appointed through a durable power of attorney can make these otherwise overwhelming dilemmas much less problematic.

Some basis for determining and documenting patient intent even in the absence of an appointed agent is very important. It is increasingly important to document patients' wishes on the chart. If the patient has a living will (despite the question of whether living wills are valid in your state), it still can serve as a reasonable indication of patient intent and should be attached to the chart. While the judiciary has provided us with ingredients to assist us in decision-making, problems still may arise when a specific designee or agent to act in the patient's interest has not been appointed. Since living will legislation has been notoriously ineffective in guaranteeing patient rights appointing, a legal agent through a durable power of attorney can minimize a great deal of ambiguity offering many advantages over a written directive. From the patient's viewpoint, an agent would help to assure that an incapacitated patient receives treatment in accordance with his/or her own wishes. Also, the appointment of an agent, unlike a living will, is respected. The agent could ask questions, assess risks and costs, speak to friends and relatives of the patient, consider a variety of therapeutic options, ask the opinion of other physicians, evaluate the patient's condition and respects for recovery, in short, engage in the same complex decision-making process that the patient would undertake if he were able. Thus an agent could extend the scope of the patient further than a written directive by making decisions consistent with the patients' values in situations he might not have specifically foreseen. Also, an agent would provide someone to enforce the patient's treatment preferences as well as permit the patient to appoint someone he trusts to represent his interest. Unlike a living will, an agent gives doctors someone to talk to who is empowered to make decisions (Fowler, 198 ).

Even when a clear agent is not established, going out of your way to determine patient intent and documenting it on the chart supercedes reasonable care and, accordingly, provides excellent insulation against potential liability. It also insures better exercise of control by the patient and retains decision-making within the institution.

While removal of feeding supports, failure to administer life-prolonging antibiotics and transfusions is an uneasy and novel area of concern, it is important that administers become involved with dealing with these issues in a timely fashion to better accommodate their patients and residents and minimize the uncertainty and ambiguity that arises in the absence of a specific policy. An understanding of the guidance offered by the legal legacy, developing contingency plans and encouraging appointment of durable agents is much more sensible applying a tourniquet measure after the fact, which more often than not, inhibits a speedy and sensible resolution.

REFERENCES

Schloendorff v Society of N.Y. Hospital, 211 N.Y. 125 105 N.E. 92 (1914).
In re: Quinlan, 70 N.J. 10 355 A.2d. 647 (1976).
Superintendent of Belchertown v. Saikewicz, 370, N.E. 2d. (1977).
Matter of Dinnerstein, 6 Mass App 380 N.E. 2d. 134 (1979).
Matter of Colyer, 99 Wash 2d. 114 (1983).
Matter of Spring, 380 Mass. 629 405 N.E. 2d. 115 (1980).
Eichner v Dillon, 420 N.E. 2d. (1981).
Fowler, Mark, Appointing an Agent to Make Medical Treatment Choices, Columbia Law Review, Vol 84:985, p. 996, (1984).
In the Matter of Conroy A-108, Decided Jan. 17, 1985 and Syllabus to the Matter of Conroy, Jan. 17, 1985 A-108. See also Matter of Conroy, 486, A.2d 1209 (New Jersey, 1985).
Barber vs. Superior Court, 137 Cal. App. 3d. 1006, 195 Cal. Reporter 484 (1983).

ALZHEIMER'S DISEASE:  LEGAL ISSUES

Coleman E. Klein

General Counsel
Alzheimer's Disease and Related Disorders Association
Detroit Area Chapter

When a person is diagnosed as suffering from Alzheimer's Disease, the
first thoughts of that person and his or her family are properly and understandably oriented toward medical care and support.  A companion concern,
generally addressed later, is that person's diminishing ability to continue
to effectively administer his or her legal and financial affairs as the
disease progresses.  It is the purpose of this discussion to review some of
those problems and the more common methods of resolving them.

WILLS

A "will" is a written document prepared and signed with certain formal-
ities (which vary from state to state) which provides for the disposition of
a person's assets (other than jointly held assets with right of survivorship), the payment of debts, the custody of minor children and the arrangement of other aspects of the person's affairs upon death.  The decedent's
assets are distributed to those persons named in the will, called "beneficiaries", immediately upon the decedent's death, after paying all debts and
taxes chargeable against the decedent's estate.

In the absence of a will, the decedent's beneficiaries are determined by
the laws of the state in which the decedent was domiciled at death.  Thus, a
decedent's assets will be distributed to persons who may not be the ones the
decedent would have preferred to have received them.  Such an unintended
result can be avoided if the decedent had executed a will.

Wills vary in both substance and form, depending upon the needs and
desires of the one making the will.  One basic requirement common to all
wills, however, is that the person making the will have "testamentary capacity" at the time the will is made.  To have testamentary capacity under
Michigan law, "an individual must be able to comprehend the nature and extent of his property, to recall the natural objects of his bounty, and to
determine and understand the disposition of property which he desires to
make."  In re Sprenger's Estate, 337 Mich 514, 521, 60 NW2d 436 (1953).
However defined, an Alzheimer's victim may lose his or her testamentary
capacity at some point as the disease progresses.

If no will was ever made, one should be prepared so that the person's
wishes will be carried out at death.  When an existing will predates the
diagnosis of Alzheimer's Disease, the will should be reviewed to assure that

it will effectively accomodate the victim's intentions as influenced by his or her awareness of the disease. Immediate consideration of the preparation of a new will or the review of an existing will cannot be overemphasized. A delay beyond the point where the victim retains the testamentary capacity to make or revise a will could result in the victim's being left without a will altogether or being encumbered with a pre-existing will that does not adequately meet the needs of either the victim or his or her family.

Since title to the assets a decedent may own (other than jointly held assets with right of survivorship, however denominated) at the time of the decedent's death must be transferred to those who will receive them, probate courts (or courts having probate-type powers) are involved in the administration of decedent's estates (those involving wills as well as those without wills) and the distribution of the decedent's assets. This estate administration is commonly referred to as "probate".

TRUSTS

Simply stated, a "trust" is a legal relationship, typically in written form, that provides for the administration and distribution of assets subject to the trust for the benefit of certain people. The person creating the trust is referred to as the "settlor". The one administering the trust is called the "trustee", who is either an individual or a financial institution such as a trust company. The ones benefiting from the trust are called the "beneficiaries". The trust is created when the settlor transfers legal title to some or all of his or her assets to the trustee, who thereafter administers those assets for the beneficiaries according to the rules which the settlor has provided in the trust agreement. Those rules include the identification of the beneficiaries (which may include the settlor), when and how much each beneficiary will receive and the circumstances authorizing those distributions. The settlor may also reserve the right to revoke or amend the trust for any reason.

The settlor must be mentally competent in order to create, revoke or amend a trust. The definition of mental incompetency varies among the states. In Michigan, it includes "a substantial disorder of thought or mood which significantly impairs judgment, behavior, capacity to recognize reality, or ability to cope with the ordinary demands of life." Michigan Compiled Laws Section 330.1400a. (Mental Illness). Thought should be given as soon as possible following a diagnosis of Alzheimer's Disease to the creation, amendment or revocation of a trust, if desired, while the victim still is mentally competent to do so.

Trusts may be incorporated in wills, to become effective upon the settlor's death, in which case they are referred to as "testamentary trusts". Trusts which are intended to be effective prior to death are referred to as "inter vivos" or "living" trusts.

Much has been written about the perceived evils and expense of the probate process and ways to avoid it. Many of those concerns are frequently exaggerated. Nevertheless, one or more properly drafted inter vivos trusts into which all of the decedent's individually owned assets have been transferred prior to death may avoid probate. That is because probate is involved in the administration of assets (other than jointly held assets with right of survivorship) which a decedent owned at the time of his death. If all assets are transferred to an inter vivos trust prior to death, however, no probate may be necessary since the inter-vivos trust, rather than the decedent-settlor, legally owns those assets upon death. There is simply nothing for the probate court to do. Testamentary trusts do not avoid probate since, as previously explained, they are included in the will and typically receive their assets from the decedent-settlor's probate estate upon death.

Unlike a will, which requires the immediate distribution of all of a decedent's assets upon death, a trust permits the distribution of assets to be deferred for considerable periods (subject to certain legal limitations) extending beyond the settlor's death in order to accomplish the settlor's objectives. Deferred transfers of assets are frequently desired where the ones to whom the settlor wishes to transfer those assets are minor children or others in whom the settlor prefers not to place ownership of a large value of assets at once. The income from the assets retained in the trust, as well as some or all of those assets themselves, will be distributed at such times and in such amounts as the settlor has provided in the trust agreement.

Trusts thus offer much greater flexibility in the management of assets than do wills alone. An inter-vivos trust may designate the settlor as the sole initial trustee and a successor trustee in the event that the settlor becomes mentally incompetent. This arrangement permits the settlor to exclusively manage and control his or her own trust assets until becoming mentally incompetent, with an orderly, automatic transition upon incompetency to the pre-determined successor.

Third parties may refuse or be reluctant to recognize the successor trustee's authority absent a judicial determination of the settlor's mental incompetency. Since one of the primary purposes of an inter-vivos trust under these circumstances is the avoidance of probate proceedings, that objective thus may not be achieved. The settlor may, however, desire such a judicial determination to prevent the settlor's premature loss of control over the trust's assets where a bona-fide dispute between the settlor and the successor trustee exists as to the incompetency. If that is the case, the trust agreement can require that judicial determination as a pre-condition of the successor trustee's exercise of authority.

Alternatively, both the settlor and one or more co-trustees may be designated to serve simultaneously, with each trustee alone (or in combination) having full power to make trust decisions at all times, including the period during which the settlor-trustee is mentally competent. Since the co-trustee's powers are not dependent upon the settlor-trustee's incompetency, third parties should not have the same reluctance to deal with the co-trustee(s) if and when the settlor-trustee becomes incompetent. It will be noted, however, that the settlor does not thereby maintain exclusive control over the trust's assets while he or she is competent.

POWERS OF ATTORNEY

A "power of attorney" is a written agreement in which one person, called the "principal", delegates certain powers and authority to another, called the "agent". It permits the agent to manage one or more of the principal's affairs when it is either inconvenient or impossible for the principal to personally manage them. Powers of attorney may only be created while the principal is not "legally incapacitated". Legal incapacity includes mentally incompetent persons under the laws of many states, including Michigan. Michigan Compiled Laws Section 700.8(2). It must therefore be reiterated that prompt consideration be given to the creation of a power of attorney before that occurs. Powers of attorney may be used for limited or broad purposes, depending upon the principal's desires. They are classified as "non-durable" or "durable".

The agent's authority under a non-durable power of attorney normally expires at the earliest of (1) the time designated for expiration in the power of attorney, (2) the revocation of the power of attorney by the principal and notice thereof to the agent, and (3) the principal's death or legal incapacity.

A durable power of attorney differs from a non-durable power of attorney in that the durable power does not terminate upon the principal's legal incapacity. In fact, even the principal's death will not terminate the agent's authority under a durable power until the agent becomes aware of the death. For that reason, a durable power of attorney is a very flexible, convenient and common method of providing for the management of an Alzheimer's victim's affairs, particularly after the victim has become legally incapacitated because of the progression of the disease. The use of a durable power of attorney is also used to avoid the necessity of the court's appointment of a conservator upon the principal's becoming legally incapacitated, thus saving time and expense.

Durable powers of attorney are very useful in managing a principal's financial affairs, particularly banking. Its use extends beyond mere banking, however, and includes virtually everything that the principal, if competent, could lawfully do of a financial nature. There are certain restrictions, however. Durable powers of attorney do not relate to some financial matters that are of such a personal quality that they may only be exercised by the principal. Examples include the making of wills and gifts (although many legal scholars reserve judgment as to whether gifts are of such a personal nature as to preclude inclusion in a power of attorney). The laws of the state governing the durable power of attorney must be consulted in order to precisely define the scope of the power.

In the event that the principal becomes legally incapacitated and a conservator is appointed by the court, the conservator has the power to revoke the durable power of attorney in many states, including Michigan. If the conservator does not elect to revoke, however, the agent thereafter accounts directly to the conservator of the legally incapacitated principal, rather than to the principal.

Durable powers of attorney must be carefully drafted to comply with the laws of the jurisdiction authorizing them. For example, Michigan Compiled Laws Section 700.495 provides that a durable power of attorney that is to be immediately effective must state that "this power of attorney shall not be affected by disability of the principal" or words of similar effect. Such a provision immediately confers power upon the agent although the principal still has legal capacity.

There are undoubtedly many people who prefer to retain exclusive power over their affairs until they become legally incapacitated. A properly drafted durable power of attorney accomodates that desire. The preceding Michigan statute, similar to those in other states, provides for what is known as a "springing" power which does not confer any power on the agent until the principal becomes legally incapacitated. The words "this power of attorney shall become effective upon the disability of the principal" or similar language would be substituted for that contained in the preceding paragraph. The power thus "springs" into existence upon the principal's legal incapacity.

The use of a springing durable power of attorney, however, requires a determination of the principal's legal incapacity. The durable power may provide that such a determination be made by one or more doctors. Nevertheless, third parties may understandably be reluctant to deal with an agent under a springing power where the third party is insecure about the legal conclusiveness of that determination. The agent may thus be forced to obtain a judicial determination, thus incurring the very expense and delay which the durable power of attorney was designed to avoid. A non-springing durable power of attorney which, by definition, does not require a finding of legal incapacity as a precondition of its use, may thus be preferable.

Durable powers of attorney have been extended to matters that are not financial. For example, durable powers have been used in making medical decisions for an incapacitated principal, such as when or if to consent or withhold consent to medical treatment. Matters of placement of an incapacitated principal in a nursing care facility or admission to a hospital are frequently included in durable powers of attorney. The inclusion of these non-financial, traditionally personal, powers has also caused concern among some members of the legal community since there is little, if any, law in many jurisdictions as to their propriety and effectiveness. For that reason, agents operating under durable powers of attorney containing such authority may find third parties reluctant to recognize that authority even though it is literally contained in the power. The alternative to such reluctance is to seek the appointment of a guardian over the principal in court proceedings; the guardian would thus presumably then have the authority to make those personal decisions. Although the principal's intent in explicitly including such personal powers in a durable power of attorney was to avoid those legal proceedings, they may nevertheless be unavoidable in those cases where third parties refuse to recognize them.

It was previously noted that the power to make gifts may be outside the scope of a durable power of attorney. It is possible, however, for the durable power to empower the agent to transfer the principal's property administered under the durable power to an inter vivos trust previously created by the principal. That would hopefully avoid probating those assets which are initially outside the trust or which the principal may not have owned until after incapacity. This may be distinguishable from the making of a gift since the principal (as the settlor of the trust), rather than the agent, has provided for the ultimate disposition of the property which the agent transfers to that trust.

CONCLUSION

The appointment of a trustee or agent involves the appointing person's deep and abiding trust of the one to whom those powers are given. Serious thought should therefore always be given to the designation of someone who will always faithfully use those powers with the best interests of the appointing person constantly in mind.

Space limitations do not here permit a more extensive review of the subjects of wills, trusts and powers of attorney, not to mention estate planning and tax saving possibilities. Similarly, space does not permit the discussion of medical, hospital and custodial benefits offered under the Social Security (SSI) laws and the related but complex subject of an Alzheimer's victim's divestiture of assets within certain time periods in order to avoid dissipating personal assets for his or her medical and maintenance purposes while lawfully maintaining eligibility for governmental assistance for those expenses. These topics are mentioned, albeit in passing, because of their great importance.

This discussion is merely a beginning; legal counsel should be consulted for an elaboration and implementation of the concepts previously discussed. It is nevertheless hoped that this broad overview will assist the reader in obtaining a general awareness of the legal ramifications affecting those suffering from Alzheimer's Disease and the planning possibilities which are available to them.

CLARIFYING WHO DECIDES


David C. Hollister

June, 1985


INTRODUCTION

My interest in the issue of medical decision-making for those incapable
or incompetent to control their own health care grew out of the prolonged
dying process of my grandfather.  The victim of a heart attack and
subsequent stroke, my grandfather lay for months in a health care setting he
resented, partially paralyzed, depressed and in and out of periods of
incompetency.  He had communicated his wishes to my grandmother, making it
clear he was not to be sustained in a vegetative or inhumane state.  He
asserted his rights, trying unsuccessfully to remove the intravenous tubes
from his arms.  Health care personnel responded by binding his arms to the
side of the bed.

My father and I attempted to intervene on behalf of my grandfather, but
were told we had no right to authorize the withholding or withdrawing of
treatment.  The hospital personnel and physicians made it clear that the law
did not allow third-party decision-makers to authorize the withholding or
withdrawing of treatment.  Although sympathetic to the family's desires,
they would be at substantial risk in acceding to our wishes and,
consequently, continued the defensive and prolonged medical treatment.

On returning to Lansing, I convened an interdisciplinary task force to
explore the complex medical, social, legal, ethical and economic questions
surrounding this issue.  Represented on the task force were physicians,
lawyers, nurses, hospital administrators, philosophers, clergy, teachers of
death and dying, senior citizens, housewives, students and other concerned
citizens.  The year was 1975--the beginning of a decade-long effort to
guarantee decision-making rights to ill and dying patients.

The task force undertook two basic tasks:  1) to decide if there was a
compelling need for legislation; and, if so, 2) to draft legislation which
most appropriately addressed the need.

Over a period of eighteen months, a consensus developed among task
force members that a compelling need for legislation did, indeed, exist.
Rapidly expanding medical technology was not only creating modern medical
miracles, but was also crossing the fine line of saving lives into the
frightening reality of prolonging the dying process.  The old concept of
informed consent no longer adequately applied to many medical situations,

where people were sustained on life-support equipment or were otherwise
incapacitated, without the ability to control their own health care.

Barry Keene, author of the recently enacted California Natural Death
Act, came to Michigan for two days to meet with the task force, various
health care providers and interest groups, and to participate in a public
forum on Death and Dying. The task force also met with Robert Veatch,
author of "Death and the Biological Revolution" and Senior Staff Director at
the Institute of Society, Ethics and Live Sciences, Hastings-on-the Hudson,
New York. Although both Assemblyman Keene and Dr. Veatch recognized the
need for legislatures to clarify the law in this area, they provided
substantially different approaches.

The California Natural Death Act is based on the concept of a living
will. An adult can voluntarily sign a "directive to the physician" which
will instruct the physician to stop treatment under the following
conditions: 1) if a physician determines the patient to be terminally ill;
2) if the patient faces imminent death; and 3) if the treatment offered
only "artificially prolongs the moment of death". If all three thresholds
are reached, the physician is required to stop treatment or face assault
charges.

The "directive" is advisory if signed by the principal when in good
health, but binding if signed 14 days after being diagnosed as terminally
ill. In either case, the physician is held harmless and not liable for
withholding or withdrawing treatment. Pregnant women are not covered by
this law. In effect, the California legislation tries to anticipate the
health care crisis and prescribe a decision ahead of time.

Dr. Robert Veatch encouraged the task force to consider a broader
approach--clarifying who would make health care decisions at any time a
person is incapacitated and unable to direct his/her own health care. He
believes that a trusted individual chosen by the principal to make health
care decisions would more likely assure that the patient's wishes would be
honored. This third-party decision-maker (agent) would make all the
decisions a principal could make if conscious and competent, provided the
decisions are reasonable and in the best interests of the principal.

The task force members considered both approaches, agreeing that,
whichever strategy was embraced, the legislation would have to meet the
following criteria:

1) The legislation must incorporate the doctrine of consent,
   self-determination and privacy of the individual, while at the
   same time acknowledging the crucial role of the physician.

2) The legislation must be flexible enough to meet the uniqueness of
   each individual's health crisis.

3) The legislation must improve upon the ad hoc decision-making
   process that now functions, but which is not sanctioned in law,
   and often violates the wishes of the patient.

The task force rejected the "California Model" for two reasons: it 1)
violated the principle of flexibility, and 2) only minimally protected the
patient's rights.

The "Veatch Approach" was chosen because it accomplishes all three of
our principles: 1) it keeps paramount the right of consent, while keeping
the physician central to decision-making; 2) it is flexible enough to meet
the uniqueness of each health crisis; and 3) it significantly improves upon

the present ad hoc decision-making process. Further, this approach is sensitive to pro-life concerns by keeping the State neutral on the question of continuing or discontinuing treatment. It is not "right to die" legislation. Rather, it is a bill dealing with the procedures by which decisions regarding treatment are made. It addresses the question: "who will make decisions regarding medical treatment on behalf of patients who cannot do so for themselves?" It does not address the question: "what will the decision be?" That decision is left to the previously designated agent and the physician.

Under Michigan law today, a conscious, competent adult has the right to accept or reject medical treatment. This right of consent is well-established in law and is based upon the doctrine of privacy and self-determination. No physician can treat an individual without first obtaining consent. The right to privacy is clearly protected in law. However, should a patient become incapable of making decisions, the law no longer has guarantees, protections or procedures to assure that the patient's wishes and rights are respected.

On December 7, 1977, I introduced HB 5778, the Medical Treatment Decision Act. This legislation was drafted by the task force following the recommendations of Dr. Veatch. It provided a mechanism to assure that the clear, legal rights one has while conscious and competent are also protected while one is incapable of making decisions.

CONFLICT IN LEGAL PRINCIPLES

> No right is held more sacred, or is more carefully guarded
> by the common law, than the right of every individual to
> the possession and control of his own person, free from
> all restraint or interference of others, unless by clear
> and unquestionable authority of law.
> 141 U.S. 250 (1891)

In 1914, Justice Cardozo noted that

> Every human being of adult years and sound mind has a right
> to determine what shall be done with own body; and a surgeon
> who performs an operation without his patient's consent,
> commits an assault, for which he is liable in damages.
> Scholeondorff v. Society of N.Y.

The principle of freedom and self-determination, especially in matters as critical as life and death, is fundamental in our legal system. The crucial legal decision whhich set the standards for "informed consent" in the 1960's was Natanson v. Kline. Kansas Supreme Court Justice Alfred Schroeder declared:

> Anglo-American law starts with the premise of thoroughgoing
> self-determination. It follows that each man is considered to
> be master of his own body, and he may, if he be of sound mind,
> expressly prohibit the performance of life-saving surgery, or
> other medical treatment. A doctor might well believe that an
> operation or form of treatment is desirable or necessary but the
> law does not permit him to substitute his own judgment for that
> of the patient by any form of artifice or deception.
> Natanson v. Kline   186 Kansas (1961)

Natanson v. Kline further stated that physicians must ensure that the patient's consent to treatment is an informed consent without which there is no contract. The court held that a physician would be liable for an unauthorized treatment if he affirmatively misrepresents the nature of the operation or has failed to point out the probable consequences of the course of treatment. The court went on to establish the criteria which must be met in order to achieve informed consent:

1) The physician must inform the patient of the treatment proposed, including the attendant risks.

2) The physician must obtain the patient's consent before administering any treatment.

3) The patient's consent must be given voluntarily and with knowledge of the nature, extent and reasonably foreseeable consequences of the proposed treatment.

When the patient is fully conscious and aware of the attendant circumstances, his right of self-determination is legally the strongest. In Erickson v. Delgad (1962) a New York Court upheld the patient's right to control his own body and allowed him to refuse a blood transfusion which placed him in danger of death. The court asserted that our system of government permits the individual to freely make a medical decision, so long as he is competent to render such a decision.

Our society has recognized that patients have the right to control their medical care even though this right is not absolute. The courts have intervened on occasions when the state had a compelling interest to override a patient's wishes. Generally, however, a conscious, competent adult has the right to accept or reject medical treatment.

This right to refuse treatment is founded on the court's interpretation of self-determination and privacy. As noted by Justice Brandeis in his dissent in Olmstead v. United States:

> The makers of the Constitution sought to protect Americans in their belief, their thoughts, their emotions and their sensations. They conferred, as against government, the right to be left alone, the most comprehensive of rights and the right most valued by civilized man.

While this right of consent is clear and well-established, another legal principle is at work which at times contravenes the right of consent--the contractual relationship between a physician and patient.

The physician/patient relationship has been held to confer a contractual duty upon the physician to render assistance to his patients. That duty continues, in the absence of an agreement to the contrary, for as long as the case requires (Ricks v. Budge, 1937).

Since the physician/patient relation is contractual in nature, it may be analyzed through the traditional framework of offer and acceptance. The patient, as the offerer, communicates the offer to the physician by seeking his/her services, usually by walking into the physician's office. The physician, as offeree, may accept the offer or refuse it categorically. However, if s/he decides to treat the patient, s/he had, in effect, accepted the offer and a contract is formed. ("'Living Will': the Right to Death with Dignity?" John G. Strand, Case Western Reserve Law Review, Vol. 26:485).

Absent some agreement to the contrary, once the physician accepts the patient's offer, whether by words or by action, the law imposes a duty on the physician to continue treatment as long as it is required. (Johnson-vs-

Vaughn 370 S.W. 2nd 591, 153; Lee v. Dewbre 362 S.W. 2nd 900; Gray v. Davidson 15 Was; McManus v. Donlin 23 Wisc. 2nd 289). Even if the patient has a flat EEG reading and no chance of recovery, the physician may be obligated to keep the respirator going indefinitely (Fletcher, Supra. note 17 at 26). If the patient were injured by the physician's failure to perform in accordance with this agreement, the physician could be held criminally liable and the injured patient could recover for breach of contract.

The strict requirements of a contract law are somewhat relaxed in certain circumstances. For example, should a medical emergency exist in which the patient is unconscious and in need of immediate treatment, common law dispenses with the requirement that the patient and physician have a contractual relationship before the physician can act. The doctrine of "implied consent" sanctions the medical treatment in such an instance (Jackouach v. Yokom 212 Iowa 914,237, NW 444; Wells v. Mcghee 39 So 2nd 196).

The legal "Catch 22" becomes apparent. The doctor's contractual duty to provide treatment can come in conflict with the wishes of the patient should that patient be incapable of expressing his/her own wishes. Further, with our current medical capability, it is not uncommon for a physician to begin life support equipment with no legal way of stopping it when it is medically appropriate to do so. As John Strand concludes in his article in the Case Western Reserve Law Review:

> The physician and hospital are frequently confronted with the dilemma of providing quality medical care, yet ensuring that the patient retains the right to control medical treatment. This problem has become more complicated as technology prolongs life, while the legal status of the physician's duty to the patient in certain situations remains murky at best. The result makes neither good medicine nor good law.

In response to this serious legal dilemma, twenty-four states and the District of Columbia have enacted legislation that seeks to protect patients' rights in controlling their health care.

Decisions to withhold or withdraw treatment are being made in health care facilities every day. Because there is no clear public policy, ad hoc procedures are used. One such procedure having no legal sanction is the NO CODE policy whereby physicians, consulting with family and others, make a determination not to resuscitate an individual in a life-threatening situation. Some argue that a NO CODE policy is preferable to a legislated solution to the problem of withholding or withdrawing life supports. However, a recent attorney general's opinion from the State of Washington highlights the legal consequences of withholding or withdrawing life support from a dying patient:

> "It is clear that disconnecting a life support mechanism falls within this definition of homicide. Even the mere negligent failure to provide medical assistance where one is under the duty to do so (i.e., a parent's duty to a child or a physician's duty to his patient) may result in criminal liability for murder

> or manslaughter...

> In addition, a patient who consents or demands that a doctor act in a manner set forth in the situation described above, if unsuccessful, may be guilty of the crime of attempting to commit suicide. The physician should know that aiding or abetting a suicide is also a crime...

Therefore, under present law, an attempt to bring about death by
the removal of a life-sustaining mechanisms would constitute
homicide.  In all likelihood the crime would be that most
serious form of homicide, first degree.

> "The Right to Refuse Treatment and
> Natural Death Legislation,"  Jane A.
> Raible, Medicolegal News, Vol. 5,
> No. 4 (Fall, 1977)

Physicians caring for critically ill patients are faced with a dilemma.
If the physician ignores the expressed desires of the patient by
administering unwanted treatment, s/he may be criminally and civilly liable
for assault and battery for violating the patient's right of privacy and
self-determination.  If, however, s/he acquiesces to the patient's or the
family's demands to withhold or withdraw treatment, and the patient dies
because of the failure to provide such treatment, s/he may be civilly and
criminally liable for the patient's death.  The patient may not have been
competent to refuse the treatment, rendering the physician liable for
failure to fulfill his/her contractual duty to care for the patient.  The
physician could even be held liable for murder!  This legal quagmire is
unacceptable for both the patient and the physician and must be clarified in
law.  Legislation is essential to be certain that the patient's wishes are
honored while at the same time honoring the physician's need to maintain
high professional standards and protection from liability.


ALTERNATIVES TO A LEGISLATED SOLUTION

Living Will

Many people nationwide have signed living wills in which they direct a
physician to withhold life-prolonging procedures in the event of a terminal
illness.  Unfortunately, these wills do not have the force of law in
Michigan.  They may be honored by a trusted family physician, but only if
all concerned parties are in complete agreement.  Even with complete
unanimity, the physician is exposed to considerable liability.  The law does
not authorize the physician to break the contract with the patient by
discontinuing or withholding care.  They may be considered abandonment and
malpractice.

California's legislation is a form of living will which assures one's
wishes will be carried out if s/he signs the document ahead of time.  It
narrowly defines the conditions which, when met, compel the physician to
stop treatment.  Unfortunately, many health crises are more complex than
those outlined in the California legislation.  The document is not flexible
enough to address each individual set of circumstances.  On the other hand,
if an individual were permitted to write a more detailed and complex living
will, trying to anticipate every eventuality, s/he would run the risk of
omitting some crucial circumstances vital to the management of the patient's
health, making the living will ineffective in that particular situation.   A
more broadly written document giving little guidance would leave too much
discretion to the physician.  Again, the chances of one's wishes being
carried out are limited.

Physician as Decisionmaker

Some believe that the physician is the best qualified to make decisions
regarding health care--that legislation would interfere with the
doctor/patient relationship.

Today, only 7.5 percent of the population has a traditional family physician. Most people get their health care from clinics, HMO's, PPA's, IPA's, emergency rooms, specialists or some other form of practice. For those individuals, a personal family physician who knows and cares for the patient and is committed to carrying out the wishes of the patient is a myth.

Further, decisions concerning health care are not only medical decisions but ethical ones as well. While physicians may be highly qualified to offer options and recommendations for health care, they are not specially qualified to make the ethical decisions required in determining what kind of medical care to pursue.

To illustrate, the Massachusetts Supreme Court ruled on the case of Mr. Saikewicz, a 56 year-old man who had developed leukemia. Mr. Saikewicz had no immediate family and had lived in an institutional setting all his life. The physicians attending Mr. Saikewicz disagreed on the type of treatment which should be undertaken. One set of physicians advocated aggressive chemotherapy which would be painful, require hospitalization and be difficult for Mr. Saikewicz to understand or appreciate, but could potentially extend his life up to two years. Another set of physicians advocated palliative care which would treat the symptoms, control the pain, and let the man die in peace in a comfortable, familiar setting.

A guardian was appointed to decide what the most appropriate treatment would be under the circumstances. The decision was an ethical one, not a medical one. The guardian of Mr. Saikewicz opted for the palliative care. The decision was challenged and the Massachusetts court upheld the guardian's judgment.

Physicians may be highly skilled and knowledgeable about their technical field of expertise, but they are not ethicists. Until very recently they have not been required to have any academic exposure to the ethical implications of their work. However, in 1978 I offered an amendment to the Physician's Licensing Act requiring courses in medical ethics as a condition of relicensure. The legislation was enacted and courses on medical ethics were established statewide. Until that time, there were no requirements for medical ethics training for physicians in the State of Michigan.

Our culture traditionally has asked physicians to assume this role of ethical decisionmaker--an awesome responsibility which may, in part, account for the fact that physicians have the highest suicide and substance abuse rate of any professional group.

Finally, physicians are not legally empowered to withdraw treatment when that treatment is no longer appropriate. The decision by a physician to withdraw treatment exposes him/her to serious liability.

Family as Decisionmaker

Some persons argue that the family is best suited to make these decisions. Unfortunately, many people do not have a family able to assume the responsibility of decisionmaking. Even in instances where family members are present, a difference of opinion and absence of a legal spokesperson may only exacerbate the problem rather than alleviate it. Further, the physician is placed in a precarious legal position and must practice defensive medicine to protect him/herself. In addition, there is no guarantee that the family will know and honor the patient's wishes, which is the central value to be considered.

After six months of prayerful consideration and thoughtful deliberation, the family of Karen Ann Quinlan decided to remove life supports from their comatose daughter, but the physician chose not to honor that decision. The publicity surrounding the Quinlan case created a serious problem for physicians. Even though they might respect the family's sincerity and agree with their decision, the physicians had a contractual responsibility to Karen and to withdraw treatment would have exposed them to charges of abandonment or even murder. The physician refused to honor the parents' request and the case went to court. Eventually, the New Jersey Supreme Court ruled that a medical ethics committee (not a physician or the family) should be empowered to make those decisions. In the state of New Jersey every hospital has such a committee which includes a physician, a nurse, a hospital administrator, a lawyer, a clergy person, a social worker and a family member. Upon the committee's reaching a unanimous decision, the physician may stop treatment without being exposed to liability. In New Jersey, naming the family as the decisionmaking entity was rejected as a solution to the problem.

## Courts as Decisionmakers

The Massachusetts Supreme Court specifically rejected the physician, the family and the medical ethics committee as the decisionmaker in the Saikewicz case by directing the probate judge to be involved in cases requiring medical/ethical decisions. This solution has proved to be cumbersome and least likely to provide an expeditious resolution to the problem that a health crisis presents. Recent court cases in Massachusetts have tried to rectify this situation by limiting the types of cases which are referred to the courts.

## Third Parties (Agents) as Decisionmakers

Michigan proposed the first legislation in the United States explicitly designating a third party to be the health care decisionmaker (HB 5778 of 1977). the bill allowed an individual the right to choose a trusted individual (spouse, physician, clergy, family member) who would be legally empowered to make medical treatment decisions. The state already recognizes the authority of third-party decisionmakers when parents make health care decisions for their children and guardians make health care decisions for their wards. In both instances, the decision must be "reasonable" and in the "best interest" of the principle. The physician remains a key decisionmaker and, if concerned that the agent is not acting in good faith, may ask for the court's intervention. This procedure is presently used when physicians question the judgment of parents and guardians.

## MEDICAL TREATMENT DECISION ACT (MTDA) - A BRIEF HISTORY

The Medical Treatment Decision Act as first introduced in 1977, sought to establish in law the right of individuals to choose a trusted individual to make health care decisions on their behalf when they were unable to do so. The proposal was widely supported by physicians, nurses, hospitals, seniors and many other advocate groups. The opposition, while fewer in number, was politically astute and well-organized, representing the Michigan Catholic Conference and the Right to Life of Michigan. They argued that this legislation would open the door to other laws that would endanger the sanctity of human life--that the present system, although not perfect, is better than a legislated solution.

Even though the Medical Treatment Decision Act failed to win approval during three successive legislative sessions, it provide the context for exploring the issues related to patients' rights. The task force also explored the hospice movement and facilitated legislation to regulate hospices in Michigan (Public Act 368 of 1978). In addition, as a direct result of the work of the task force, legislation was proposed and enacted requiring physicians to take courses in medical ethics as a condition for relicensure.

PROBATE CODE REVISION

One of the criticisms of the Medical Treatment Decision Act was that Michigan law already sanctions the designation of a third party decisionmaker in the revised Probate Code of 1978. While section 495 doesn't explicitly authorize or specify how health care decisions would be made, it does reference health care and appears to give authorization for a third party decisionmaker. It does not, however, protect the health care professional who honors that request.

House Bill 4175 would have revised that Probate Code to make explicit the power, rights and responsibilities of the attorney-in-fact in making health care decisions for another. This bill does not create a new right in law but simply clarifies a right that already exists. This bill, introduced on February 17, 1983, received a favorable hearing before the House Judiciary Committee but failed to pass a vote of the full House of Representatives.

So while the Probate Code makes a general statement that one can designate an attorney in fact to make health care decisions, using the provision of the durable power of attorney, it does not spell out how this person would function, prescribe limits or protect a health care professional who honors the wishes of the third party decisionmaker. HB 4175 was designed to correct these deficiencies. This bill, though similar to the Medical Treatment Decision Act conceptually, is different in that it seeks only to clarify an existing practice and procedure, not create a new practice and procedure.

A survey of members of the State Bar verified that it is common practice to designate an attorney in fact, under the durable power provisions of the existing Probate Code, to make health care decisions when the principle becomes incompetent or incapacitated. Many attorneys have developed standard forms to use as part of wills which specify when medical care can be withheld and withdrawn. With this evidence and the testimony of doctors, lawyers, judges, health care professionals and family members who fought to assert the right of incompetent persons to die with dignity, the House Judiciary Committee overwhelmingly supported the bill and reported it out on May 11, 1983 with broad bipartisan support.

While the bill enjoyed broad support from all aspects of the medical and health care community, from attorneys, from senior citizens and others, it continued to be controversial. Smarting from the recall of two state senators and wishing to avoid further controversy, the House defeated HB 4175 and sent it back to the Judiciary Committee, where it died.

However, the issues surrounding this proposed legislation will not go away and will be addressed by the legislature or by the courts. It is my sincere hope that the legislature will forthrightly consider the complex issues involving incompetent and incapacitated patients and develop a policy which works for patients, health care professionals and other interested parties. It is in that spirit that on June 24, 1985, I introduced HB 4883.

LEGISLATIVE ADVOCACY AND ALZHEIMER'S DISEASE:

THE CALIFORNIA EXPERIENCE

Kathryn C. Rees

Rees and Associates, Inc.
Governmental Advocacy and Political Consulting
Sacramento, California

California's Alzheimer's disease legislative program is unquestionably ambitious, exciting, and innovative. While we clearly have not met all the needs of our families, we have made great strides in carving out a place in the legislative agenda. Equally important is the fact that California ADRDA has created a structure for meeting future goals. Organizations that truly succeed in the legislative arena combine the talents of a well respected legislative advocate with a finely-tuned, well-honed grassroots legislative Keyperson Program. These two inexorably interrelated components are the very undergirding of a dynamic program which achieves results. In California we have worked very hard to develop this strong interrelationship.

Rees and Associates, Inc., a legislative consulting firm, was retained in March 1984 to achieve three objectives for ADRDA during its first year before the legislature:  1) to establish ADRDA as the Alzheimer's disease presence in Sacramento, 2) to coalesce the perception of ADRDA as a unified, reasonable, credible organization, and 3) to manage legislation to ADRDA's best interest and represent ADRDA issues before the legislature. Initial attempts at representing Alzheimer's disease issues were frustrated by extraordinary confusion among legislators as to who or what organization represented Alzheimer's disease. Through the efforts of Rees and Associates working to correct this misperception, and with strong support from local ADRDA chapters, ADRDA is now viewed as a unified, reasonable, credible organization. Until establishing that base, however, little real success could be expected from other legislative efforts. The effect of informing legislators about Alzheimer's disease and the needs of families and caregivers has been dramatic. Once educated to the specific needs of the ADRDA population, most legislators responded favorably and sympathetically to bills providing services to victims and families.

The importance of joint and coordinated efforts between ADRDA and the legislative advocate cannot be overemphasized. In a time of increasing governmental regulation and a plethora of bills that have potential impact on Alzheimer's disease patients, all resources within an organization are needed to insure effective results. Legislative goals and priorities must be clearly defined and presented convincingly to lawmakers and administrators in state government. The ADRDA membership plays a vital role in grassroots lobbying. The dynamics of this relationship between family members as grassroots advocates and the professional legislative consultant's work in the state capitol is what may make the vital difference between passage or failure of critical legislation in California.

While Alzheimer's disease is certainly recognized as a major health problem throughout the nation, it's effect is multiplied in California by the percentage of older residents in the state, already large and increasing yearly. Some 200,000 to 250,000 Californians are thought to be afflicted with the disease. Estimated annual expenditures for nursing home care in the Medicaid (Medi-Cal) program alone for 1986-87 are well over $1 billion dollars. If, as predicted, 30 to 40% of those patients are in skilled nursing facilities due to complications of Alzheimer's disease, it is no wonder that lawmakers are terrified to make the fiscal commitments to handle this problem.

Our legislative work in California is varied and complex. Through the efforts of ADRDA, especially the Public Policy Committee, and Rees and Associates, some main areas of concern have been identified as priorities. We have had remarkable successes and have been able to affect legislation in areas that include, but are not limited to, the following categories:

1) The Alzheimer's Disease Task Force, created by ADRDA supported legislation, was appointed by the Governor and the Department of Aging. It's mandates included conducting a statewide conference to be held in the spring of 1986, and recommending priorities and options to the Governor, his Administration, and the State Legislature regarding Alzheimer's disease.

2) Specialized Alzheimer's Disease Day Care and Resource Centers were established through ADRDA supported legislation. There are eight centers open throughout California providing recreational and social activities, cognitive assessments, nursing and physical therapy, respite care, counseling, and referral and support services to families; and public information and training for professionals. The observations and analysis of these resource/respite care programs will form the foundation for expansion of services.

3) Adult Day Health Care legislation has provided almost $3 million dollars over the last three years which has resulted in the opening of 47 centers already and an anticipated 20 more which are in the funding process. These projects provide supervision and some skilled nursing care to Alzheimer's disease and other patients able to return home daily.

4) Respite care, both in-home and in various community settings, is being examined carefully by the California State Legislature, for Alzheimer's disease patients and other functionally impaired and frail elderly persons. Approaches vary and there are currently four legislators carrying bills that address respite care. We are constantly monitoring and analyzing these measures to determine where to place our support and how to influence the outcome of respite care legislation.

5) Relative to research and diagnosis, ADRDA supported legislation which allocated $1 million to establish six Alzheimer's Disease Diagnostic and Treatment Centers at university medical centers, with about $250,000 of that money earmarked for pure research and the remainder being allocated to the Diagnostic and Treatment Centers. The centers provide a thorough diagnostic workup of patients as well as an extensive continuum of services through case management coordinated, where possible, by the Alzheimer's Day Care Resource Centers. Additional legislation which earmarked $800,000 to pure research was passed by the legislature, but vetoed by Governor Duekmejian. Though the bill was vetoed, our strong support and hard work

on this legislation proved to ADRDA chapters and legislators our effectiveness and tenacity. Personal testimony and support letters contributed to what was a difficult passage of the measure through policy and appropriations committees and the floor of the legislature. Rees and Associates coordinated a letter writing campaign to the Governor's office upon learning of a possible veto and, indeed, hundreds of letters were sent in support and later decrying his veto. We have reintroduced a research bill and have reinstated a grassroots campaign both with the legislature and the Governor's offfice. The reintroduction of such a bill requires a renewed committment. A new climate and emerging demands for appropriations in areas like AIDS care and research make obtaining Alzheimer's disease research monies a great challenge.

6) <u>Division of community property</u>, relative to Medicaid (Medi-Cal) eligibility is also within the purview of legislation we monitor. An ADRDA supported bill, passed in 1985, addressed the issue of community property belonging to a married couple to be considered when one spouse is institutionalized. The state must amend its rules to automatically divide in half the entire community property of a married couple, making that portion of the non-institutionalized spouse's property unavailable for consideration of Medicaid (Medi-Cal) eligibility for nursing home placement.

7) <u>Tax credit legislation</u>, along with respite care and research funding, is a great priority to moderate and middle-income families who are ineligible for Medicaid (Medi-Cal), unable to afford nursing care, and caring for their family member at home. California has been attempting to pass tax relief legislation for Alzheimer's disease families since 1984. There is interest and committment to the ideology, but, as with all tax savings measures, great resistance. Our Assembly Revenue and Taxation Committees are, as a matter of general policy, opposed to all tax credit measures. Despite this drawback, there may be sufficient sentiment in the legislature to move ahead with our tax credit legislation.

8) The question of <u>insurance coverage</u> for Alzheimer's disease and long term care must be addressed. An ADRDA supported measure was passed and signed by the Governor last year, requiring the state Alzheimer's Disease Task Force to study the efficacy of insurance coverage for respite care. New legislation that we have been asked to support this year creates a pilot long-term care insurance program for members of the state retirement system. Another bill requires the Department of Insurance to conduct a feasibility study of long term care coverage.

9) <u>Legal and ethical issues</u> are also carefully monitored. Conservatorships, wills, access and safety issues, abuse reporting, and quality of care in intermediate and long term care facilities are all areas of concern to the Alzheimer's patient, family, and caregiver community. The job of monitoring legislation is complex and continuous.

Each year there has been a significant increase in bills, issues, and interests pertinent to Alzheimer's disease. As a consequence of organizational growth, visibility, and better understanding of the disease itself on the part of public officials, ADRDA is now well-positioned in California to move ahead on all fronts. However, it is imperative that we have an organized approach and that committment be continuous at all levels.

Legislative advocacy has come of age, in non-profit organizations as well as for corporations, industries, unions, and professional associations. With over 600 lobbyists registered with the California Secretary of State's office, and over 7,000 bills introduced this session, the magnitude of business conducted in the state capitol is extraordinary. Competition for access to legislators is intense. Without a designated and qualified legislative consultant acting as the "eyes" and "ears" of an organization, it is impossible to follow, much less influence lawmaking. Securing the services of a professional legislative consultant was sound planning by ADRDA in California. With the size of our full-time legislature, we could not have otherwise succeeded in passing the array of measures benefiting Alzheimer's disease families that has been realized since early 1984. Such political expertise enabled ADRDA to achieve the following results:

- Establish a political presence in Sacramento.

- Monitor regulatory development to assure proper implementation of Alzheimer's disease programs according to the intent of the legislation.

- Screen, monitor, analyze, and evaluate legislation for potential impact on Alzheimer's disease patients and families.

- Issue action alerts to notify ADRDA members of the need for support/oppose letters or personal testimony on specific legislation.

- Sponsor and co-sponsor legislation carried by authors committed to achieving our goals. Establish solid relationships with key legislators.

- Serve as an information clearinghouse for other state legislative staff and ADRDA members nationwide.

- Create a Keyperson Program to support the legislative advocate and contact legislators on key issues.


ADRDA in California must constantly work within the organization to develop a strong network which can be called upon for support on specific issues. Rees and Associates worked with ADRDA members on developing a program geared to effective grassroots lobbying. Known as the Keyperson Program, it is basically a system for identifying persons in each legislative district who become advocates for Alzheimer's disease issues with carefully planned goals, objectives, and timelines. These people must be able to communicate effectively, with integrity and diplomacy, current issues and those ADRDA positions on which action is needed. The Keyperson accomplishes these objectives by lobbying in the legislator's district as a constituent and concerned citizen. Through telephone calls, letters, and personal contacts, the Keyperson establishes an on-going relationship of trust. Once recognized as an informed, knowledgeable resource, a local "expert" on Alzheimer's disease, the Keyperson can have invaluable influence on pending legislation. Obviously these persons must be credible, informed, good communicators, reliable, and interested in the political process. It is most important that they operate within the policy parameters agreed upon by ADRDA and it's political consultant.

Last year we developed the <u>Alzheimer's Disease and Related Disorder Association Keyperson Manual and Legislative Affairs Handbook</u>, a document that outlines specifically the qualifications, responsibilities, activities, and protocols for a complete Keyperson Program. It includes sample letters and listings of key committee members. This material was presented at a workshop of California ADRDA leaders who use it as a guide for creating their own local network. The interaction between lobbying in the state capitol and what Keypersons do is ongoing with the legislative consultant who originates requests for specific action. However, the Keyperson network must be visible and active whether or not a specific legislator is involved in a specific issue.  All legislators vote on all bills that reach the floor.  Furthermore, all legislators are interested to hear from their constituents when they have done a good job.  They are also anxious to know first-hand about programs that meet social needs and will often accept invitations to visit support groups, respite centers, or to attend conferences or seminars.  The objective is to maintain constant, positive visibility.

To summarize, California's legislative program has made great strides because of the dual structure we have created: a competent, professional advocate in the capitol and a network of ADRDA members who understand the priorities and importance of governmental affairs work.  Yet, we have much to do.  In expanding our Keyperson Program beyond a few very overworked people currently serving, we must recruit many others from within chapter ranks.  ADRDA members in California, as well as across the country, must begin to view themselves not just as caregivers and family members, but as advocates for change.  Moving beyond support groups and care coordination, these people must explore their untapped potential to gain real and lasting advances.  In a political sense, what is needed is for these families to become organized and activated, to define objectives, and to articulate their needs to policymakers. This approach has proven itself within the organizations devoted to heart, cancer, and lung diseases, and is absoulutely relevant to Alzheimer's disease.  Though a comparatively small organization, through the legislative approach outlined here, ADRDA should be able to see results it would ordinarily take much larger and better financed groups to achieve.  We must not be deceived, however, into underestimating the committment, hard work, and cooperation required.

From our California perspective hiring a professional political consultant has worked effectively, not by any means as a replacement for involvement by family members, but to provide experienced management, advice, and positioning within the political process.  California's experience is one example of an effective strategy for developing and influencing public policy.  Other states may wish to adapt, adopt, or tailor portions or all of the California program depending on their own unique situations.  Creating a coordinated, cooperative relationship between ADRDA members, its leadership, and an experienced legislative advocate, as long as all work carefully to achieve clearly defined goals and strategies which have been agreed upon, will result in maximum benefits for the entire Alzheimer's disease community in California and nationwide.

A PUBLIC POLICY DESIGN STRATEGY

FOR ALZHEIMER'S DISEASE

Woods Bowman

Representative, 4th District
Illinois House of Representatives
Evanston, IL

## INTRODUCTION

I became familiar with ADRDA through a friend who invited me to a conference on Alzheimer's Disease. Over lunch one of the participants turned to me and asked, "What do we have to do to pass a bill in Illinois?" I was a bit startled because I knew the Illinois chapter did not yet have a legislative agenda. I replied that, "It all depends on what you want the bill to do."

It was an impulsive question. I am sure that, upon reflection, my companion would realize he was putting the cart before the horse. However, he was committing an additional, more sophisticated, error. His question assumed the politics of passing the legislation was independent of its substance. In fact, politics and substance are inextricably intertwined, a theme to which I will return often.

My remarks will be a mixture of analysis and case study based upon our experience in Illinois which last year passed the most comprehensive package of Alzheimer's legislation in the nation, with the possible exception of California which preceded us. I will discuss the substance of the legislation in the context of elaborating the political process which brought it about.

I do not begin with a recitation of the substance of the package because I want to impress upon you at the onset that each state is different in many ways: the needs of its citizens, the existing institutional arrangements for delivering tax supported services, the procedures of its legislative branch and its politics. In short, every legislative package must be tailor made, you cannot get bills "off the rack" and expect them to fit your needs. We in Illinois examined the California legislation and then set out in our own direction. We used the California legislation as a check list to make sure we addressed the full range of issues inherent in Alzheimer's disease and I urge you to use the Illinois legislation in the same way.

The technical aspects of the disease define the possibilities for policy. Patterns in the strivings of families as they attempt to cope with the disease define the necessity for action.

363

The first step is education. Educate yourselves, educate political leaders and educate the general public. These activities can proceed more or less simultaneously, but it helps if you start with yourselves.

## Educate Yourselves

Granted, those with Alzheimer's victims in their families know a lot about the human cost of the disease and they do not need further education in that regard. But if you want to affect public policy you need to have an easy familiarity with the technical aspects of the disease. Science still has many unanswered questions about it, but it has many working hypotheses which drive research and attitudes regarding Alzheimer's.

Familiarizing yourself with the technical aspects of the disease will help you appreciate how Alzheimer's differs from other diseases and will help you better see how existing public health policy is inadequate. For example, the nationwide pattern is for public health policy to be prevention oriented and treatment oriented. Alzheimer's appears to be neither contagious nor linked to particular life-styles, so with the current state of our knowledge, prevention is not a policy option. Moreover, there is no known cure, so at the present time treatment likewise is not an option.

Although there will be hearings held as a part of the normal legislative process, do not wait for these hearings to develop the data which will guide the initial draft of your legislation. Trial lawyers never ask a witness a question they do not already know the answer to. The purpose of the questions at trial and testimony at legislative hearings is the same -- to build a public record for decision. Hearings are intended to answer the public's questions, not your questions.

## Educate Political Leaders

Once you have a fairly good handle on the issues, you should start reaching out to legislators and begin educating them. There are two main reasons for this and neither are obvious. First, you will need to test your ideas. You may not have as good a handle on the issues as you may think. If you are not used to dealing with people in the political process, you may not fully appreciate the way they look at things and you need to be able to see the issues through their eyes if you are to have any hope of influencing them.

Second, you will have to find a sponsor for your legislation. You will need someone who does more than lend his or her name to the bills. You will need these people, of course, but it is critical that you find someone with the time, skill and political connections to work closely with you --someone who will instruct you on the nuances of the legislative process in your state, help you write the bills and plan strategy.

If you do not know any legislators in whom you can place your complete confidence, you need to go shopping. Do not ask anyone to sponsor your bills during the first discussion; wait until you have interviewed nearly everyone you want to talk to. Make sure you try to talk to the key legislative leaders and committee chairs. While you will be discussing your issue in nonpartisan terms, you must be keenly aware of the partisan nature of the legislative process. If both houses are controlled by the same party you should probably have a member of that party sponsor your bills (especially if the Governor is also of the same party). Just remember it may not be important to you who gets credit for passing the bills, but it is important to the elected officials.

There are only a couple of simple rules to follow when meeting with legislators. First, most legislators are part time and do not have large staffs, if they have any staff at all. You can and should treat them just as you would treat anyone else. Second, legislators will want to know why you are visiting them. If the meeting is exploratory, say you are asking their advice. If you are promoting a specific bill, give them the bill number and ask their support.

By having a series of meetings with legislators while the legislation is in its formative stages you can identify the legislators who are excited by your ideas and whom you feel you can trust. While it is not necessary to have a legislative leader sponsor your bills, a freshman may not have the necessary connections and insights to be an effective sponsor, either.

You can use this process of education to begin building the network of interested individuals and groups which will help later when the time comes to exert influence on the legislative process. In Illinois we held a day-long conference on the subject of Alzheimer's Disease. It was sponsored jointly by the Appropriations Committee which I chair and the medical school of Southern Illinois University. We shared the expenses of the conference and the Illinois State Medical Society chipped in by covering the cost of a concluding reception. Attendance was by invitation only; the guest list of 100 included researchers, service providers and policy makers throughout state government. Mutual interaction, which is impossible at a legislative hearing, was encouraged. Panels of experts helped focus discussion in two areas: research and family support. Before we drafted any bills, we had fairly complete answers to the key questions.

The legislative hearings which were held after the bills were introduced were used to educate legislators, to develop public awareness and public involvement and to fine-tune the language in the bills. The hearings turned up few surprises, but they proved to be indispensable. We took testimony from 100 persons and, by holding the hearings in different locations, we educated citizens in four major media markets throughout the state. The vast majority of testimony came from persons other than those at the conference, so by the time the bills went to the floor of the House, nearly 200 allies in and out of state government had been recruited and consensus had been built. As a result, no amendments were offered on the floor except some of a technical nature offered by the sponsors themselves.

To summarize: legislative hearings should conclude the process of educating legislators and the public which was begun much earlier.

Educate the Public

The conference and hearings were an important part of educating the public in Illinois, but we could not have done the job without the personal interest of one of the best known TV personalities in Chicago. Linda Yu developed a series of news features which ran throughout a whole week as part of her station's prime time news program. She followed up by covering every aspect of the legislative process.

Not only was Ms. Yu's coverage important in its own right, but the other media outlets in the Chicago area began to identify the legislation as newsworthy and coverage multiplied.

You may not be as fortunate as we were in Chicago to have a local media personality adopt Alzheimer's Disease as their personal crusade, but it need not be merely a matter of luck. Do not hesitate to lobby the media, just as you would lobby the legislature. Go to the feature editors of the major media outlets (print and electronic) and try to interest them in running stories on Alzheimer's Disease.

Before you meet with them, you should know what will pique their interest. They will be interested in the unusual characteristics of the disease, its mysterious origins and its intractability to treatment. They will want names of victims and families they can interview to provide the human dimension to their stories. They will want to know what you are doing to alleviate the problems. Here you can get some advance publicity for your legislative agenda, even if you are still in the process of developing it.

If you are successful in developing feature coverage by major media outlets in your state, do not forget to return to the same media outlets to talk to their editorial directors and try to interest them in doing editorials on the subject. Often the feature and editorial departments of the same outlet do not communicate with each other, so a story will not automatically guarantee a supporting editorial. On the other hand, if a feature story has already run or aired, you have an excellent entre' to the editorial offices you should not waste.

If you cannot stir up any enthusiasm among the major media outlets, do not despair. Make a list of all the newsletters you can think of which might have an interest in Alzheimer's Disease. Many state departments have house organs which might run stories. Quasi-governmental organizations like Health Systems Agenices and private groups like major hospitals have newsletters. Get stories in as many as you can. You may be surprised at the size of the cumulative audience of these newsletters. Also, you may be surprised how many legislators read these newsletters. Once legislators see stories in several different newsletters, they will take the issue seriously.

DEVELOPING YOUR PROGRAM

The program I have outlined for you may sound ambitious. But it is just the beginning, you still do not have a legislative program. Issues have yet to be sharpened, options identified, choices made and bills written. My remarks in this section will be devoted to some of the policy issues which we wrestled with in Illinois and I believe are common to many states.

You should classify the issues into broad categories. Each state is different, but the basic issues are similar.

First are the issues which revolve around medical and technical problems. These issues include public support for research into the causes of the disease, research into improvement of diagnostic techniques, and, of course, research to find a cure.

The second set of issues embrace availability of services to victims and their families. These issues can be subdivided into (1) creating services which do not now exist, such as supervisory care and specialized day care, (2) providing access to existing services which are targeted to other populations, such as in-home chore housekeeping and health care for the frail elderly, (3) assisting middle-income families with the financial burden.

A third set of issues involves developing public awareness establishing an administrative mechanism for incorporating new discoveries into public policy.

This breakdown of the basic issues parallels one first articulated in 1983 by Dr. Nancy Lombardo, a member of the ADRDA National Public Policy and Issues Committee. I reworked the classification slightly to focus attention on the specialization I see emerging in addressing the issues.

Because research of all kinds has long been a federally supported activity there are strong, and I believe reasonable, barriers to state involvement. After all, we want to concentrate our tax dollars on the very best research institutions in the nation; anything else would be wasteful. In fact, research is a preoccupation of the national ADRDA.

The states, on the other hand, have taken the lead in setting up service delivery systems. Regardless which human service you examine you will rarely find anything resembling a nationally administered and integrated delivery system. Here is where you can have your greatest effect at the state level: find out what service people need and get it to them.

Finally, public awareness is everybody's job. You cannot legislate public awareness and so the burden of making the public aware and shaping its attitudes falls squarely on the shoulders of private groups such as ADRDA and its local chapters. To be sure you can use the legislative process at the national and state levels as tools in this regard, but the main burden is yours to carry.

## Medical/Technical Issues

Just because the focus of research policy is at the federal level does not mean you should not consider the needs in this area and assess the possibilities for state involvement.

There is probably a niche the states can fill at relatively low cost and that is in the area of diagnosis. Alzheimer's is only one of many presenile dementias, some of which are treatable. But there is no direct diagnosis yet available. It is identified by a protracted workup through the process of elimination. It is unreasonable to expect every family practitioner and every community hospital in the nation to be equally effective in performing these arduous workups.

Therefore in Illinois we chose to strengthen our existing research centers and harness them to provide better support for family practitioners attempting diagnosis. We tied the practitioners and hospitals in our state into a new Alzheimer's Disease Assistance Network with our premier research institutions becoming Regional Alzheimer's Disease Assistance Centers and forming the focal points of the network. The network also reaches out and involves various health, mental health and social service agencies that provide referral, treatment and support services.

The Regional ADA Centers themselves will be required to have a full range of research programs, training programs for caregivers, diagnostic capabilities, and referral services.

They will be encouraged to enter into contractual arrangement with other hospitals in the state for referral of difficult to diagnose cases.

The State Department of Public Health will develop an Alzheimer's Disease Plan to help guide the formation of the network and foster its development. The plan shall be prepared in consultation with an advisory council and shall be updated every three years.

We attempted, with less success, to develop better data for research. Since a positive diagnosis of Alzheimer's Disease is possible only upon autopsy our first impulse was to require an autopsy of every person who died in a state of dementia. This approach turned out to be fraught with administrative problems, ethical problems (suppose the families do not want the autopsy performed) and political problems. We settled instead for a systematic education program which made coroners aware of the value of examining the brain tissues and made the families of Alzheimer's victims aware of the importance of attending to the necessary paperwork early so the autopsy would be performed immediately upon death without a time-consuming and traumatic decision making process occurring at the time of death.

I wanted to go further and require a release form to be signed before services would be rendered by the Regional ADA Centers, but for a variety of reasons that seemed an unwise approach. I mention it only to give you an idea of the range of ideas we considered before we settled on our final product.

## Availability of Services

Upon review of existing services we discovered that some needed services were not being offered by anyone, or at very few locations: respite care, specialized adult day care, crisis intervention, etc. We developed one bill to provide for a program of matching grants to social service agencies to develop experimental programs and another bill which set up an interagency task force which would be in a position to identify service gaps and provide a resource to the Department on Aging, the grant administrator, with useful information as it went about the business of developing new services.

In another bill we established a system of financial incentives for nursing homes to address the special needs of Alzheimer's victims.

But there were many existing services already in place which our research showed were not available to all Alzheimer's victims because of different barriers. For example, our extensive system of in-home chore housekeeping and health care services is targeted at either elderly or permanently disabled populations. The criteria for getting access to these programs include an age and disability screen. If the Alzheimer's victim is younger than 65 years of age, they cannot qualify, so we lowered the age at which our Department on Aging could provide service to Alzheimer's victims and made sure that the Department of Rehabilitation Services had a mandate to provide service to still more youthful victims regardless of the fact that Alzheimer's Disease is not otherwise considered in law to be a "disability".

There were other barriers to gaining access to these programs as well. A test of service need had to be applied and passed. This test had been designed with the physical needs of people in mind. As one of our witnesses put it, "The screen tested if a person has the physical capacity to pick up and use a broom unaided, but not whether they had the mental capacity to know which end of the broom to use." As you know, many Alzheimer's victims are physically healthy, this is part of the unique tragedy of Alzheimer's. We had to redefine the screening criteria to enable these people to gain access to an existing and much needed service.

We also recognized the financial barriers confronting middle income families in obtaining nursing home placement. As you know, neither private insurance nor medicare pays for extended stays in nursing homes. Medicaid does, but it is means tested and the entire household must become destitute before Medicaid financing is available. We passed a bill which permits families to divide their assets between married couples and for the victim's interest in the family home to be transferred to his or her spouse and thereby protected from the Medicaid "spend down" requirement. We also extended this protection to those persons availing themselves of means-tested in home care programs.

Private insurance is a tougher nut to crack. One cannot very easily require insurance companies to create a product which does not now exist and to sell it at a reasonable rate. In an attempt to prod the private insurance industry into taking action we established a task force under the Department of Insurance to research the matter. If they adopt an aggressive posture and recommend the creation of certain products and show how these products might be reasonably priced, we can use these results to challenge the industry. There are some big ifs here, but it seemed worth a try.

Public Awareness

It is difficult to legislate a program of public awareness, but we tried to work it into several of the bills. When we established the Regional ADA Centers we required they establish a system of referral to all support services. We provided for education of county coroners regarding Alzheimer's disease. We established the interagency task force and authorized it to hold public hearings. We set up the insurance task force. These are all a part of the public education picture.

The legislature has an on-going interest in Alzheimer's Disease, too. The Committee on Aging in the House may well hold additional hearings in two or three years to review the statewide plan called for in one bill and the insurance task force report called for in another.

CONCLUSION

This section is called CONCLUSION, but there can be no real conclusion to public policy formation, especially in an area which is constantly changing as new knowledge of the disease and its incidence is acquired and as public attitudes about the disease undergo a quiet revolution.

Once legislation is passed, the real work begins. The first task is to make sure the Governor signs the legislation. If there has been little contact with the Governor's office or any of the executive agencies during the legislative process, this may pose a problem. That is why we in Illinois invited the Governor's staff and his department heads to a conference early in the development of the legislation. We were thus able to anticipate problems and by the time the legislation reached his desk, there was no question that he would sign it. In fact, he had a well-publicized bill signing ceremony.

But this is not all, a department charged with new responsibilities may not have the same vision as the originators of the legislation. The rules and regulations drawn by the departments to implement the new laws may be narrow and stultifying. There may not be adequate funding in future budgets. In short, one cannot take anything for granted. There must be adequate followup especially in monitoring the activities of all entities which have been charged under the new laws. What the law gives the rule can take away.

It will be necessary to monitor and evaluate the policy outcomes over a period of several years. As advocates you should establish a committee to see to it. If you have developed the issue thoroughly up to this point, your group will be considered a "major player" by policy makers in government. As a major player its views will be solicited before any major change is effected in Alzheimer's Disease policy in the future. As a major player its members will have access to the policy makers in government.

As a major player your advocacy group will have a responsibility to be knowledgeable about technical breakthroughs in diagnosis and treatment and to be sensitive to new problems which emerge as older problems are solved.

PUBLIC POLICY AND LONG TERM CARE:  DOMESTIC

AND INTERNATIONAL PERSPECTIVES

Mary S. Harper

National Institute of Mental Health
U.S. Department of Health & Human Services
Rockville, Maryland

ABSTRACT

Public policy for long term care in the U.S. is institutionally oriented. Less than half of L.T.C. is publically financed. There is no national
policy for L.T.C. Public policy for L.T.C. does not include the homeless
elderly, the uninsured, uninsurable elderly, and the near poor elderly just
about the poverty line with assets. Reimbursement for L.T.C. by Medicare/
Medicaid is in favor of acute care. Public policy does not reward the eight
million unpaid family caregivers of services to the elderly. L.T.C. in
other countries is more community based than the U.S.A. and the government
assumes greater responsibility for the financing.

The major impacts in shaping the delivery and cost of health will be
long term care. This country is experiencing a demographic revolution. It
is graying, and the elderly clearly dominate the health field as consumers.

Long Term Care Service needs increase with age. Actually 5600 people
celebrate their 65th birthday each year, that is about 2.0 million persons
celebrated their 65th birthday in 1984. In the same year, about 1.4 million
persons 65 or older died resulting in a net increase of over 560,000 (1550
per day) Over 12 percent of the U.S. population is 65 years or older (29
million in 1984). The number of older Americans increased by 2.3 million or
10 percent since 1980 compared to an increase of 4 percent for the under 65
population (AARP-1985).

Since 1900, the percentage of Americans sixty five and over (65+) has
tripled (4.1 % in 1900 to 11.9% in 1984) and the increased nine (9) times
from 3.1 million to 28.0 million) (Aging in America 1985-1986).

The older population itself is getting older. IN 1984, the 65-74 age
group (16.7 million) was over seven times larger than it was in 1900, by the
75-84 age group (8.6 million) was eleven (11) times larger and the 85+ age
group (2.7 million) was 21 times larger.

In 1984, persons reaching 65 had an average life expectancy of an
additional 16.8 years (18.7 for females and 14.5 years for males).

A child born in 1984 could expect to live to 74.7 years, about 27 years
longer than a child born in 1900.

According to Scalon & Feder (1984), health care expenditure in 1984 was $333.4 billion ($1365 for each person) of this amount $120 billion was spent for personal care for the 29 million elderly Americans 65 and older.

Long Term Care (LTC) is the fastest growing segment of the U.S. health care industry. Revenue of the most visible LTC providers – nursing homes – topped $24 billion in 1981, more than five (5) times their 1970 level.

What makes someone part of the LTC population is not a particular diagnosis or condition but the need for supportive service over an extended period. Supportive services for this population addresses a broad range of health, social and personal care needs of individuals who for one reason or another have never developed or have lost some capacity for self care. Long term care includes persons under 65 as well as persons over 65 (Meltzer et al., 1981).

The LTC population include:

|  | No. of Homes -Beds | No. of Residents |
|---|---|---|
| Nursing and Related Care Homes Fuller (1983) | 26,817 with 1,508,732 beds | 1,378,702 |
| Residential Facilities Sirrocco (1985) | 8,030 with 133,335 beds | 114,704 |
| Adult Day Care |  | 13,500 |
| Board and Care Homes Newcomer & Stone (1985) |  | 1,500,000 |
| Single Room Occupancy (SRO) Hotel/Homes, Minkler & Querbo (1985) |  | 1,700,000 |
| Mentally Retarded (Note 1 million are elderly) Hauber, et al., (1984) |  | 2,800,000 |
| Acute Hospital: Older Patients Rovner (1986) |  | 12,000,000 elderly admitted to 5800 acute hospitals in the USA last year. |
| Non-instructional elderly with one or more chronic condition with limitations & needs help with one or more of the basic activities of daily living Fuller (1983) |  | 3,600,000 (2.7 million are age 65+) |
| Mentally Ill, Goldman, et al., (1981) |  | 1,200,000 (0.8 million in community) |
| Penal institutions, Goldman, (1981) Note: The percentage of persons 65 years of age and older inmates increased by 3.8% in 1960 and 4.8% in 1970. |  | 10,0000 |

|  | No. of Homes -Beds | No. of Residents |
|---|---|---|
| Home heath care<br>Note: 65-70% of the home health care beneficiaries are elderly<br>Contemporary Long Term Care | 8000 agencies serving 2,000,000 individuals | |
| Respite Care, McFarland (1985) | No official count | |
| Hospice Care<br>Note: There are 935 operating hospice programs and 4120 are in the planning stage according to the national hospice organization (NHO) Scanlon & Feder (1984) | No official count | |
| Homeless GAO (1985) | | 2,000,000+<br>(50% are elderly) |

Therefore, I am saying that there are at least twenty million elderly people in long term care in the U.S.A. Seventy to 85% of the LTC in the community is provided by the family and 75% of the institutional care is provided by nursing aides or para professional staff. Many of the aides are either poorly trained or have no training at all. There is a beginning trend for community colleges to offer preservice training in one semester for aides. Some nursing homes and home health care agencies have exemplary training programs. According to the American Health Care Association (1984) there are 64,315 full time nurse employees, 86,044 licensed practical nurses and 462,900 nursing aides.

With this size population there are numerous implications for public policy. The financing, organization, administration, and the provision of LTC service for the elderly is a costly, complex, and critical area of public policy.

Policy formulation is the determinant of both the impact of LTC and of the shape of the practice. However, practitioners and policy formulators have not taken the matter of LTC seriously, except for monetary policy which determines what services are delivered.

Policy is both formal and functional, formal policy may be something on paper while functional policy determines what gets defined as LTC problems, and what priority is given in terms of informing the public about the availability of LTC services. What is policy? Dye (1972) in his book defines policy as, the authoritative allocation of values for the whole society. Public policy in this sense is a projected program of goals, values and practice. Public policy may be regulative, organizational, distributive and extractive. The formulation of policy is a process of the interaction of the factors of want, demand, support and regulation. From this point of view policy determines the goods or services to be rendered, and the scope of services delivered. Policy allocates values and is itself a reflection of values.

A recent observation made by a leading state politician, Lamm (1984) stated; "the terminally ill elderly has a duty to die and get out of the way" - is reflective of some of the values and attitudes about the elderly, which are frequently reflected in public policy.

Estes (1979) sees the genesis and growth of public policy for aging as stemming from the manner in which society in general and the helping professions in particular have chosen to define the issues of aging in the U.S.A. She sees much of what America has done is to define the elderly as a problem.

In the U.S.A., the central problems of older people are those of isolation, disengagement, individual pathologies, poverty, loneliness and assorted functional incapacities. Estes argues that having defined the issue in this a manner, policy makers preferred solutions which centered around integrating, socializing and other wise assisting older persons in adjustment and accommodating themselves to the larger society. Estes further states that a number of "health professional-service domains through which they maintain themselves by defining the needs of the elderly in ways congruent with their professional requisites. Much of the performances cluster around creating a passive and dependent relationship for the elderly.

If aging policy means a intentional, coherent overall plan about what the United States should do about the elderly citizens, then the U.S.A. does not have a social policy on old age. Rather, the activity pursued by successive governments (federal, stat, county and local) on behalf of elderly citizens are outcomes, both direct and indirect, of many often times fragmented programs. Some of the programs specify the elderly as a target group; others aim at the larger society but benefit the elderly. Many programs have developed unsystematically and frequently with little regards for those already existing. A partial explanation for this overlapping often results from responses to "invested" interest groups and their "pressure" on congress. However, there does exist an ad hoc federal inter-agency committee on research in aging, whose function is the prevention of duplication of programs and the encouragement of more collaboration between agencies/programs.

Although policies and programs affecting LTC services for the elderly have been examined by congressional committees, the Congressional Budget Office, state agencies, the Public Health Service, General Accounting Office (GAO), Health Financing Administration (HCFA) and other offices with the Department of health and Human Services, and by a number of able individuals and groups outside of government, many basic problems remaining unresolved. Particularly vexing has been the continued increase in long term care cost; the lack of adequate community or in-home care alternatives to institutional care paid for by Medicare/Medicaid, questions of fiscal capacity, the relationship of federal, state and local governments, lack of access to LTC for the underserved, "ineligibles for Medicare/Medicaid, lack of access for some of the Medicaid eligible, fragmentation/lack of continuity of care, and chronic problems that have made sound policy decisions more difficult.

There are still questions about quality assurance (structural, process and outcomes). Sybert and Weiss (1985) report that there are thirty (30) inspections by different regulatory agencies (federal and state) each year, and 600 federal regulations and equal number of state and local level government patient care policies, staff qualifications, physical plant conditions, life and fire safety codes, patient rights, capital improvements, new constructions and reimbursements.

Politics, economics and social structure have far more to do with the role and the status of the elderly than does the aging process and its effects on the individual. Most important are economic, politics, particularly relating to employment, health and retirement. It must recognize that 50% of health care is politically determined and not by health care professionals/providers. Health care is on the major

determinant of health. As result of Lalonde's study (1974) of the National
Health Insurance in Canada, he learned that providing access to health care
and improving the quality of care were not the most effective steps toward
improving the health of the population. After examining the major factors
affecting health, Lalonde grouped these factors into four (4) categories,
namely,

*Human biology
*Environment
*Life style
*Health care organizations, and he posed five
  policy intervention strategies namely:

Health promotion
Health research
Disease prevention
Health regulations
Health care, as well as social components

It would seem to me that the focus of public policy would be toward the
five strategies above. Instead, health public policies are focused on
institutional care, reimbursement and the medical practitioners. This is
unfortunate, because 95% of the elderly are in the community and 80% of the
care is provided by the family – unfortunately with little consultation,
supervision or monitoring by a health professional. One of the strategies
of LTC is the frequent absence of medical and nursing supervision/
monitoring. One recent study in California (1981) found that the physician
spent less than a half minute per day with the average nursing home patient.
Flagle (1978) reported that the registered nurse spent 12 minutes per day in
a skilled nursing facility (SNF) and only 7 minutes per day in an
intermediate care facility (ICF). In Fries & Cooney (1983) study, they
found that the nursing aide spent 104 minutes with the most intense group of
patients (patients who were incontinent, needed bathing, feeding etc.).

Health care is no longer the primary domain of the health providers.
There are over 48 business/health care coalitions who have undertaken a
variety of strategies to control health care cost, lobby for health
programs, policies, legislation and monitor the implementation of public
policy (Greenmen, 1983).

The office of Technology Assessment identified some of the major conditions, and diagnosis of the elderly in LTC institutions/non-institutions.

Dementia
Urinary
Hearing impairment
Osteoporosis
Osteoarthritis
Depression
Cardiovascular Disease
Cander
Hypertension
Bronchitis & Asthma
Dizziness
Confusion
Feelings of hopelessness
Cognitive impairment/decline
Cancer

Most of the conditions above are chronic conditions for which there are no
known cause and a great deal of uncertainty about the care, treatment or
cure. Yet, most of our public policies address acute conditions, acute care

and institutional care. Eighty percent (80%) of the elderly have one or more chronic conditions. The kind of condition which there are no cure and advice on changing of life style may be as effective as some of the medications taken. Chronic illness has overtaken acute illness as the major health concern and as the prime cause of dysfunction for people of all ages.

Strategies for LTC

1. To delay the onset of preventable disease in healthy adults

2. To lengthen the period of functional independence in those elderly with chronic disease, and

3. To improve the quality of one's later life.

There are three major shifts in federal policy which will directly affect LTC of the elderly.

*A significant reduction in federal expenditures for domestic and health programs.
Note: In the September 1985 issue of Today's Nursing Home the LTC leadership organization reports that $40 billion have been cut from the Medicare budget in the past five years and it is proposed that $55 billion will be cut from Medicare and $1.3 billion from Medicaid in the next five years. The elderly are already spending 15% of their income on health care cost, which will increase to 18.9% of their income by 1990.

*Decentralization of program authority and responsibility to states, particularly through block grants.
Note: Decentralization has brought about a lot of diversities and some inequities in public polices. States are having a hard time to maintain and expand their present LTC services with budget cuts. At risk of not having access to quality care are such groups as the uninsured, the socially isolated, the poor, and racial/ethnic minorities.

*Deregulation and greater emphasis on market forces and competition to address the problem of continuing increases in the cost of medical care.

As a strategy for improving LTC services, many states are forming coalitions around reimbursement for LTC, wage stability, research centers, Alzheimer's research centers, establishing clinical units for Alzheimer's disease and for AIDS patients (Acquired Immune Deficiency Syndrome).

The federal policy shifts come at a time when many states and local governments are experiencing fiscal strain or fiscal crises due, in part, to the rapid rise in expenditures for the medical indigent and the imposition of limitations on, and even reductions in tax revenues. In the short term, changes at the state level, particularly limitations in medical expenditures, are likely to have the most profound effect on medical care of the elderly. These changes will most likely include reductions in Medicaid eligibility both in scope of benefits as well as tighter controls on hospital, nursing home and physician reimbursement. Geiger (1980) observe that conditions for the elderly have grown worse since the middle of the 70's and noted that "social policy currently portends a decade of disaster for the health of older Americans regardless of our ultimate actions in the area of medical care".

Although the elderly are major consumers of health care and social services, the integration of these two systems of care (institutional and non-institutional) have never been a focus of public policy. The result has been two systems of care offering multiple, parallel, overlapping and noncontinuous services.  Neither the medical care system nor the social service system (the hospital nor the community) is wholly adequate in addressing the elderly's needs for support.  Because of the multiple conditions and illness, the elderly need multidiscipline, multiservice approaches in acute and LTC settings and effective care management.  Medicare was enacted in 1965 as one appropriate response to the acute medical needs of the elderly.  TEFRA (Tax Equity and Fiscal Responsibility Act of 1982) may well be one response to LTC needs of the very old elderly.  The diagnostic related group (DRG) driven reimbursement formula encourages the release of acute care admissions as quickly as possible.  In all to many instances, it has been a matter of discharge quicker and sicker.  The development of non-acute or step down services is a major option to accelerate the movement of patients from the in-patient bed to a community setting in a responsible way.  TEFRA/step down services offer a spectrum of institutional, community or home services.  Short term step down services may be provided by a general hospital in the form of a rehabilitation unit.  Any skilled nursing facility may be the setting for convalescent care which may include rehabilitation services, meals on wheels, home health care or foster care programs.

The average length of stay in LTC facility is 2 years, yet the policy makers seem to think of LTC in terms of 10 to 20 years of health care services.  The elderly needs short-term long term care (STLTC) and long term long term care (LTLTC).

STLTC facilities would include hospitals, skilled nursing facilities (SNF) out patient, hospice care, day care and rehabilitation hospital home health care (HHC).  Among the elderly persons who experienced SNF stays in 1977, 53.7% (600,000 admissions) stayed less than 90 days, whereas 46.3% stayed 90 days or more (U.S. DHHS, 1979).  Over on (1) million older persons use medicare - reimbursed HHC services annually (Weissert, 1985).  The STLTC serves the temporarily needy, frail elderly, who returns to the homes (39.8%) or are admitted to the hospital (23.5% or die (21.2%).  At least 1.7 million elderly are already involved in STLTC.

The LTLTC facilities serve the more permanently disabled, frail elderly who generally require long term services that is more socially and functionally oriented as compared to the more medically-oriented STLTC.  Ten to 18% of the elderly need a case manager to coordinate, moniter and mobilize their services.  Public policy must reflect the levels of LTC needed by the elderly.  We must not build facilities and staff them as if the resident will be there for long periods of time.  Such consideration will be cost savings and cost effective.

According to the March 6 issue of the New York Times (1986) some of the public policies governing Medicare/Medicaid reimbursement policies have created an unusual situation in which 30 female nursing home residents in New York City have sued their husbands for support in family court.  This is because the state law provides that such support payment cannot be included by Medicaid when it calculates how much a couple "assets and retirement income can be taken."  One resident sued her husband for support after 51 years of marriage.  He had only $400 per month and food stamps to live on.  This amount should be calculated when considering Medicaid eligibility, however, if she successfully sues her husband, this amount is exempt from calculation of Medicaid eligibility.

The family provides 75 to 80% of the non-institutional care.  There is no explicit policy on the family or even family care for disabled relatives at any stage of life, the impact of current policy and programs on the elderly of family members is indirect, inconsistent and unplanned.  With the growth of the elderly population and the shrinking of public funds, there has been a clamoring to draw the line between family responsibility and public responsibility for the care of the elderly. In response, some policy makers are apparently willing to shift greater responsibility to the family, and given states virtual license to hold families financially responsible if their spouse, child or parent is a Medicaid patient in a nursing home. In a recent survey, 27 states said such a policy was under consideration. Three states said that the concept was considered and dropped. Buchannan (1984) reports that the attorney general in Idaho, released an opinion on March 23, 1984 indicating that the law "is inconsistent with federal law regulating the use of Medicaid funds". Schorr (1980) found in a survey of kin contribution to the care of Medicaid patients in Pennsylvania, that half of the contributors had an annual income of $5400 or less and the other half had an income of $12000 or less annually. The family responsibility/LTC law could hardly be construed as an "incentive" for these families. Other evidence in federal policy effort to provide incentive for family care support of impaired members is the use of the tax system in home care as stated by Perlman (1982). In 1954, it became possible for families with specific income levels to deduct from their income tax a limited amount for expenses incurred in the care of a disabled spouse or dependent. In 1975 tax law was amended so that a tax credit of 20% of the care cost was substituted for the tax deduction. Although some adjustments were made, this tax credit is seen as only useful to families who have higher taxable incomes and not for families with Medicaid patients.

The elderly in LTC are heav users of over 35 regular services (legal counseling, care by the orthopedic surgeon, clinical services, podiatrist, optician, meals on wheels, etc.). Therefore, the elderly sometimes are receiving services from 9 to 12 different clinics. In some instances receiving medications or treatment create iatrogenic conditions. Therefore, public policy should minimize fragmentation and promote continuity of care as through the social health maintenance organization S/HMO or single point entry where a case manager coordinates/monitor all appointments and activities, including hospital care, outpatient, daycare, home health care, hospice, respite, etc.

## Chronological Age and Social Policy

In view of the increasing number of four and five generation families; middle aged families with three and four children in college, faced with inflation and "cuts," both parents working because of necessities and sharing the expenses of one or two parents in a nursing home costing $2000 to $3000 per month, "Aging as a criterion for focusing public policy programs" is an issue frequently addressed in the policy arena. The "yuppies" are questioning many of the "entitlement" and "transfer funds" services available at tax payers expenses, and "exemptions" of the elderly etc. There is an organization entitled, Americans for Generational Equity Association. They had a congressional hearing in April 1986 in Washington. I raised this as a recurring public policy issue for you to keep in mind when establishing and/or evaluating public policies for the aging/elderly in these days of scarce public resources. Therefore, some of the questions relevant for policy formulation, which we may ask include:

1. How meaningful is age as age criterion for defining eligibility?

2. In identifying target populations for service programs we must specify the characteristics of the elderly for whom the program and policies are aimed, i.e., frail elderly, low-income elderly, elderly living alone, or the unserved/underserved elderly.

3. What are some of the advantages and disadvantages of using need rather than age or a combination of need and age as a criteria

for service programs?  What are the implications for societal and demographic change?

The current issue that confronts policy workers is the value of designing policy and programs for persons of a certain age or for those with a particular need (e.g., disability income).  The advantages and disadvantages of age targeted policies/programs have been widely debated by Estes (1979); Chenbaum et al., (1983); and Neugarten (1982).

Morris (1982) has discussed a number of programmatic options that are involved in targeting benefits to handicapped or chronically limited persons in LTC.  All are based on the notion of shared responsibility between family and the state.  The first option is the use of demographics or an aid – in – attendance allowance in which the disabled person is paid a flat monthly fee regardless of income level, the advantage is the built-in-equity.  However, the monthly fee would only supplement care-cost expenditures to a limited degree (i.e., the fee would be in all likelihood inadequate).  Another advantage of the allowance is that the disabled person has complete control over care or services and can pay informal caregivers for assistance.

Despite the fact that the U.S. policy has historically been individual-focused, some gerontologists (Morris & Levitt, 1982) have argued that it is essential to develop a social policy that is family-centered.  The reasons are that families are the major providers of services to the non-institutionalized impaired elders, and unless policy begins to bolster family care-giving, it will decline in prevalence or have untoward effects on American families.  Unless the family efforts are supported and strengthened by policy and programs, family caregivers will be overtaxed.  As a result, the care provided by kin to the impaired relative will deteriorate (e.g., neglect, abuse) the family will deteriorate with concomitant "hidden social cost" (e.g., mental illness, stress and strain, substance abuse, delinquency) or the impaired relative will be placed in an institution which is the highest cost care modality.

Some of the policy options for financing LTC include:

Options

    Tax credits for families
    Reverse annuity mortgages
    New federal program to cover long-term care
    Extension of Medicare to cover social services
    Individual Retirement Accounts (IRAS) for long-term care
    Increase in co-payments for medicare
    Enforcement of family financial responsibility
    A voucher system for Medicare
    Increase in deductibles for Medicare
    Increase the age of Medicare eligibility
    Increased LTC insurance

Private financing of LTC has increased.  Categories of private insurance include (U.S. DHHS/OAS, 1985).

    *Individual LTC insurance
     (12 insurance companies covering 50,000 individuals)

    *Group LTC insurance
     (coverage for 800,000 workers and dependent totaling 2.2 million people)
    *Prepaid LTC insurance (e.g., S/HMO, elder plan of New york City,

Kaiser, Portland, Ultra care for Medicare recipients)

## Barriers to Private Financing

*Annuity rigidity
Only 15% of elderly are on pension.  1/2 annuity are fixed monthly
payment.

*Illiquid assets - elderly may have home as asset but this is essential
for their housing.

*Loans and regulation incentives to divest.  Medicaid and estate
tax requires divestment.

## Public Financing of LTC include

Medicare and Medicaid finance two thirds of the cost; nursing home
expenses totalled $25 billion with 42% of costs of such coming from two
programs (40% form Medicaid and 2% from Medicare).  About %13 billion in
nursing home expenditures are paid by the private sector, insurance is
expected to pay only $287 million.  The per capita health costs for the
elderly is estimated at $4200 in 1984 including $1900 for hospital care and
$880 for nursing home costs.

To assist with policy directions, a recently established group entitled
National Committee for Future Health Policy is headquartered in Washington,
D.C. with Dr. Carl Eisdorfer as the president and Charles H. Edwards execu-
tive director.

## Some Research Questions/Issues raised by the Committee include

1.  What are some of the emerging theories of state budgeting and
policy implementation by analyzing the shifts in legislative and
administrative decision making under conditions of state discretion and
constrained fiscal capacity?

2.  Identification of the key state policies that contribute to the
service, supply, population demands, public program expenditures and
utilization outcomes.

3.  Establish formula for reimbursement for LTC according to treatment
outcomes.

4.  Identification of the potentially tractable maniputable policy
variables that might be considered for adoption at federal or state levels
that are likely to affect desired expenditures and utilization outcome.

5.  What are the incentives for nursing homes to admit outliers
(patients requiring heavy duty cars at higher cost) and the uninsured,
ineligibles for Medicare/Medicaid?

6.  What impact will altering Medicaid eligibility for nursing home
care have on utilization of expenditures for these services?

7.  What impact does the availability supply of health providers (both
institutional and non-institutional) a have on access to and costs of care
provided to public beneficiaries?

8.  What effect can expansions in home and community services be expected to have on institutional costs?
9.  How will the current state fiscal crises affect state policies with

respect to health and social programs for the elderly?

10. Have changes in prospective payment systems, of reimbursement policies for public programs had any measurable effect on program costs?

11. How are expansions or contractions in one program, say SSI, likely to affect other programs for the elderly such as Medicaid?

12. What is meant by the term "nursing home bed shortage" and what are the policy implications of such a shortage?

13. What implication does the presence of excess demand for nursing home care have for the costs associated with expanding non-institutional long term care services?

International Issues & LTC

In 1950, the United Nations estimated there would be approximately 200 million persons 60 years of age throughout the world. By 1975, this figure had increased to 350 million. The United Nations (UN) projections to the year 2000 indicate that this number will increase to 590 million, and by 2025 to over 1,100 billion, That is a 224% increase since 1974 as compared to the 102% increase in the rest of the population. The greatest increase will be in the less developed countries.

A doubling of the size of the population age 65 and over took place between 1950 and 1980 in developing regions. According to projections for the future, elderly populations in developing regions will increase at a faster rate than in the developed region, leading to a situation where the majority of individuals age 65 and over (approximately 57% in the year 2000) are in developing countries.

According to Siegel & Honaver (1983) and Orial (1982) the number of octogenarians in the world are:

China 25 million
India 10.6
USSR 10.1
USA 7.1
Japan 5.9

A pattern of governmentally assured personal social services for the elderly evolved late in the developed countries, where industrialization brought in its wake an increase in the gross domestic product (DP) and a change in family and social relations. Despite the dispersion of the family, the significant role of the family in the case of the elderly re-mains.

There is a trend in the less developed countries (LDC) toward migration of the younger people to cities for employment and better living conditions. In most countries except the Latin American countries, the elderly is frequently left in the rural areas with their grandchildren. Transportation and health services are scarce in the rural areas.

By and large, the elderly are cared for at home. The family is the primary caregiver who is generally financed by constant attendant allowances (Home Care Worker). The number of home helps reported in selected countries grew steadily between 1970 and 1973 from 118,718 to 281,409. On a rank order basis, Great Britain and Sweden clearly provide the most home help and Australia, Italy and Israel and Austria have the fewest.

In Denmark - 18% of the population over age 65 is reported to be childless

In Italy, 40% of the elderly live alone.

In Japan, 74% of the elderly live with their children (generally the oldest son.)

In the less developed countries there are few organized health services for the elderly by the government, therefore there are very few, public policies. The very few health services which do exist are operated by private volunteer groups such as the Salvation Army, Lions Club, etc.

The World Health Organization (WHO) (1980) has developed a widely used numerical system, the International Classification of Disease (ICD) to classify acute health problems in its study of morbidity and morality. Recognizing the growing importance of chronic health problems in modern society, the commission on chronic illness suggested that the adaptation and widespread use of a consistent and comparable technology were essential to improve the meaning and usefulness of information collected about individuals with chronic, disabling conditions. More recently, the WHO (1980) has developed an International Classification of Impairments, Disability, and Handicaps (ICIDH). The purpose of the ICIDH is to provide a conceptual framework for the collection and standardization of data relevant to policy and to monitor the progress of chronic and disabling conditions in individuals and groups. The ICIDH clarifies the meaning of many frequently used (and all too frequently misused) concepts common to the practice of rehabilitation. The use of the ICIDH will enable us to do collaborative cross national research in LTC.

## Dementia Internationally

Cross nationally, it has been estimated that approximately 5% to 8% of persons 65 and over suffer from severe dementia. The fact that dementia increase steeply with age is of interest to policy makers since the very old population is the fastest growing segment of the older population practically everywhere and requires more health services.

WHO (1980) has projected that we will see a 100% or more increase in dementia in the less developed nations between 1975 and 2000. Although the corresponding increase projected for the more developed nations is smaller, around 50%, it is nonetheless stunning.

In the U.S.A. and the United Kingdom, at least twice as many persons with severe dementia are being cared for at home as well as in all long term care facilities. In continental Europe, studies indicate that only 1/5 of the elderly with severe forms of mental disorders, including dementia are placed in institutions (Gibson, 1984).

Although most dementia patients live in the community, persons with dementia comprise the majority of elderly found in LTC settings in many nations. In Japan, for example, 5.2% of the elderly in psychiatric hospitals suffer from dementia as do 27% of those in special care nursing homes. Similarly, in Israel, 50% of the elderly who are institutionalized in psychiatric facilities are victims of dementia. It is also estimated that dementia represents about 50% of all institutionalized elderly in France and in the U.S.A. In France, one study indicates that dementia represents about 40% of the residents in nursing homes and 90% of those in specialized geropsychiatric settings. It must be remembered that families seek institutionalization as a last resort. In many of the hospitals in the less developed countries, a member of the family remains with the patient if she/he is confused, wandering and "troublesome."

There are very few community resources, patient education and family counseling.

In Japan, the "Association of Family Members Caring of Confused Persons" was established in 1979 in Kyoto. They now have 24 prefectures in Tokyo. Alzheimer's groups exist in Britain and Canada.

Day care in Sweden has special programs for dementia patients such as day care hospice attached to the nursing home.

In Britain, community psychiatric nurses provide assistance in the home for dementia patients and their families. An organization in Europe entitled, "Age Concern" has established an intensive domiciliary care service for dementia patients who live alone. Such a program enables the patient to stay home. A staff of 3 aides are available on a flexible work schedule.

One issue is whether to integrate the dementia patient with the non-dementia patients. A study in Britain suggests a ratio of about three (3) confused to every mentally alert residents in TLC can be absorbed without difficulty for other patients and staff.

In the Netherlands, care for their dementia patients is in psychogeriatric nursing homes. Japan's "Advisory Committee on Public Health," has recommended a public policy on dementia.

Several countries have organized regional conferences around common issues in LTC such as manpower needs and use, cost containment, collaborative research.

In many countries disability and constant-attendant allowances for the elderly constitute another approach to the provision of social services, mainly through adjustment in income through adjustments in income policy. Forty seven (47) countries (excluding the United States, Canada and Federal Republic of Germany) have some form of constant-attendant allowance. To be eligible on must:

*Need attendance by another adult for at least part of the day because of a medically certified disability.

*(Usually but not always) meet means-tested income requirement. Payments may be geared to prior earnings or at a fixed flat rate sum.

In New Zealand, persons caring for disabled older relatives are not entitled to four weeks of paid vacation per year by the government. The older person is either placed in suitable accommodations or given care in the home. They frequently will use LTC for short term stays (respite).

In Sweden there are the night attendants, who work either or all three shifts in the home when the elderly person qualifies. Chores including monitoring medication, bathing, giving medication, toileting and turning patients.

In 1982, 124 nations sent delegates to the UN sponsored world assembly on aging. I had the privilege of participating in the development of a world plan of action for the elderly. We developed a policy framework of a aging which can be summarized in twelve/phrases:

Namely -

*Equality
*Independence
*Free choice
*Home care
*Accessibility to public services
*Cohesion between generations
*Mobility
*Productivity
*Self care
*Mutual help
*Family care

Recommendations from the world assembly on aging included:

*Involvement of the family in decisions and services;

*Development of a strategy to enable the elderly to lead indepen-
dent lives;

*Initiation of day-care measures to prevent social isolation and lone-
liness;

*Support of relatives who care for the terminally ill;

*Participation of the aged in the development and functioning of health
care services;

*Intensified efforts to develop home care to enable the elderly to
remain in their home communities.

I would like to close my presentation by sharing with you six basic
principles of health care delivery by David Werner.

1. Health care is not only everyone's right, but everyone's responsibility.

2. Informed self care should be the main goal of any health program or
activity.

3. Ordinary people provided with clear, simple information can prevent
and treat most common health problems in their homes – earlier, cheaper, and
often better.

4. Medical knowledge should not be the guarded select few, but should
be freely shared with everyone (at their level of comprehension).

5. People with little formal education can be trusted as much as those
with a lot. And they are just as smart.

6. Basic health care should not be delivered, but encouraged.

In summary, the United States does not have a national policy on long
term care, Long term care is the fastest growing aspect of health care
delivery serving almost 20 million people and it deserves a national policy
which will focus on quality of care, continuity of care, institutional and
non-institutional care, cost effectiveness, family/patient education/coun-
seling, chronic and acute care, manpower development and retention, less age
discrimination and more focus on the functional capacities/limitations of

the elderly, physical as well as mental illness, and less drug misuse/
abuse/over prescribing of drugs.

Basically, LTC in the U.S.A. is institutionally oriented; however,
there has been a 196% increase in home health care since the use of the
Prospective Payment System (PPS).

Fourth-one percent of long term care is financed by the general public,
3% by commercial insurance and 52% by the elderly and their family. L.T.C.
basically lacks continuity and the quality of care ranges from poor fair –
fairly good.

There are eight million informal caretakers, who provide 75% to 90% of
the non-institutional care and this help is not recognized in public policy.

Seventy five to 85% of the institutional care is provided by nursing
aides. Only 17 states require licensure of these aides.

There is no consistent public policy on quality of care standards in
home health care. According to the Commission on Elderly People Living
Alone (1986) over 8 million elderly Americans live alone. A majority (52%)
of the elderly over 85 years of age live alone and are high risk of institutionalization if not provided with HHC and a support system.

A study by the Villers Foundation (1986) found thirteen percent (13%)
or 3.5 million elderly are below federal poverty line (5156), (23% are
female head of family and 31% are black elderly). Public policy should
accommodate the poor, the uninsured and the uninsurable.

Willging (1986) of the Nursing Home Association reports that less than
one third of nursing homes have even sought Medicare certification.

To succeed, health policies must ensure the involvement and participation of the aging themselves. Programs must be flexible and appropriate,
giving the individual's chance to say how their needs should be met when
possible. the family should be involved in the planning, implementing and
evaluation of a health care program as a rule.

REFERENCES

Aging America: Trends and Projections 1985–86 edition, U.S. Government
      Printing Office, Washington, D.C., 1986.
A Profile of Older Americans: American Association of Retired Persons,
      Washington, D.C., 1985.
Burmeister, R. and Warner, S.J., 1984, "Long Term Care Administration:
      Past, Present and Future," American Health Care Association Journal,
      5:15.
Brody, S.J., 1984, "DRG-the 2nd Revaluation in Health Care for the Elderly."
      Journal of the American Geriatric Society, 32:676.
Buchannan, R.J., 1984, "Medicaid: Family Responsibility and Long Term Care"
      Long Term Care Adminstration Journal, 12:19.
Chenbaum, W.A., 1983, Shades of Gray: Old Age, American Values and Federal
      Policies Since 1920, Little Brown & Co., Boston.
Commission on Elderly People Living Alone, MD., 1985.
Dye, T.R., 1972, Understanding Public Policy, Prentice Hall, New Jersey.
Enhrenreich, B., and Enhrenreich, H., 1971, The American Health Empire:
      Power Profits and Politics, Vintage Books, New York.
Estes, Carroll L., 1979, Aging Enterprise, Jassey-Bass Publisher, New York.
Ester, C., and Lee, P.R., 1981, Policy Shifts and Their Impact on Health
      Care for Elderly Persons, The Western Journal of Medicine, 8:511.

Facts in Brief on Long Term Care, American Health Care Association, Washington, D.C., 1984.

Flagle, C.D., 1978, Issues of Staffing: Long Term Care Activities, in: "Nursing Personnel and the Changing Health Care System" M.L White, ed., Ballinger, Cambridge.

Fuller, B.A., 1983, Americans Needing Help to Function at Home, U.S. Dept. of Health & Human Services, National Center for Health Statistics, Hyattsville.

Fries, G.E., and Cooney, L., 1983, A Patient Classification System for Long Term Care, Health Care Financing Administration, Hyattsville.

Geiger, H.J., 1980, "Elder Health & Social Policy: Prelude to a Decade of Disaster,: Generations, 4:11.

Gibson, M.J.S., 1985, Older Women Around the World, The American Association of Retired Persons, Washington, D.C.

Gold, B., 1979, United States Social Policy in Old Age: Present Patterns and Predictions, in: "Social Policy, Social Ethics," B. Neugarten and R.J. Havaghurst, eds., University of Chicago Press, Chicago, 1979.

Goldman, H.., Gattonzi, A., and Taube, C., 1981, "Delivery and Counting the Chronically Mentally Ill: Hospital and Community Psychiatry, 37:1011.

Hauber, F.A., Bruininks, H., Hill, B.K., Larkin, K.C., Scheerenberger, R.C., White, C.C., 1984, National Census of Residential Facilities: A 1982 Profile of Facilities & Residents, American Journal of Mental Deficiency, 89:236.

Greenman, B.W., 1983, Business/Health Care Coalition in Profile, Institute For Health Planning, Madison.

Home Health and Long Term Care: Contemporary Long Term Care, 1985.

Homeless: A complex Problem and the Federal Response, Washington, D.C., G.A.O., 1985.

Lalonder, M. 1974, A New Perspective on the Health of Canadians, Ottawa.

Lamm, G., Elderly React Sharply to Remark to Lamm About a "Duty to Die," Washington Post, March 29, 1984.

Lee, P.R., 1982, Health Policy and the Aged, in: "Annual Review of Gerontology and Geriatrics, C. Eisendorfer, ed., Springer, New York.

Lee, P.R., 1980, "Health Policy Issues of the Aged: Challengers for the 1980's," Generations, 4:40.

Meltzer, J. and Farrow, F. and Richman, H., Policy Options in Long Term Care, University of Chicago Press, Chicago.

Minkle, M. and Quervo, B., 1980, "SRO: The Vanishing Hotels for the Low Income Elderly, Generations, 4:40.

Morris, R., 1982, "Caring for Vulnerable Family Members: Alternative Policy Options", Home Health Care Quarterly, 3:244.

Morris, R., and Levitt, T., 1982, Issues of Social Service Policy, in: "International Perspectives on Aging, Population Challenges," Nations - United Nation & Press, Geneva.

McFarland, L.G., 1980, "Respite Care", Generations, 4:44.

National Council Monitor: A Publication of the National Council of Health Centers, Washington, D.C., 1984.

Neugarten, B., 1982, Age or Need? Public Policy for Older People, Sage, Beverly Hills.

Newcomer, R., and Stone, R., 1985, "Board and Care Housing", Generations, 5:38.

Oriol, W., 1982, Aging in all Nations, National Council on Aging, Washington, D.C.

Pasmore, E., 1980, International Handbook on Aging: Contemporary Development and Research, Greenwood Press, Westport.

Perlman, R., 1982, "Use of Tax System in Home Care: A brief Note", Home Health Care Service Quarterly, 3:280.

Private Financing of Long Term Care: Current Methods and Resources, U.S. Dept. of Health & Human Services, Office of the Assistant Secretary for Planning and Evaluation, Washington, D.C., 1985.

Rovner, S., "Medicare: The Cost Cutting", Washington Post, January, 1986.

Scanlon, W.J. and Feder, J. (1984), "Healthcare: Financial Management," Journal of the Healthcare Financial Management Association, 6:1-9.

Schorr, A., (1980). "Thy Father and Thy Mother", A Second Look at Filial Responsibility and Family Policy, U.S. Dept. of Health & Human Services, S.S.A.

Selby, P. (1982), Aging 2000: A Challenge for Society, NIP Press Limited: Boston, MA.

Siegal, J.S. and Hoover, S.L. (1983), International Trends and Perspectives: Aging. International Research Document No. 12, Dept. of Commerce, Washington, D.C.

Sirrocco, A. (1985), An overview of the 1982 National Master Facility Inventory Survey of Nursing and Related Care Homes, National Center for Health Statistics, Hyattsville.

State of California, California Health Facilities Commission Long Term Care Effectiveness Standards Task Force Sacramento, Calif, Unpublished Data, 1981.

Sullivan, R. "Nursing Home Cost Force Elderly to Sue Spouses" New York Times, March 6, 1986.

Sybert, M. and Weiss, H. (1985), "Gaining The Upper-Hand in the Survey Process," Contemporary Long Term Care, 11:45

Technology and Aging in America, OTA-BA 265, Office of Technology Assessment, Washington, D.C., 1984.

Tax Equity and Fiscal Responsibility Act, Public Law No. 97-248, 1982.

U.S. Department of Health & Human Services, National Center for Health Statistics, Series 10, Hyattsville, 1980.

U.S. Department of Health and Human Services, Public Health Service, National Center for Health Statistics, (1979) National Nursing Home Survey: 1977 Summary of the United States. Vital and Health Statistics, Series 13, No. 43, p. 62.

Weissert, W.G. (1985), Estimating the long-term care population: Prevalence rates and selected characteristics. Health Care Financing Review, 6(4): 83-92.

Who Scientific Group of Epidemiology of Aging. Technical Report Series 796, 984, Geneva, 1983.

World Health Organization Technical Report Series 706. The Uses of Epidemiology in the Study of the Elderly, Geneva, 1984.

CONTRIBUTORS

Harvey J. Altman
Department of Psychiatry
Wayne State University School of Medicine
Detroit, MI 48202

Beverly A. Baldwin
School of Nursing
University of Maryland
Baltimore, MD 21201

Raymond T. Bartus
Department of CNS Research
Medical Research Division of
American Cyanamid Co.
Lederle Laboratories
Pearl River, NY 10965

Virginia Bell
Sanders-Brown Research Center on Aging
University of Kentucky
Lexington, KY 40536

Paul E. Bendheim
Institute for Basic Research in
Developmental Disabilities
Staten Island, NY 10314

David C. Bolton
Institute for Basic Research in
Developmental Disabilities
Staten Island, NY 10314

Dorothy Booth
College of Nursing
Wayne State University
Detroit, MI 48202

Jeffrey Borenstein
Department of Psychiatry
New York University Medical Center
New York, NY 10016

Rep. Woods Bowman
Fourth District
Illinois House of Representatives
Evanston, IL 60201

Dorothy H. Coons
Institute of Gerontology
The University of Michigan
Ann Arbor, MI 48109

Mary J. Curle
Renaissance Health Care
Detroit, MI 48237

Pamela G. Dawson
Sunnybrook Medical Center
University of Toronto
Toronto, Ontario, Canada M4R 1T3

Reginald L. Dean
Department of CNS Research
Medical Research Division of
American Cyanamid Co.
Lederle Laboratories
Pearl River, NY 10965

Richard L. Douglass
Departments of Family Medicine and
Community Medicine
Wayne State University School of Medicine
Detroit, MI 48202

Steven H. Ferris
Department of Psychiatry
New York University MEdical Center
New York, NY 10016

Judith A. Floyd
Department of Nursing
Wayne State University
Detroit, MI 48202

Emile Franssen
Department of PSychiatry
New York University Medical Center
New York, NY 10016

Donald M. Gash
Department of Neurobiology and Anatomy
University of Rochester School of Medicine
Rochester, NY 14642

Samuel Gershon
Department of Psychiatry
Wayne State University School of Medicine
Detroit, MI 48202

Anastase Georgotas
Department of Psychiatry
New York University Medical Center
New York, NY 10016

Christine Gmeiner
Department of Nursing
Lafayette Clinic
Detroit, MI 48207

Barry Gurland
Center for Geriatrics and Gerontology and
Long Term Care Gerontology Center
Columbia University
New York, NY 10032

Robert E. Harbaugh
Section of Neurosurgery
Department of Surgery
Dartmouth-Hitchcock Medical Center
Hanover, NH 03756

Mary S. Harper
National Institute of Mental Health
U.S. Department of Health and Human Services
Rockville, MD 20857

Leonard L. Heston
Department of Psychiatry
University of Minnesota
Minneapolis, MN 55455

Lorraine G. Hiatt
Consultant in Environmental
Psychology/Gerontology
New York, NY 10024

Susan Hicks
Renaissance Health Care
Detroit, MI 48237

Rep. David C. Hollister
Michigan House of Representatives
Fifty-Seventh District
Lansing, MI 48909

Mary M. Jirovec
College of Nursing
Wayne State University
Detroit, MI 48202

Harold R. Johnson
School of Social Work
The University of Michigan
Ann Arbor, MI 48109

Zaven S. Khachaturian
National Institute on Aging
Bethesda MD 20205

Coleman E. Klein
General Council
Alzheimer's Disease and Related
Disorders Association-Detroit Area Chapter
Southfield, MI 48076

Karen Linnell
Renaissance Health Care
Detroit, MI 48237

Mary Martinen
Alzheimer's Disease and Related Disorders Association
Detroit Area Chapter
Southfield, MI 48076

Lambert McGuire
School of Social Work
University of Pittsburgh
Pittsburgh, PA 15260

Michael P. McKinley
Departments of Neurology and
Biochemistry and Biophysics
University of California, San Francisco
School of Medicine
San Francisco, CA 94143

Marcia L. Morris
Department of Psychiatry
University of Minnesota
Minneapolis, MN  55455

Betty M. Morrison
School of Education
The University of Michigan
Ann Arbor, MI 48109

Howard J. Normile
Department of Psychiatry
Wayne State University School of Medicine
Detroit, MI 48202

Gregory F. Oksenkrug
Department of Psychiatry
Wayne State University School of Medicine
Detroit, MI 48202

Linda R. Phillips
College of Nursing
University of Arizona
Tucson, AZ 85721

Patricia Prinz
Sleep and Aging Research Program
American Lake VA Medical Center
Clinical Research Center
University Hospital
Department of Psychiatry
University of Washington
Seattle, WA 98195

Stanley B. Prusiner
Departments of Neurology and
Biochemistry and Biophysics
University of California, San Francisco
School of Medicine
San Francisco, CA 94143

Kathryn C. Rees
Rees and Associates, Inc.
Legislative Advocacy Governmental Affairs
Sacramento, CA 95814

Barry Reisberg
Geriatric Study and Treatment Program
Department of Psychiatry
New York University Medical Center
New York, NY 10016

Susanne S. Robb
School of Nursing
University of Pittsburgh
Pittsburgh, PA 15261

Dennis Robbins
The LeVine Institute on Aging
of the Jewish Home for Aged
West Bloomfield, MI 48033

Stacy Salob
Department of Psychiatry
New York University Medical Center
New York, NY 10016

Carl Salzman
Department of Psychiatry
Massachusetts Mental Health Center
Harvard Medical School
Boston, MA 02115

Barry Siegel
Department of Psychiatry
Wayne State University School of Medicine
Detroit, MI 48202

Emma Shulman
Department of Psychiatry
New York University Medical Center
New York, NY 10016

Gertrude Steinberg
Department of Psychiatry
New York University Medical Center
New York, NY 10016

John Toner
Center for Geriatrics and Gerontology and
Long Term Care Gerontology Center
Columbia University
New York, NY 10032

M. Vitiello
Sleep and Aging Research Program
American Lake VA Medical Center
Clinical Research Center
University Hospital
Department of Psychiatry
University of Washington
Seattle, WA 98195

Gaynell Walker-Burt
Michigan Department of Mental Health
Lansing, MI 48926

Ann Whall
School of Nursing
The University of Michigan
Ann Arbor, MI 48109

Herman J. Weinreb
Laboratory of Bacteriology and Immunology
The Rockefeller University
Department of Neurology
New York University Medical Center
New York, NY 10021

Donna L. Wells
Sunnybrook Medical Center
University of Toronto
Toronto, Ontario, Canada M4R 1T3

Henry M. Wisniewski
Institute for Basic Research in
Developmental Disabilities
Staten Island, NY 10314

Mary O. Wolanin
University of Arizona
Tucson, AZ 85721

Multi-infarct dementia, 213, 250

Networking, 279–284
Neurofibrillary tangles, 61, 87–89,
        90, 91, 92, 102, 103, 131,
        134, 135, 136, 144, 185, 187
Neuronal transplants, 100, 165–168
Norepinephrine, 2, 52, 102, 106,
        109, 148, 166, 167, 168
Nucleus basalis, 91, 92, 100, 101,
        102, 103, 109, 117, 131,
        134, 143, 167, 168, 186

Paired helical filaments (see
        Neurofibrillary tangles)
Parkinson's disease, 87, 88, 91–92,
        99, 109, 165, 166, 185, 211
  incidence, 51–53
  incidence of dementia in, 87, 91
Patient management, 191–194, 201–
        207, 213–217, 219–223, 225–
        232, 235–245, 249–257, 267–
        270, 271–276
Physostigmine, 100, 186
Plaques, 61, 72, 75, 81, 87–88, 90,
        91, 102, 131, 135, 136, 143,
        185
Power of attorney, 335, 336, 338,
        343–345
  durable, 343, 344–345, 355
  non-durable, 343–344
Primary care
  physicians, 191–194
Prion, 75–83
Private duty nursing, 205–206
Probate, 342–343, 345, 354, 355
Pseudodementias, 29, 34, 35, 45,
        46, 47–50, 51, 53–54, 210
Psychosis, 1, 2, 3, 4, 5, 6, 33
Psychostimulants, 171, 172, 178
Public policy, 347–355, 357–360,
        363–369, 371–385

Raphe nuclei, 102, 144, 145–146,
        147, 148
Receptors, 99, 100–101, 103
Respite care, 188, 193, 199, 203,
        206, 207, 222, 274–275, 300,
        331, 333, 358, 373, 378, 383
Rhythms, 262–263

Sandoz Clinical Asessment Geriatric
        (SCAG), 6–7
Scopolamine, 99
Scrapie, 75–83, 88, 89–90
Self-determination, 335–339, 343–
        345, 347, 348, 349–350, 351–
        352
Septum, 131
Serotonin, 2, 52, 102, 106, 109, 166
  and Alzheimer's disease, 143–144,

Serotonin (continued)
  and Alzheimer's disease
        (continued) 146, 148, 149
  and learning and memory, 145–147,
        148
  receptors, 102, 145, 148
  and sleep, 147
Sleep, 147
  and apnea–hypopnea activity, 116
  stages of, 259–260
Somatostatin, 106, 187
Striatum, 99, 101, 144
Substantia nigra, 91, 99–100, 101,
        144
Support groups, 287
Surrogate informants, 210–211

Thalamus, 144, 146
Third-party payment, 201, 202, 204,
        206, 207, 359, 369
Trisomy-21, 69, 90, 91
Trust, 342–343, 345
Tyrosine hydroxylase, 100

Vasoactive intestinal polypeptide,
        106

WAIS, 48, 177
Wandering, 4, 10, 213–217, 249–257,
        261, 263, 272, 274, 275,
        287, 311, 322, 383
Will, 341–343, 345, 359

397